Diseases of the Small Intestine in Childhood

Diseases
of the Small Intestine
in Childhood

Second Edition

John Walker-Smith MD (Syd), FRCP (Ed), FRCP (Lond), FRACP.

Consultant Paediatrician, St Bartholomew's Hospital, London;
Senior Lecturer in Child Health,
The Medical College of St Bartholomew's Hospital
and The London Hospital Medical College at
the Queen Elizabeth Hospital for Children, London;
Honorary Consultant Physician, Hospitals for Sick Children, London.
Formerly Staff Physician in Gastroenterology,
Royal Alexandra Hospital for Children, Sydney, Australia.

With a Foreword by

A. M. Dawson MD, FRCP (Lond)

Consultant Physician, St Bartholomew's Hospital, London

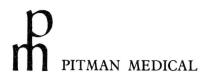
PITMAN MEDICAL

LSNR J IM

First published 1975
Second edition 1979

Catalogue Number 21 4196 81

Pitman Medical Publishing Co Ltd
P O Box 7, Tunbridge Wells,
Kent, TN1 1XH, England

Associated Companies

UNITED KINGDOM
Pitman Publishing Ltd, London
Focal Press Ltd, London

CANADA
Copp Clark Pitman, Toronto

USA
Fearon Pitman Publishers Inc, San Francisco
Focal Press Inc, New York

AUSTRALIA
Pitman Publishing Pty Ltd, Melbourne

NEW ZEALAND
Pitman Publishing NZ Ltd, Wellington

British Library Cataloguing in Publication Data
Walker-Smith, John
    Diseases of the small intestine in childhood.
    —2nd ed.
    1. Intestine, Small—Diseases
    2. Pediatric gastroenterology
    I. Title
    618.9′23′4   RJ456.S57   78-40761

ISBN 0-272-79533-X

Text set in 11/12 pt VIP Plantin, printed and bound
in Great Britain at The Pitman Press, Bath

Contents

To Elizabeth, Louise, Laura and James

Foreword

It is a great pleasure to write a foreword to the second edition of this book. Its early appearance and the translation of the previous edition into other languages is undeniable proof of the success and value of the first edition.

Dr Walker-Smith is to be congratulated on bringing his text up to date in the simple clear style that has been the hallmark of his monograph. There is a nice blend of basic physiology, pathology and the practical aspects of the diagnosis and management of children with disorders of the small gut, which so obviously represents his personal experience. What a refreshing change from the over-documented annotated bibliography that often passes for a textbook.

It is a fascinating read for the adult physician and fast becoming a must on the shelves of paediatricians.

A. M. DAWSON
Royal Hospital of St Bartholomew
London

Acknowledgements

A number of colleagues gave helpful advice concerning the text of the first edition and I should like to acknowledge my debt to Dr A. M. Dawson, Dr B. Dowd, Mr J. S. Dickson, Dr N. E. France, Professor C. B. S. Wood, Dr C. Murray, Dr M. Boyce, Dr M. Rossiter, Dr A. Kilby, Dr A. Ferguson, Dr M. Shiner, Dr D. Silk, Dr J. Chessels, Dr M. Harrison, Miss D. Francis, Dr J. Hilpert, Dr M. Araya and Mr L. Greaves.

In preparation of the second edition several of the above have continued to provide very useful advice, particularly Dr Anne Ferguson and Dr N. E. France. In addition, the following colleagues have rendered great assistance Mr A. Phillips, Dr P. E. Manuel, Dr C. Campbell, Dr P. Aggett, Dr E. Guiraldes, Dr E. dePeyer and Dr S. Avigad and Mr A. W. Middleton. I am again grateful to Dr D. Shaw who selected the X-rays for illustration and, also, Mr A. Phillips for electron micrographs.

I should also like to express my thanks to Professor C. C. Booth, who first inspired me to take an interest in small intestinal disease, and then to Professor T. Stapleton and the staff of the Institute of Child Health in Sydney where my studies in small intestinal disease in children first began. I am also indebted to Professor R. Walsh and Dr Helen Walsh who did so much to encourage me at that time. I also would like to acknowledge the especial debt I owe to Dr A. M. Dawson and his team at St Bartholomew's Hospital who have done so much to foster paediatric gastroenterology. I must also record my continuing debt to the European Society for Paediatric Gastroenterology and Nutrition who have done much to stimulate interest in small intestinal disease in childhood, and would especially like to record my thanks to Professor Jean Rey, Dr J. Visakorpi and Dr D. H. Shmerling who have been a great source of help and inspiration.

I am also greatly indebted to my secretary Mrs E. Lister who has worked so hard on the manuscript of the second edition.

Finally, I would like to record my thanks to my wife and family who have been so understanding in the time given up to write this book.

Preface

During the four years that have elapsed since the first edition of *Diseases of the Small Intestine in Childhood* was written there has been a remarkable expansion of knowledge in this area. This is in large measure due to the increasing awareness of the importance of small intestinal disease among children, particularly in the developing world where diarrhoeal disease continues to have such a high prevalence and, indeed, continuing mortality. As a consequence increasing research is being undertaken in this field, and in view of the rapid increase in knowledge a new edition was felt to be necessary to take into account these recent developments.

In the first edition, the preliminary exciting work on the identification of stool virus particles by electron microscopy in children with acute gastroenteritis was referred to briefly. In this edition, a completely new section is devoted to rotavirus gastroenteritis and also to the other viruses, now identifiable in the stools of children with acute gastroenteritis. It is remarkable how much information, quite unknown until 1973, is now available in this area. Yet it is obvious that a great deal more research requires to be done; for example, the relative importance of rotavirus infection in the genesis of diarrhoea in the developing world is still far from clear.

Throughout this new edition increasing attention is given to immunological studies, and in the introductory chapter a new account is given of the immunological function of the small intestine. This reflects the increasing importance attributed to immunological factors in genesis of small intestinal disease.

The importance of cow's milk protein intolerance in paediatric gastroenterology is reflected by the new work in this field, especially the diagnostic role of serial small intestinal biopsies in relation to milk withdrawal and challenge. The chapter on this malady has been considerably expanded.

The increasing problem of Crohn's disease in childhood, during the past five years, has led to more space being devoted to this subject including a discussion of improved diagnostic techniques and a review of current management.

The close relationship between nutrition and small intestinal disease is emphasised throughout the book and has been given more emphasis in this edition.

The author hopes these additions will greatly increase the value of the book to those for whom the first edition was primarily designed, and that readers will continue to find it easy to read and a useful source of up-to-date references.

Finally, the author once again, would like to express his sincere thanks to his colleagues at St Bartholomew's Hospital and the Queen Elizabeth Hospital for Children, especially to the junior staff of the gastroenterology department at the Queen Elizabeth Hospital for Children who have done so much to help and advise in the writing of this edition.

J. A. Walker-Smith,
Royal Hospital of St Bartholomew,
London, July, 1978.

Preface to the First Edition

The development of specialities within paediatric medicine such as paediatric gastroenterology has been slower than in adult medicine but with the development in recent years of new diagnostic techniques which are safe and readily available for use in children, this specialisation is now rapidly occurring. The number of published texts which deal specifically with these developments so far, has been very limited and this book aims to go some way towards meeting this deficiency in the field of paediatric gastroenterology.

The small intestine is the principal organ of absorption in the body and so abnormality of this organ may have far-reaching consequences for the child's physical well-being and general development by virtue of malabsorption of vital nutrients. Thus knowledge of diseases of this organ and their consequences plays a most important part in paediatric practice.

Diseases of the small intestine have been selected for this publication as there has been a considerable amount of new work in this field in recent years. Much of this has not yet appeared in standard paediatric texts and is at present only available in medical journals, yet this group of disorders is a most important one and accounts for a large proportion of gastroenterological disease seen in childhood. As an example of this, during one twelve month period from 1 July 1967 to 1 July 1968 over 1,100 children were admitted to the Royal Alexandra Hospital for Children, Sydney, with a major disorder of the small intestine. While the great majority of these children suffered from gastroenteritis, there were also many suffering from conditions such as giardiasis, coeliac disease, meconium ileus, malrotation, congenital atresia, strongyloidiasis and intestinal lymphangiectasia. This illustrates that disease of the small intestine occurring in childhood should be regarded as a major part of the whole field of paediatrics.

Many of the clinical observations made in this book are based on the author's experience of gastroenterology at the Royal Alexandra Hospital for Children, Sydney, Australia, and St. Bartholomew's Hospital and the Queen Elizabeth Hospital for Children, London, England. For convenience in the text, these hospitals are referred to with slightly abbreviated titles without mentioning their city of origin, I have attempted however, also to summarise current opinion and the results of research from many centres throughout the world.

The purpose of this book is thus to provide a review of diseases of the small intestine in children with emphasis upon a discussion of their causes, clinical manifestations and the newer techniques which are used in diagnosis as well as modern methods of management, particularly those which are dietetic.

Attention has been focused on the commoner and more important diseases of the small intestine in children as seen in Britain and Australia and less attention has been devoted to the less common diseases. However, a bibliography is attached to each chapter for further reading. Each bibliography is not intended to be comprehensive, but rather aims to indicate those articles which the author has found to be a useful source of reference and which he commends to the reader for further study.

It is hoped that this book will be of value to the consultant paediatrician and paediatric surgeon as well as to the paediatric registrar and house officer as a practical guide to their understanding of these diseases. It is also intended for those adult physicians, gastroenterologists and surgeons who wish to survey the clinical spectrum of disease of the small intestine in childhood; a spectrum of disease different from that seen in adult life. When the same disease occurs in both children and adults, the different manifestations in the two age groups is emphasised. It is hoped that general practitioners, medical students, dietitians, and members of the nursing profession may find this book a useful source of reference.

Finally the author would like to express his appreciation to his colleagues at the three hospitals mentioned above for their help and encouragement which has led to the production of this book.

J. A. WALKER-SMITH
Royal Hospital of St Bartholomew
London July 1974

I

General Introduction

DEVELOPMENT OF PAEDIATRIC GASTROENTEROLOGY

Diseases of the small intestine have long afflicted children. Gastroenteritis and cholera, disorders which have their principal effect on the small intestine, have through the ages had a high prevalence and mortality among infants and children. They continue to do so today in the less fortunate parts of the world, but small intestinal disease is also an important health problem among children of all countries.

Many individuals over the past century have added to the knowledge of these diseases, but only in the last 25 years have certain centres become especially associated with the development of paediatric gastroenterology. Reviews of paediatric gastroenterology in the journal *Gastroenterology*, in 1967 and 1970, and the formation of the European Society for Paediatric Gastroenterology in 1968, have drawn attention to these developments and have led to a wider recognition of the diversity and importance of paediatric gastroenterology and, in particular, small intestinal disease in children.

In recent years there has been a much wider understanding of the physiology and pathology of the small intestine in man. This has been due: firstly, to new laboratory techniques, notably those using preparations of animal small intestine, and secondly, to the development of sophisticated methods of investigating small intestinal structure and function in man, such as small intestinal biopsy and small intestinal perfusion.

A great deal of this new investigative work has been done in adults, but increasingly more and more observations are being made in children. As a result, the body of knowledge available concerning the small intestine, its structure and function both in health and in disease in childhood has enormously increased.

Of particular importance in the development of paediatric gastroenterology was the demonstration by Sakula and Shiner in 1957 of a flat, small intestinal mucosa on biopsy of the small bowel of a child with coeliac disease. The subsequent confirmation of this observation in large numbers of children with coeliac disease by many other investigators, and the development of a safe intestinal biopsy capsule as a diagnostic tool in paediatric practice, led to a great surge of interest in small intestinal disease in children and played a major part in the development of paediatric gastroenterology as a legitimate specialty within paediatrics.

There is still a real danger that when specialists concentrate on one organ or on one restricted branch of medicine that they may neglect the whole individual. As the function of the small intestine impinges so much on the function of so many other organs, those clinicians who interest themselves in this organ and its diseases should be particularly aware of the principles and practice of general paediatrics. It is equally true that the general paediatrician should have a real understanding of diseases of the small intestine and their management.

FUNCTION OF THE SMALL INTESTINE

The small intestine is the principal organ of absorption in the human body and complete resection of the small intestine is not compatible with life. It is thus a vital organ whose continuing healthy function is a major determinant for the continuing good health and normal development of the growing infant and child.

The small intestine has a number of important functions. These include:

1. The onward passage of the ingested food bolus
2. Continued digestion of this bolus
3. Absorption of the digested nutrients into the blood and lymph vessels
4. An important immunological function including the production of secretory immunoglobulins
5. A regulatory role in protein metabolism
6. Secretion of hormones

Disease of the small intestine may manifest as a disruption of one or more of these functions. Interference with the first of these produces the various syndromes of complete or incomplete small intestinal obstruction. Interference with the remaining functions characteristically produces diarrhoea, usually with failure to thrive, but there may also be systemic abnormalities, i.e. there are associated disturbances of organs outside the alimentary tract secondarily affected by disease of the small intestine. Indeed, a child with primary small intestinal disease may present with systemic symptoms alone and with no symptoms of gastrointestinal disturbance, e.g. a child with coeliac disease may present only with shortness of stature.

There is inadequate space to review all these functions here, but it is appropriate to mention some aspects of particular clinical importance and discuss them briefly.

Site of Absorption

Knowledge of the site of absorption of various nutrients from the small intestine (Fig. 1.1) is of importance in understanding the various disturbances of absorption that may occur when lesions of the small intestinal mucosa chiefly affect the proximal small intestine (e.g. coeliac disease), the distal small intestine (e.g. Crohn's disease), or the whole length of the small intestine (e.g. tropical sprue).

Important differences in function between proximal and distal small intestinal function are listed in Table 1.1.

Table 1.1
Functional differences between jejunum and ileum

	Jejunum	Ileum
Absorption of sugar	+ +	+
protein	+ +	+
fat	+ +	+
Bicarbonate	absorb	secrete
Vitamin B_{12}	−	+
Bile salts	−	+
Water and electrolyte absorption	'glucose-dependent'	'glucose-independent'

Courtesy Dawson, 1974.

Mechanisms of Absorption

Knowledge of the mechanisms of absorption of nutrients may have important clinical relevance to the understanding of small intestinal disease, and to illustrate this point the mechanisms of fat and protein absorption will be briefly discussed here. Absorption of other nutrients is discussed in appropriate chapters.

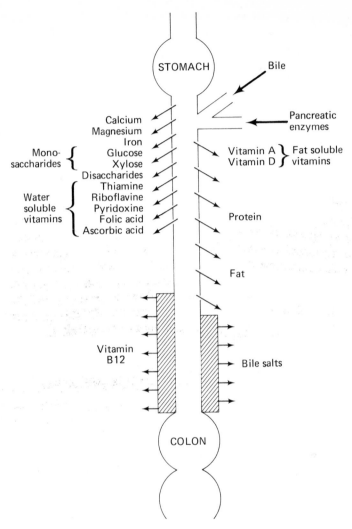

Fig. 1.1   Sites of absorption from the small intestine. (Permission of Booth, 1968.)

Fat Absorption

The fat in the diet of man includes triglycerides, cholesterol, and fat-soluble vitamins. Triglycerides, the major source of dietary lipid, are tri-esters of glycerol, i.e. they consist of three molecules of fatty acid esterified to glycerol. Fatty acids are described as long, medium or short, depending upon their chain length, and they may be saturated or unsaturated, depending upon the presence or absence of a double bond.

In man, most dietary triglycerides contain long-chain fatty acids (LCT), the most important of which are the mono-unsaturated fatty acid, known as oleic acid, containing 18 carbon atoms, and the saturated palmitic acid containing 16 carbon atoms. Medium-chain triglycerides (MCT) contain fatty acids of 6 to 12 carbon atoms in length and do not constitute more than a minor proportion of normal dietary lipids.

Three of the fatty acids are generally known as essential fatty acids (EFA). These are linoleic acid, linolenic acid, and arachidonic acid. Linoleic acid usually accounts for most of the essential fatty acids in a normal diet. In fact, most foods contain small quantities of linoleic acid in the cell walls, e.g. cereals 0·5 per cent. When an artificial diet is introduced consideration of dietary deficiency of essential fatty acids must be given, especially in babies where it has been suggested that 2 to 4 per cent of dietary energy should be provided as linoleic acid. In breast milk, 7 per cent of the fatty acids are linoleic acid.

Medium chain triglyceride preparations do not contain EFA unless specifically added.

Dietary triglycerides are hydrolysed within the lumen of the small intestine by the pancreatic enzyme lipase in the presence of bile salts. Fatty acids and monoglycerides so produced form, with the aid of bile salts, mixed micelles chiefly. Micelles are water soluble polymolecular aggregates which have detergent properties. Mixed micelles are essential for the absorption of fat soluble nutrients. Bile acids form micelles when their concentration reaches a certain critical value. In man this is of the order of 1–2 mM.

Thus, the products of pancreatic lipolysis, bile salts and lecithin form mixed micelles. It is probable that absorption of the bulk of lipids takes place from this micellar phase. The exact mode of mucosal uptake was controversial until Strauss, in 1966, provided unequivocal evidence that the major products of intraluminal hydrolysis are absorbed into the enterocytes by passive diffusion from bile salt micelles.

Once long chain fatty acids (chain length of C 16 to 18) and monoglycerides are absorbed into the cell, re-esterification to tri-glycerides occurs. These triglycerides are then surrounded by a coating of protein, cholesterol ester, and phospholipid to form chylomicrons which appear in the lymph and then are transported to the blood via the thoracic duct.

Most triglycerides in the diet are long chain, but medium chain triglycerides (chain length C 6 to 12), which are present in special infant milks such as Pregestimil, are absorbed by a different process. These acids have a greater water solubility than the long chain fatty acids. They are hydrolysed more rapidly and are not as dependent on pancreatic lipolysis. Once absorbed into the epithelial cell they are not re-esterified but go straight to the liver via the portal vein. Thus, medium chain triglycerides are absorbed more rapidly and efficiently. Beta-lipoprotein is necessary for chylomicron formation.

In certain conditions this sharp division between the mode of fatty acid transport related to chain length may not always apply; for example, in biliary obstruction some long chain fatty acids are transported via the portal vein.

Disease of the small intestine may disrupt the normal process of fat absorption in a number of ways and knowledge of these simple physiological principles helps in understanding these disturbances.

Diseases of the small intestine that interfere with fat absorption include the following:

1. Deficiency of conjugated bile salts as occurs in the stagnant loop syndrome (*see* Chapter 10).
2. Decreased uptake of fat as occurs with reduction in absorptive area, e.g. in massive resection of the small intestine (*see* Chapter 11) and in association with mucosal damage, e.g. coeliac disease (*see* Chapter 4).
3. Deficiency of chylomicron formation, e.g. abetalipo-proteinaemia (*see* Chapter 12)
4. Deficiency of transport of chylomicrons via the thoracic duct, e.g. intestinal lymphangiectasia (*see* Chapter 12).

The management of fat malabsorption in such disorders is to correct the primary disorder, when possible, by appropriate treatment, e.g. coeliac disease with a gluten-free diet, but when this is not possible (e.g. massive intestinal resection) by the substitution of medium chain triglycerides (MCT) for long chain triglycerides in the diet. This may considerably reduce the severity of the steatorrhoea. Proprietary milk feedings that contain MCT include Portagen and Pregestimil (*see* Appendix).

Protein Absorption

Normally, in childhood, the digestion and absorption of dietary and endogenous protein is very efficient. Protein is hydrolysed within the

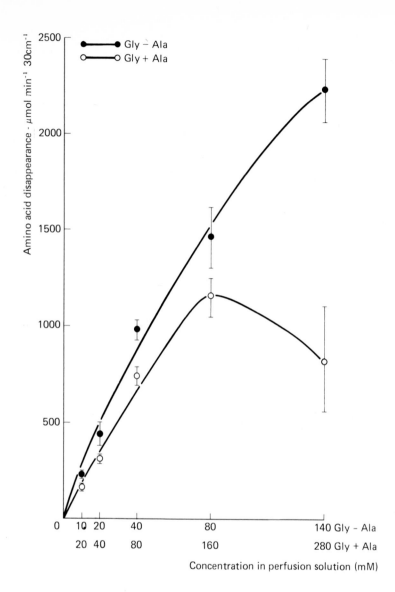

Fig. 1.2. Comparisons of intraluminal disappearance rates of amino acids during perfusion of 30 cm segments of human jejunum with test solutions containing glycyl-L-alanine (Gly-Ala, closed circles) or equivalent equimolar concentrations of glycine + L-alanine (Gly + Ala, open circles). Values are mean ± SEM, n = 4 or more.

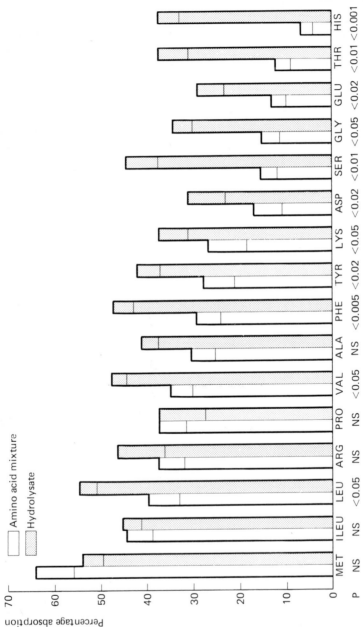

Fig. 1.3. Absorption of individual amino acids from a hydrolysate of lactalbumin and an equivalent amino acid mixture. Open columns = amino acids mixture. Shaded columns = hydrolysate. Significance of difference between the absorption of individual amino acids from the amino acid mixture and hydrolysate is also given, NS = nonsignificant. (Permission of Fairclough.)

lumen of the duodenum and proximal jejunum to a mixture of small peptides and free amino acids which are presented to the mucosa for absorption (Silk, 1976).

The results of studies of intestinal amino acid transport performed in normal subjects as well as in patients with inherited disorders have shown that there are at least four group-specific carrier-mediated transport systems that mediate absorption of (1) the neutral amino acids; (2) the dibasic amino acids and cystine; (3) the dicarboxylic amino acids; and (4) proline, hydroxyproline and glycine.

Until recently it was assumed that complete hydrolysis of protein to free amino acids was required before absorption took place. During the last few years, however, it has been clearly shown in man that unhydrolysed di- and tripeptides are also absorbed by carrier-mediated transport systems. As Fig. 1.2 shows, the mechanisms involved in the absorption of free amino acids and peptides are quite distinctive, as over a wide range of concentrations the net absorption of amino-acid residues from the dipeptide glycyl-L-alanine (Gly-Ala) occurred significantly faster than when equivalent concentrations of the constituent free amino acids (Gly + Ala) were perfused (Silk, 1977). Whether or not all dipeptides and tripeptides are absorbed by a single or multiple peptide carrier-mediated transport system remains to be elucidated. Once absorbed, the peptides are hydrolysed by cytoplasmic peptidases and the liberated free amino acids enter the portal circulation. The faster absorption of bound peptide rather than free amino acids has now been shown for many individual di- and tripeptides. When absorption of amino acids from a partial enzymic hydrolysate of lactalbumin consisting predominantly of small peptides was compared with absorption from its equivalent free amino-acid mixture during intestinal perfusion experiments, most amino acids were found to be absorbed to a greater extent from the hydrolysate solutions (Fairclough, 1978), Fig. 1.3.

In addition, greater plasma amino-acid increments were observed, after oral administration of a partial enzymic hydrolysate of fish protein, than of its equivalent free amino-acid mixture (Silk et al., 1976). In the light of these findings there is now reason to believe that partial enzymic hydrolysates of protein, consisting predominantly of small peptides that are relatively hypotonic, may be preferable to synthetic L-amino acid mixtures as part of elemental diets used in the oral management of protein malnutrition. The relevance of this to childhood disorders is currently being investigated. The rare disorders of intestinal malabsorption of free amino acids are described in Chapter 12.

Secretory States of the Small Intestine

It is obvious, then, that malabsorption of ingested nutrients such as fat or protein is a major consequence of small intestinal disease. Not only may there be malabsorption in such disease states but there may also be an abnormal secretion of fluid and electrolytes into the small intestinal lumen.

Small intestinal secretion represents the balance between the influx of fluid and the outflux of fluid from the small intestinal mucosa. It is important to realise that some absorption may still continue even when there is net secretion.

In order to understand sodium and glucose absorption, conventional thinking at present is of a three-compartment model for sodium transport in relation to the surface mucosa: (1) Small intestinal lumen, (2) Enterocyte, (3) Extracellular space.

Normally, sodium and glucose from the lumen cross the brush border down an electrical gradient. In the enterocyte, the level of sodium is lower than it is in the lumen. This low level is maintained by the action of Na^+K^+ ATP-ase which pumps sodium up an electrical gradient into the lateral extracellular space outside the enterocyte. Thus, there is a hypertonic solution in the lateral extracellular space. Na^+K^+ ATP-ase is probably identical with the sodium pump.

A number of disorders in which there is secretion into the small intestine are now recognised (Table 1.2).

Table 1.2
Causes of secretory states

Cholera
Gastroenteritis (i) some strains of *Escherichia coli* (cholera infantum)
(ii) Viral gastroenteritis.
Intractable diarrhoea
Coeliac disease

There is now good evidence that the crypt is the site of secretion in cholera mediated by adenyl cyclase.

Immunological Function of the Small Intestine

The vital absorptive role of the small intestine has been universally accepted for many years, but although it has been known for some time that the lamina propria of the small intestine contains large numbers of plasma cells as well as lymphocytes, and that Peyer's patches consist of lymphoid tissue, it has only been widely appreciated in recent years that the small intestine has a major immunological function.

Before discussing in detail the available information concerning the immunological function of the small intestine it is necessary briefly to review some basic concepts concerning the lymphoid immune system in man. This is a truly adaptive system which recruits both specific humoral and cellular immune defences. It brings these to bear where needed, and at the same time it creates a reserve of memory cells, against future demands (Holborow and Lessof, 1978). Both the humoral and cellular components of the normal immune response to antigen are dependent upon adequate numbers of functional lymphocytes. Humoral immunity is mediated principally via immunoglobulins synthesised by plasma cells which are, in turn, derived from a lineage of differentiated lymphocytes originating from a stem cell in the bone marrow. These lymphocytes are known as B cells, i.e. bursa dependent cells. This name comes from embryological and phylogenetic studies, no bursa equivalent having yet been identified in man. Cell-mediated immunity depends upon other lymphocytes and also macrophages. The lymphocytes are known as thymus dependent or T cells and are concerned principally with the development of delayed hypersensitivity reactions (*see* chapter 5), but T cells are also concerned with humoral immunity. Indeed, it appears that the humoral response is regulated by two opposing sets of T lymphocytes. First, there is the group of helper T cells, which induce specific antibody production by B cells (IgA production is dependent upon helper T cells), and secondly, there is the group of suppressor T cells which suppress the activity of the helper lymphocytes. These two groups bear antigens determined by immune response genes. Helper T cells bear an antigen called I-A and suppressor T cells an antigen called I-J. Both T and B cells are found within the small intestinal mucosa. In man, it appears that B cells predominate.

At present it is believed that in man there are two types of lymphoid tissue, namely, central and peripheral. In the central lymphoid tissue, haemopoietic stem cells differentiate into mature lymphocytes, with receptors, which are capable of specific recognition of antigen. In man there is only one discrete central lymphoid tissue, namely, the thymus, whereas in the bird there are two such tissues, the thymus and the Bursa of Fabricius. In man, the stem cells differentiate into the T cells in the thymus, and the B cells, at first, in fetal life, in the fetal yolk sac, then the liver, followed by the spleen and, in the adult, in the bone marrow. Both classes of lymphocytes (T and B cells) after differentiation, in their place of origin, migrate via the bloodstream and the lymph, to populate the peripheral lymphoid tissues, seldom returning to their place of origin.

Peyer's Patches

The aggregated lymphoid tissue of Peyer's patches are concentrated in the lamina propria. They were first described by J. C. Peyer in 1667. Embryologically, they are well developed by about the fifth month of fetal life and progressively increase in size and number as gestation proceeds, and after birth. This continues till about the age of 12 years (Cornes, 1965). While in the adult they are characteristically found in the ileum, in childhood they extend proximally into the jejunum and into the duodenum. Thus, such lymphoid aggregates may be found on proximal small intestinal biopsy in childhood. Isolated lymphoid follicles may also occur as well as these larger aggregates that contain several follicles.

Lymph follicles form dome-like swellings from the surface of the gut, giving a characteristic appearance with the dissecting microscope (Fig. 1.4).

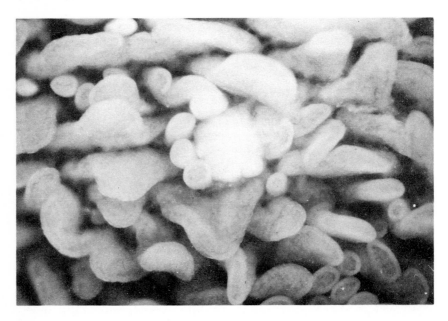

Fig. 1.4. Dissecting microscope appearance of a single lymphoid follicle surrounded by finger and leaf-like villi in a small intestinal biopsy.

Normally, the primary immune response to an antigen is influenced by the dose of the antigen as well as by its physical properties and the route of administration. Also of critical importance is the immune status of the host which, in turn, is influenced by both age and heredity as well as by adjuvant or immunosuppressive agents in the environment (Ferguson, 1976).

Normal immunity is a state of heightened responsiveness to an antigen due to one or more immunoglobulin classes of antibody and/or to specific cell-mediated immunity, thereby, often conferring protection against any invasive or pathogenic effects of the antigen.

Tolerance is a specific non-reactivity of lymphoid cells to an antigen. This is the normal response to antigen contact in early fetal life. The usual responses to feeding an antigen after birth are the local secretion of IgA antibody and a systemic state of tolerance to that antigen.

The gastrointestinal tract has a unique immunological function because it is capable of responding to bacteria and macromolecules of dietary origin within the gut lumen by a local response, as distinct from the systemic antibody response (Walker and Hong, 1973). Indeed, the gut lymphoid tissue is principally a defence mechanism against the onslaught of intraluminal antigens of whatsoever sort.

The small intestine contains two sorts of lymphoid tissue. First, there is aggregated lymphoid tissue (Peyer's patches) part of the so-called gut associated lymphoid tissue (GALT). Second, there is the diffuse distribution of plasma cells and lymphocytes within the lamina propria, as well as the lymphocytes between the epithelial cells lining the villus surface (intra-epithelial lymphocytes). There is now good evidence that the aggregated lymphoid tissues are the principal sites of initiation of immune responses, whereas the other cells spreading diffusely throughout the lamina propria are largely effector cells carrying out immune responses. The earlier view that the aggregated lymphoid tissue was the equivalent of the Bursa of Fabricus in man has now been refuted (Parrott, 1976).

The lymphoid cells of such an aggregate are separated from the intestinal lumen only by the overlying epithelial cells (0·3 μm). This epithelium immediately above the lymphoid follicles of Peyer's patches is different from the epithelium found elsewhere along the small intestine. It not only contains large numbers of intra-epithelial lymphocytes with few goblet cells but the epithelial cells themselves are cuboidal rather than columnar. Owen and Jones (1974) have called some of them M cells because of their distinctive ultra-structural appearance. They have luminal surface microfolds rather than microvilli, and they have a thin rim of cytoplasm with relative abundance of organelles suggesting an active vesicular transport system. These cells are tightly joined together. Thus, the reticulum formed by these M cells allows cells from the lymphoid series to approach the gut lumen very closely without being lost into the lumen.

The anatomy of Peyer's patches in relation to its B and T cell content in the mouse has been carefully studied (Fig. 1.5) and is

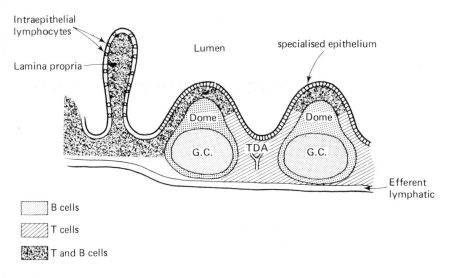

Fig. 1.5. Diagram of Peyer's patch structure in the mouse. G.C. Germinal centres. TDA thymus-dependent area. Permission of Prof. D. M. V. Parrott and W. B. Saunders Company Ltd., from *Clinics in Gastroenterology*, **5**, 211.

probably similar in man. The patches consist of circumscribed collections of B lymphocytes, the lymphoid follicles and diffuse lymphoid tissue, the interfollicular zone, populated mainly by T-lymphocytes. These lymphoid structures have no afferent lymphatics to carrying antigen to them. Indeed, it is now clear that antigen enters these patches via the dome epithelium. The evidence for this is the demonstration of passage of soluble and particulate antigen and intact bacteria in experimental animals and the demonstration of micropinocytotic capabilities in man (Owen and Jones, 1974). Absence of effector cells permits antigen entry here but also, as a direct result, may make the gut-associated lymphoid tissue more susceptible to invasive pathogenic bacteria. Indeed, there is some evidence that bacteria may specifically adhere to the surface of lymphoid follicles in the small intestine (Phillips *et al.*, 1978).

Diffuse Lymphoid Cells

Turning to the lymphoid content of the rest of the small intestinal mucosa, at birth this mucosa is normally devoid of lymphoid cells, i.e. these appear later in development than do the lymphoid aggregates. In

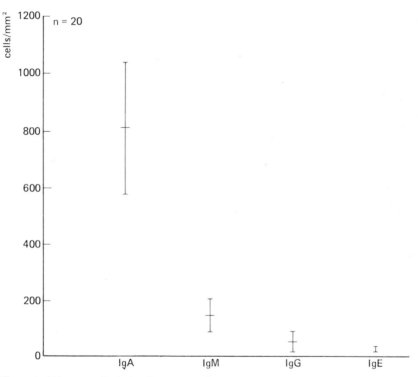

Fig. 1.6. Diagram of relative frequency of plasma cells containing immunoglobulins of individual classes of lamina propria of small intestinal mucosa. (Permission of Kilby.)

the mouse, lymphocytes and plasma cells are seen in the lamina propria around 10 days of life. Members of the T and B cell types that appear in the small intestinal mucosa are not the small T and B lymphocytes, which are the major constituents of blood lymph and peripheral lymphoid organs, but are differentiated descendants of these cells, originating from the circulating blood.

The effector cells of the B series in the lamina propria are chiefly IgA—secretory plasma cells but there are also IgM, IgG and IgE secreting plasma cells. Their relative frequency are shown in Fig. 1.6.

It is likely that the T cells are represented chiefly by the intra-epithelial lymphocytes (Ferguson and Parrott, 1972) but some are also found in the lamina propria, where they may have to interact in some way to function. Macrophages may be an important link in this interaction. Both T and B cells entering the gut are in the form of activated immunoblasts and there they differentiate into the effector cells.

Parrott has outlined the current hypothesis for the maturation journey of B blast cells from Peyer's patches to populate the lamina propria (Fig. 1.7). The final maturation of B blast cells to typical

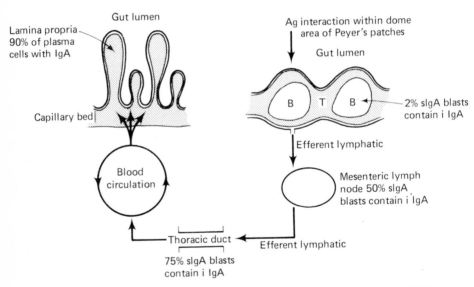

Fig. 1.7. Diagram of scheme proposed by Parrott for 'maturation journey' of B blast cells from Peyer's patches, where only two per cent of the blasts with surface IgA (S IgA) contain intracytoplasmic IgA (iIgA) through the mesenteric lymph node (50 per cent iIgA) and thoracic duct (75 per cent iIgA) to their ultimate destination in the lamina propria where 90 per cent of plasma cells are actively producing IgA (Data from Guy-Grand, Griscelli and Vassali, 1974). (Reproduced by permission of Prof. D. M. V. Parrott and W. B. Saunders Co. Ltd. from *Clinics in Gastroenterology*, 5, 211.]

plasma cells occurs within the lamina propria but in the lymph 75 per cent may already be able to form IgA, and in the mesenteric lymph nodes 50 per cent.

Thus, the main function of this gut-associated lymphoid tissue is to propagate the immune response as widely as possible by means of mobile effector precursors. Put another way, Peyer's patches fire off into the intestinal lymph cells that migrate into the lamina propria and there synthesise IgA.

In the Peyer's patches, the lymphocytes are primed before recirculating and homing to the lamina propria. The stimulus for homing is unknown. It appears to be only partially dependent on antigen in the gut lumen as it can occur in the absence of antigen. Once in the lamina propria it is postulated that, under the influence of intraluminal antigen, primed effector cells are inhibited from returning to the blood stream. However, it is clear that they can go to the gut even if there is no antigen in the gut. The effector cells in the gut are the intra-epithelial lymphocytes (probably T cells) and a mixture of T and B lymphocytes in the lamina propria. Once in the lamina propria, B lymphocytes mature, probably under antigen stimulus, and become immunoglobulin secreting plasma cells, mainly of the IgA cell class but also of IgM, both of which act as secretory immunoglobulins. A few cells of the IGG and IgE cell series are also present (*see* Fig. 1.6).

T cells probably travel also by mesenteric and thoracic lymphatics (Cebra *et al.*, 1977) to reach the lamina propria. There they appear to have some protective function. Until recently, little emphasis has been placed upon the function of T lymphocytes in the small intestinal mucosa, but Katz and Rosen have reported intractable diarrhoea in patients with T cell deficiency and Ferguson and MacDonald (1977) have emphasised their destructive potentiality. Whatever the role of T and B cells may be in the mucosa it is clear that they have become sensitised to intraluminal antigen in Peyer's patches.

Immunoglobulin Secretion

For some time now it has been known that immunoglobulins with antibody function are present in the intestinal secretions and also in extracts of faeces (coproantibody). Heremans and his co-workers had identified the isotope of immunoglobulin we now know as IgA in the serum in 1959. Then Tomasi and colleagues in 1965, showed that immunoglobulins in the intestinal secretions differed in their structure from those found in the blood. They found secretory IgA to be the predominant immunoglobulin in the secretions of the gut and also in human milk. Secretory IgA is both structurally and antigenically distinct from that found in the serum. Secretory 11S IgA is a dimer of two molecules of serum IgA linked by secretory piece. Secretory IgM is particularly important when there is a deficiency of IgA. Halpern and Koshland (1970) later found a distinct polypeptide called J-chain in secretory IgA and also IgM. IgM has 5 subunits linked by a J-chain, synthesised by lymphocytes. (Fig. 1.8).

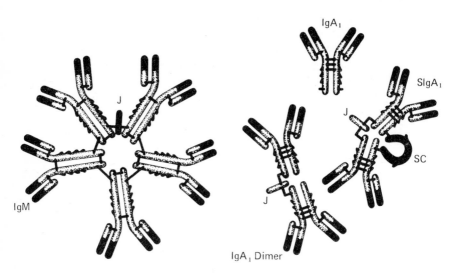

Fig. 1.8. Models of immunoglobulins. Immunoglobulin M containing 5 subunits held together by disulphide bonds J-chain. Immunoglobulin A with monomer, dimer with J-chain and secretory IgA containing: both J-chain and secretory component. (Reproduced by permission of Nestlé Research News from Ballabriga, Hilpert and Isliker, 1974/5.)

IgA plasma cells produce dimeric IgA to which is added J-chain and secretory piece, a glycoprotein synthesised by the golgi apparatus of the epithelial cell. This renders IgA resistant to protein digestion either by pancreatic enzymes or by bacterial enzymes. Thus, plasma cells, by secreting IgA antibodies, play a major role in preventing antigen entry across the small intestinal mucosa. These antibodies appear to be effective simply by complexing with antigen in the small intestinal lumen. They can neutralise specific toxins, diminish adherence of bacteria to mucosal surfaces, and so lessen the probability of bacterial colonisation of the gut as well. The presence of such secretory IgA antibodies within the small intestinal lumen is, of course, dependent not only upon their local production in plasma cells but also to their passage across the barrier provided by the epithelium of the mucosa of the small intestine or of that of an intestinal gland.

Serum immunoglobulin levels must not be regarded as necessarily reflecting increases or decreases of small intestinal immunoglobulin production because the immune function of the gut is largely independent of the systemic immune system. Only in hypogamma and agammaglobulinaemic states do serum levels reflect small intestinal immunoglobulin secretion.

The presence in the serum of IgG antibodies to a food constituent implies that immunogenic molecules must have been absorbed from the lumen of the small intestine, then passed via the lamina propria and the lymph or portal circulation to the systemic circulation, where they are phagocytosed and processed by macrophages in the spleen and lymph nodes, followed by secretion by plasma cells of specific antibody to the antigen into the serum. Serum IgA antibodies may have a similar origin but they could arise by secretion by IgA immunoblasts during traffic in lymph and blood (Ferguson, 1976). Small amounts of antibody to food antigens, e.g. cow's milk, may be found in the serum of normal children (Fig. 1.9). The proteins of

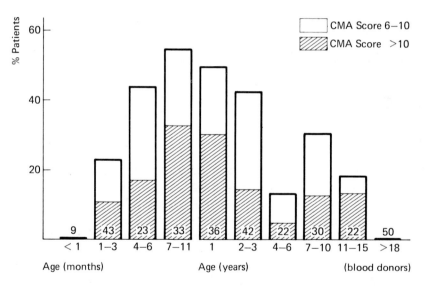

Fig. 1.9. The influence of age on serum antibodies to cows' milk, in children investigated for possible gastrointestinal or allergic disease (coeliac patients excluded). The cows' milk antibody (CMA) score is derived from the sum of scored titres of antibody to the five cows' milk proteins—1 in 16 scores 1, 1 in 32 scores 2, etc. Percentage of patients with scores of 6 to 10 and >10 are shown for each age group, and the number of patients is indicated at the foot of each column. (Reproduced by permission of Ferguson from Ferguson A., 1976.)

cow's milk are thymus-dependent antigens, i.e. co-operation between T and B cells is required for subsequent antibody production by B cells. The presence of serum precipitins to food antigens such as cow's milk protein does not indicate clinical intolerance. High titres are evidence of very high antigen dosage, e.g. undigested proteins in cystic fibrosis, or of undue permeability of the small intestinal epithelium, e.g. coeliac disease, but are not diagnostic of allergy to the food.

Antigen Entry

Although it is often assumed that the gastrointestinal tract provides an impenetrable barrier to the uptake of antigen despite the massive exposure to antigen that its large surface area, especially that of the small intestine, affords, it is now known that the mucosal barrier to antigen entry may be incomplete even in healthy individuals, especially in infancy. In man, pinocytosis of antigen has been observed morphologically, and this may be especially important in the neonate, but there is evidence that it may occur throughout life.

First, adsorption occurs, i.e. interaction between large molecules and cell surface, and secondly, invagination (endocytosis). Intracellular digestion then takes place within lysosomes and any remaining intact antigen is extruded by exocytosis. Normally, after immunisation to a particular antigen occurs in early infancy, absorption is reduced (Walker, 1976). Local IgA antibodies form complexes with antigen and so interrupt pinocytosis of macromolecular antigens by the intestinal absorptive cells (immune exclusion) (Fig. 1.10).

Early studies suggested that estimation of coproantibodies were useful for the diagnosis of coeliac disease and food allergy, but it is now clear that although higher levels than those found in control children occur in these disorders their estimation is not diagnostically useful. Normal children can mount a local humoral immune response to foods. Most coproantibody is IgA, while most serum anti-food antibody is IgG. There is no evidence of cell mediated immunity to foods in normal humans.

Secretory IgA also interferes with adherence of micro-organisms to epithelial surfaces. IgA is unable to activate complement of the classical pathway, but can do so via the alternate pathway. Its precise role against bacteria and viruses is still not clear. Animal studies have shown that protein feeding reduced subsequent protein absorption but that tolerance also occurred to protein actually absorbed, i.e. the development of antigen exclusion and antigen tolerance occurred

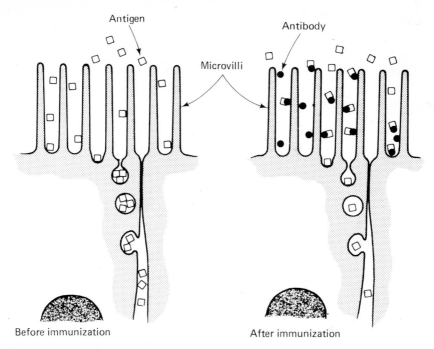

Fig. 1.10. Diagram of antigen absorption via the enterocyte before and after local immunisation. (Reproduced by permission of Dr Walker from Walker, W.A. and Isselbacher, K. J. from *Gastroenterology*, 67, 531.)

simultaneously (Swarbrick, Stokes and Soothill, 1979). Tolerance may, in fact be more important than antigen exclusion in preventing damage. Thus, nature appears to diminish antigen absorption as much as possible but, when it does occur, it ensures that a state of tolerance exists so as to avoid a damaging response. The individuality of the responsiveness of this local immune system has been shown in the experimental animal by Swarbrick, Stokes and Soothill (1979), who have shown genetic variation in antigen handling by the gut. Indeed, those workers have shown experimentally; first, that antigen is absorbed intact; secondly, that oral immunisation reduces subsequent absorption; thirdly, that oral immunisation induces systemic toler-ance; and fourthly, that there is genetic variation for antigen handling.

The gut is unique in having a local immune system independent of the systemic antibody system. How relatively important this local immune system is in the prevention of antigen absorption as compared to non-specific factors such as intestinal mucus and epithelial cell permeability itself remains uncertain. In addition, the systemic immune system also has an important role because systemic immunisation to a gut antigen occurs, and it is important to remember that ingestion of oral antigen may lead not only to local sensitisation but also to a systemic immune response, whether it be immunisation or tolerance.

SMALL INTESTINAL PERMEABILITY

The small intestinal mucosa provides several anatomical barriers to the passage of substances from the lumen of the gut to the blood capillaries. These include the glycocalyx, the microvillous membrane, the basal lamina of the enterocyte (*see* chapter 3), and the capillary endothelium. The overall permeability of the mucosa is determined by the permeability of each of these barriers.

In physiological terms, the permeability of a membrane to a substance is related to absorptive rate and concentration. Permeability is of critical importance for rate of absorption. In the absence of a specific active transport system, the absorption rate of a solute is a function of membrane permeability (passive permeability).

A 'pore hypothesis' has been put forward to account for the permeability characteristics of the gut for a variety of substances. Physiological studies in adult man suggest that the pore size in the jejunum have an 8 Å radius, and in the ileum a 4 Å radius (Fordtran *et al.*, 1965). This pore hypothesis suggests that large molecules may not pass through the membrane, but physiological studies suggest molecular shape may also be important as some large molecules such as polymers can get across the gut membrane.

At present, study of permeability in small intestinal disease states is somewhat confusing because some observers have suggested that permeability is decreased in coeliac disease (Fordtran *et al.*, 1967) whereas others have suggested that it is increased (Menzies, 1972).

Passage of substances across the gut may also come about by different mechanisms, e.g. via extrusion regions at the tip of the villus or by pinocytosis (*see* Fig. 3.24). These mechanisms may be particularly important for macromolecular absorption, e.g. protein antigens.

PHYSIOLOGICAL MECHANISMS INFLUENCING BACTERIAL FLORA OF THE SMALL INTESTINE

The alimentary tract plays a major role in influencing its own bacterial content (Harries, 1976).

1. *Gastric Juice*. Hypochlorhydria predisposes to cholera, and in

adults post-gastrectomy patients have a higher incidence of bacterial enteritis. Thus, the acid secretions of the stomach appear to have a protective role against bacterial effects in the small intestine. Children with chronic malnutrition have hypochlorhydria and this may contribute to bacterial overgrowth of the small intestine found in such children.

2. *Small Intestinal Motility*. Peristalsis is vitally important in keeping the lumen of the small intestine relatively sterile. Impaired motility may produce overgrowth of the small intestine by bacteria producing the stagnant loop syndrome.

3. *Small Intestinal Immune Systems*. IgA antibodies produced by the small intestine are known to combine with antigen, neutralise some viruses and toxins, and so play a role in gut defences. Thus, secretory IgA appears important, yet children with selective IgA deficiency do not have overgrowth of bacterial flora within the small intestinal lumen, whereas patients with hypogammaglobulinaemia have overgrowth with anaerobic bacteria in the small intestine (Brown et al., 1972). Hindocha and Harrison (1977) have found that 15 (29 per cent) of 51 children admitted to a gastroenteritis unit had low or low normal serum IgA levels on admission. Transient IgA deficiency in infancy has been described as a predisposing factor for infantile atopy (Taylor et al., 1973). It is possible that such a temporary infantile immunodeficiency may lead to poor antigen exclusion and so predispose to bacterial and, possibly, viral enteritis, as well as sensitisation to food protein as a sequel. However, the true role of immunodeficiency in bacterial enteritis and its sequelae awaits elucidation.

BACTERIAL COLONISATION OF THE SMALL INTESTINE

Bacterial colonisation of the small intestine and its relationship to disease of the small intestine is an important one. In 1969, Gracey, Burke and Anderson described the 'contaminated small bowel syndrome' where culture of small intestinal contents grew abnormal amounts of aerobic and or anaerobic organisms. The possible importance of such colonisation in relation to monosaccharide malabsorption is discussed in chapter 7 and in relation to neonatal surgery in chapter 9. Its importance in the chronic diarrhoea associated with protein-energy malnutrition remains a vexed question. Gracey (1977) has reviewed this subject. Three main issues arise—First, does the finding of significant bacterial contamination of the small intestine in such children as he has described in Indonesia relate to impaired immune function resulting from malnutrition? Second, is it the consequence merely of living in a grossly contaminated environment, as he has established in Indonesia? Third, does the abnormal microflora affect intestinal function? These questions remain unanswered. The author believes that the presence or absence of a small intestinal mucosal abnormality in these children is the factor of critical importance.

SMALL INTESTINE AND NUTRITION

It is also appropriate in this introductory chapter, to observe that while small intestinal disease may often present with secondary nutritional deficiency it is true that primary nutritional deficiency may compound and even cause small intestinal disease, e.g. children with protein-energy malnutrition may secondarily have an abnormal small intestinal mucosa (see chapter 12) and infants with under-nutrition who develop acute gastroenteritis, are more liable to develop delayed recovery thereafter (see chapter 6).

This interrelationship between small intestinal disease and nutrition is particularly germane to the question of the ideal form of infant nutrition, because the mode of nutrition may exert an important influence upon the genesis of small intestinal disease. The author agrees with many clinicians, notably Dr Cicely Williams, that breast feeding is the ideal form of nutrition for the human infant (Williams, 1962). It is clear that the promotion of breast feeding would go a long way towards a reduction in the continuing mortality and morbidity from small intestinal disease in early infancy, especially in developing communities, but also to an important extent in developed communities.

Table 1.3
Some virtues of breast milk in relation to small intestinal disease

Some protection against gastroenteritis.
Bottle-fed infants have higher mortalities in epidemics of gastroenteritis.
Hypernatraemic dehydration is rare in breast fed infants.
Protection against food allergy.

The virtues of breast feeding from the viewpoint of small intestinal disease stem from the nutritional composition of breast milk and its immunological properties. Modern artificial feeding has gone a long way towards mirroring the nutritional composition of mother's milk but no amount of modification of cow's milk protein can convert it into human milk protein, nor can artificial feeding provide the immunological properties of breast feeding. It is possession of these immunological properties that gives breast feeding its greatest advantage, namely, the protection it affords against infection.

Human colostrum and breast milk contain abundant humoral factors as well as macrophages and lymphocytes (both T and B cells), all of which are important in providing such protection. The IgA content of breast milk with its specific antibodies against strains of enteropathogenic *Escherichia coli* is an important protective mechanism against enteritis due to such strains of *E. coli*. Goldblum *et al.*, (1975) have shown that there is transfer of sensitised lymphocytes from the mother's gastrointestinal tract to her mammary gland leading to the specific anti-*E. coli* antibody secretion of breast milk. They have shown that human colostrum contains numerous cells that produce such IgA antibody specifically against the O antigens of commonly encountered strains of enteropathogenic *E. coli*. This antibody provides passive immunity to protect the infant's gastrointestinal tract from organisms his mother has previously encountered. Breast milk also contains large amounts of an iron-binding protein, lactoferrin (Bullen, Rogers and Weigh, 1972). This protein has an important bacteriostatic effect and the combination of lactoferrin and specific IgA antibody has a synergistic bacteriostatic effect on *E. coli*.

The presence of antibodies to rotavirus in breast-milk has also now been shown (Simhon and Mata, 1978), and breast milk as well as cow's milk contains a non-antibody virus inhibitor (Matthews *et al.*, 1976).

Evidence has also been produced that cell-mediated immunity may be acquired by breast feeding. It has shown that breast-fed infants may passively acquire T-cell responsiveness to a specific antigen by ingestion of breast-milk (Schlesinger and Covelli, 1977). Whether this responsiveness is transmitted via a soluble transfer-factor-like substance or via intact cells in mother's milk, is not yet clear. There is also a higher content of C_3 and C_4 components of complement in breast milk. C_3 binds with IgA and inhibits adherence of *E. coli* to the small intestinal mucosa. It also has a much higher content of lysozyme than does cow's milk.

The normal flora of the gut plays an important part in the resistance to gastroenteritis provided by breast-feeding. Breast feeding is associated with a preponderance of lactobacilli in the colon in the presence of an acid pH. Thus, stools of breast-fed babies have an acid pH, low counts of *E. coli*, and high counts of lactobacillus bifidus, whereas bottle-fed infants have more alkaline stools with large numbers of *E. coli* and a few lactobacilli. The acid pH of the breast fed infant's stool is probably related to a physiological malabsorption of lactose in these babies (Counahan and Walker-Smith, 1976).

Thus, a number of important factors present in breast milk account for the protection breast feeding provides against gastroenteritis, particularly that due to enteropathogenic *E. coli*. This protection, however, is not complete (*see* chapter 6), nevertheless bottle-fed infants have higher mortalities than breast-fed babies in epidemics of gastroenteritis. Harfouche (1970) found diarrhoea rates to be ten or more times higher in bottle-fed babies, and mortality from gastroenteritis was five to ten times greater than in breast-fed babies. In addition, when breast-fed infants do develop gastroenteritis, hypernatraemic dehydration is rare.

Finally, there is evidence that breast feeding for the first three months of life in the infants of families with atopic disease who develop transient IgA deficiency may prevent the development of allergy including cow's milk protein intolerance (Taylor *et al.*, 1973).

Thus, there is firm evidence that breast-feeding is biologically superior to any other form of nutrition for the human baby. Nevertheless, when a mother does elect to bottle feed her infant she should do so without undue anxiety. Although modern artificial feeding will not give her baby the protection against infection that breast feeding provides, if the mother takes particular care with hygiene and has nutritional advice concerning the most appropriate type of artificial feeding for her infant, she can bottle feed her baby with some degree of confidence.

Modern technology has, in fact, led to a considerable improvement in the cow's milk based artificial feedings now available for babies. Low solute feedings, whose composition is closer to breast milk than it is to cow's milk in regard to sodium, calcium, phosphorous and protein content, are preferable to partly modified milk formulae with their high solute loads, particularly of sodium. Such high solute feedings are associated with the development of hypernatraemic dehydration, a significant complication of infantile gastroenteritis (*see* chapter 6). Fortunately in Britain, following the recommendations of the Department of Health and Social Security in their report entitled 'Present-day Practice in Infant Feeding', high solute milks have almost passed out of use, for infants under six months.

Nevertheless, bottle feeding is a more complicated technique than simple breast feeding. Continuing attention to hygiene is vital when an infant is bottle fed, especially in tropical countries where the environment may be heavily contaminated bacteriologically.

SMALL INTESTINE AND THE PSYCHE

Finally, in this chapter, we must discuss the possibility that the child itself and its relationship to its mother and family may be overlooked by those caring for children with small intestinal disease. Indeed, small intestinal disease often does have important emotional consequences for the child and its family and the recognition of this is a vital part in understanding such disease. The converse may equally be true, that emotional disorders may have important effects upon the small intestine, although this is less well understood.

Katz (1971) has commented upon the close interreaction between mother and child, on the one hand, and alimentary function of the child, on the other. He observes that few areas involving mother–child transactions are more loaded with emotional content than is alimentation. It has been known from time immemorial just how closely a mother is involved in her baby's feeding, digestion and elimination. It is also known how closely a baby's emotional life is lived through his gastrointestinal tract. This close relationship between emotions and alimentary function continues throughout childhood and adolescence into adult life. Although, it is perhaps less obvious in the older individual, this intimate relationship has been recognised since the time of Beaumont and his classical observations in the nineteenth century, but only more recently has it become widely accepted that disturbed alimentary function itself may profoundly alter an individual's emotional state.

Katz believes that studies of baby-gut-mother transactions serve to counteract deeply ingrained prejudice that an event is either primarily physical with some psychological effects, or primarily psychological with some physical effects. The farther one goes back in human developmental studies, the less clear becomes any distinction between what is psychological and what is physical. In other words, the less clear becomes the division between events happening to the handling environment, i.e. the mother, and events happening to the baby itself.

Clinicians who are concerned with small intestinal disease in childhood must, therefore, have a close appreciation of the importance of these factors if they are to understand disturbances of small intestinal function, particularly in infants but also in older children.

2

History Taking and Physical Examination

HISTORY TAKING

A careful history is the most vital step in the investigation of children with small intestinal disease. This is because the history will usually give a firm clue as to the diagnosis and also provide an indication of the most appropriate investigations that should be undertaken.

There are two aspects to this history taking. First, there is the narrative history concerning the child's illness from its onset up to the present, and second, there is the specific interrogation concerning the child's symptoms and past history.

As in most paediatrics, the child's mother is usually the main source of the history of the child's illness. However, in the older child, useful information may be obtained from the child himself. In the neonate no history may be available at all. The father and other members of the family who may be present at the time of interview may also prove to be useful sources of history, as small intestinal disease, for example gastroenteritis, may affect more than one member of the family. In this way vital information may be obtained.

A detailed dietary history is of particular importance in children with this group of disorders, especially a dietary history of the early weeks of life. Exact details of which feeding or feedings the infant has been given should be recorded as well as the time of introduction and nature of solids that have been introduced into the infant's diet. It is, of course, self-evident that the clinician himself should be aware of the composition of the various infant feeding formulae that are generally available and some data concerning this is presented later. The relevance of the child's early dietary history in an analysis of the child's illness is provided by the example of coeliac disease, which cannot be considered a diagnostic possibility unless the infant has been exposed to gluten. Gluten in Britain is usually given first as rusks or as cereal products.

It is often important to take a history on more than one occasion as all the available details may not have been collected on the first occasion. The initial interrogation may lead the parents, on reflection, to recall additional relevant information and such information may only be revealed by a second interview. In addition, the results of an initial investigation of the child may suggest a further line of enquiry not previously pursued.

The symptoms and signs of small intestinal disease in children can largely be placed into three broad groups, namely—

1. those symptoms and signs that direct immediate attention to the alimentary tract, i.e. gastrointestinal symptoms; for example, diarrhoea, vomiting, abdominal pain, abdominal protuberance and anorexia
2. those clinical features due to nutritional disturbance and growth and developmental slowing, such as failure to thrive and weight loss, shortness of stature and delayed development, as well as the various deficiency states such as anaemia, rickets, oedema, tetany and skin changes
3. clinical features due to the disturbance of water and electrolyte balance

Some symptoms, such as the emotional disturbance that characterises coeliac disease, may not readily fit into these groups.

Chief Symptoms

The principal symptoms that may occur in children with small intestinal disease will be briefly discussed here but a fuller account of the symptoms in individual disease entities is given in later chapters.

Diarrhoea

Diarrhoea is the frequent passage of loose stools. This is the commonest symptom of disease of the small intestine in childhood. Perhaps surprisingly, there is sometimes difficulty in recognising its presence usually due to failure to take an adequate history or to examine the stools. On the other hand, an erroneous diagnosis of diarrhoea may sometimes be made in a breast-fed infant. This is because it may not be appreciated that for about the first three weeks of life breast-fed infants often pass loose stools which may number up to ten or twelve a day. Such loose stools may be passed for longer than three weeks in some infants; indeed, they may be passed until the time when solids are introduced into the infant's diet. The stools of a breast-fed infant may, on occasion, be bright green in colour and strongly resemble those seen in gastroenteritis, but once solids are added to the infant's diet or even a small amount of cow's milk as a complement, the stools will immediately become firmer in consistency.

The first point to establish about diarrhoea is whether it is an acute or a chronic problem and then whether it is associated with any other symptoms. In children with acute diarrhoea the frequency and severity of the diarrhoea are both of much importance as this information may give a guide to the infant's likely stage of hydration. Diarrhoea becomes chronic when it lasts more than two weeks.

In relation to chronic diarrhoea, it is most important to determine whether it is associated with other symptoms such as failure to thrive. Its time of onset and relation to changes in the diet, e.g. the change from breast feeding to bottle feeding, may give a useful clue to diagnosis. The nature of the stools, such as whether they are watery, as occurs in infants with sugar malabsorption, or bulky and pale, as occurs in children with steatorrhoea, should be determined. An enquiry should always be made concerning the presence of blood in the stools, as may occur in infants with intussusception and some children with bacterial enteritis.

Vomiting

It is sometimes difficult to distinguish posseting from true vomiting in the infant. Posseting is the bringing up of small amounts of milk particularly at the time of winding. True vomiting in infancy should always be considered as a significant symptom. The presence of bile in the vomitus, particularly in the neonate, should be regarded as highly suspicious of intestinal obstruction. Acute vomiting often accompanies diarrhoea as part of the syndrome of acute gastroenteritis. Chronic or intermittent vomiting may also be associated with diarrhoea as occurs, for example, in children with a malabsorption syndrome.

Abdominal Protuberance

Abdominal protuberance occurs commonly in children with small intestinal disease and may on occasion be the presenting symptom of a child who has coeliac disease. Abdominal protuberance may, however, occur in any child with malnutrition and can be almost a universal finding among young children in some developing countries.

Intermittent abdominal distension may be associated with episodes of incomplete small intestinal obstruction.

Abdominal Pain

The presence of abdominal pain in the young infant may be suggested when there is a history of episodes of drawing up of the legs coupled with screaming. Such episodes are typical of children who have an intussusception. Although in the adult abdominal pain may be a clear-cut symptom of active disease, in the school-age child it is not often associated with organic small intestinal disease. Crohn's disease is an important, albeit uncommon, cause of abdominal pain in such children but in general abdominal pain is not a common symptom of small intestinal disease in childhood.

Failure to Thrive

When an infant presents with failure to gain weight or grow according to expectations, one of the many causes of this syndrome is small intestinal disease. The circumstances that precede the onset of failure to thrive must be determined and these may be a valuable clue as to the diagnosis, for example post-enteritis syndrome, where there is a clear history of gastroenteritis preceding the onset of the infant's failure to thrive.

It is particularly important to determine the caloric intake of such infants because a low caloric intake *per se*, i.e. 'under-feeding', in these circumstances may provide a simple explanation for failure to thrive, particularly in early infancy.

Emotional Symptoms

Irritability and emotional disturbance are a common occurrence in infants and children with small intestinal disease and the close link between the 'emotions' and the 'motions' has already been implied.

The relationship between the onset of these symptoms and symptoms of alimentary disturbance is an important part of the history.

PHYSICAL EXAMINATION

Although there may be little to be found on physical examination of a child with small intestinal disease, very useful information may at times be obtained from careful physical examination. The first step is general inspection of the child without any clothes, preferably at first standing up, in the case of a toddler and older child. Standing the child and examining him naked is an important stage in examination as abdominal distension and wasting around the pelvic and shoulder girdles may otherwise be overlooked. A photograph of the child's general appearance is also useful as a record and should be taken whenever possible as a basis for future comparison. A careful measurement of the child's weight and height is essential, and this should be recorded on a percentile chart together with earlier measurements when these are available (Fig. 2.1). Such information in Britain and Australia is readily available from the Infant Welfare and Baby Health Clinic cards, which most mothers will possess. Single measurements of height and weight may be misleading but such serial measurements may give information of diagnostic significance. All body systems should be examined carefully, but examination of the skin, particularly for signs of dehydration in the young infant, may be useful. Examination of the skin may also give an indication of loss of weight and malnutrition. The abdomen should be given careful attention. Abdominal distension, tenderness and the presence of abdominal masses should be looked for in every case. The signs to be particularly sought in the child should be apparent from the history and it is not proposed here to give a detailed account of all the possible abnormalities that might be found on physical examination. The physical features of each particular disorder of the small intestine are discussed in their appropriate chapters.

Simple examination of the stool may give very useful information and should be part of the physical examination whenever possible. Detailed laboratory examinations of the stool are discussed in chapter 3.

This initial clinical assessment of children presenting with gastroenterological symptoms will usually suggest two or three disorders that need to be considered as diagnostic possibilities. Those tests most

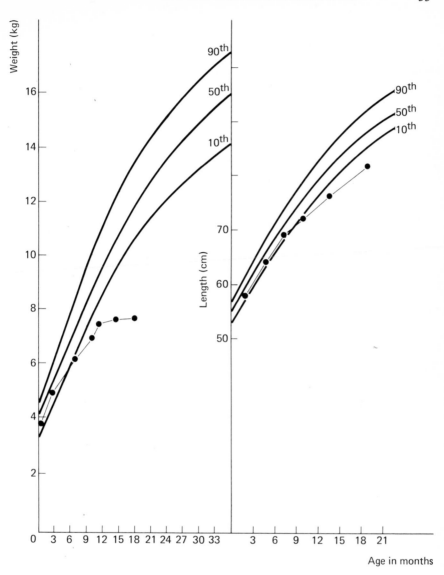

Fig. 2.1. Percentile chart of an infant with failure to thrive.

relevant to these disorders should then be performed. This approach is far more productive than running a screen of investigations in order first to demonstrate the presence of malabsorption, and then having shown malabsorption to be present, to consider its possible causes, as used to be routine practice in paediatrics in the past and still is sometimes in adult gastroenterology. In paediatric gastroenterology, when a particular entity seems likely on initial clinical assessment, the relevant specific diagnostic test should be performed, e.g. small intestinal biopsy if coeliac disease is suspected, or sweat electrolytes if cystic fibrosis appears probable.

3

Techniques of Investigation

The small intestine may be investigated in a number of ways, which are listed in Table 3.1.

ANATOMICAL

Radiological

Evidence of anatomical abnormality of the small intestine may be obtained by X-ray studies. This subject has been reviewed by de Silva (1971), but for more detailed accounts the reader is referred to texts on paediatric radiology.

Small Intestinal Obstruction

Plain antero-posterior X-ray films of the abdomen, with the child in supine and upright positions, are indicated whenever there is clinical evidence of small intestinal obstruction. Table 3.2 indicates some of the diagnoses that can be made with a plain X-ray of the abdomen in these circumstances.

Duodenal obstruction with the characteristic 'double bubble' (Fig. 3.1) may be diagnosed very simply preoperatively by plain X-ray of the abdomen. The farther down the obstruction occurs in the small intestine the greater the number of dilated loops of intestine that can be seen. Infants with meconium ileus may have a characteristic 'soap bubble' appearance due to an admixture of gas and of meconium on plain X-ray of the abdomen. When perforation has occurred, free gas will be seen in the peritoneal cavity and when it has taken place in intrauterine life, pneumoperitoneum and peritoneal calcification due to meconium peritonitis may be observed.

Table 3.1
Investigations of the small intestine

ANATOMICAL	Radiological	plain X-ray abdomen barium studies
	Endoscopy Technetium scan Laparotomy	
MORPHOLOGICAL	Small intestinal mucosal biopsy	dissecting microscope light microscope electron microscope
	Autopsy studies	
FUNCTIONAL	Enzyme assay and histochemical studies of mucosal biopsies	
	Absorption studies	fat/sugar/protein
	Detection of deficiency states secondary to small intestinal disease e.g. iron deficiency folic acid deficiency rickets	
	Investigation of distur- bances of water and electrolyte balance	
	Investigation of bile salt metabolism, including ^{14}C glycocholate breath test	
	Lactose hydrogen breath test	
IMMUNOLOGICAL	Serum immunoglobulin levels	
	Immunological class of plasma cells in biopsies of small intestinal mucosa	
	Food protein antibodies	
	Lymphocyte function	
BACTERIOLOGICAL	Stool culture	
	Duodenal aspirate culture	aerobic anaerobic
PARASITIC	Examination of duo- denal juice for *Giardia lamblia* and *Strongyloides stercoralis*	
VIRAL	Stool and duodenal fluid examination with electron microscope for viruses	

Table 3.2
Diagnoses possible on plain X-ray of abdomen

Duodenal stenosis or atresia
Jejuno-ileal obstruction
Meconium ileus
Intestinal obstruction with perforation
Milk plug syndrome

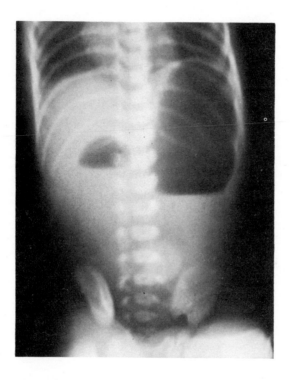

Fig. 3.1. Complete duodenal obstruction with gaseous distension of stomach and duodenum: 'double bubble'.

The place of barium studies in the further investigation of children with small intestinal obstruction is controversial. De Silva at the Royal Alexandra Hospital suggests that barium sulphate is the most satisfactory media in these circumstances and states that water soluble contrast may be dangerous in infants.

A barium study in a child with duodenal obstruction may reveal a diaphragm with an opening outline by barium. When such a study in a child with small intestinal obstruction reveals that the duodeno-

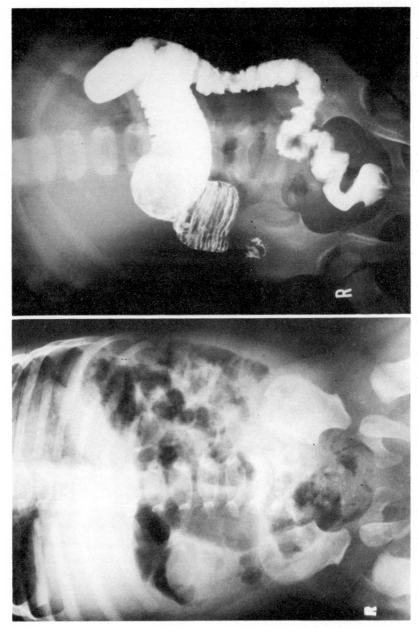

Fig. 3.2. Plain X-ray of the abdomen of an infant with an intussusception and a barium enema outlining the intussusception.

jejunal flexure is to the right of the mid-line, the cause is most likely to be a volvulus or a peritoneal band.

A barium enema may give useful information in children with distal small intestinal obstruction; for example, the demonstration of an abnormally placed large intestine, suggesting the diagnosis of malrotation. A barium enema in infants with meconium ileus may reveal filling defects in the large and small intestine caused by meconium plugs.

A barium enema may also be used as a diagnostic and as a therapeutic technique for children with intussusception (Fig. 3.2).

Malabsorption Syndromes

Plain X-rays of the abdomen of children with malabsorption may often reveal a dilated small and large bowel. Barium studies characteristically reveal dilatation of the small intestine and segmentation and fragmentation of the barium column. Dilatation is the most characteristic finding in coeliac disease. Haworth *et al.* (1968) studied the radiological appearances of the small bowel in 78 children with malabsorption due to coeliac disease, and 42 children with malabsorption due to other causes at the Queen Elizabeth Hospital. They concluded that dilatation of the small bowel as measured both on plain X-rays of the abdomen and barium studies was an extremely reliable indication of coeliac disease. The advent of safe, reliable and readily available techniques of small intestinal biopsy has, however, led to measurement of small intestinal dilatation being abandoned as a diagnostic technique for coeliac disease in childhood.

Thickening of the mucosal folds may be found in intestinal lymphangiectasia and lymphosarcoma, but lymphosarcoma may also cause displacement of loops of the small intestine or a local enlargement of glands may compress part of the small intestine; for example the duodenum (Fig. 3.3).

In the older child, if barium is combined with lactose, such a meal may be a useful way of diagnosing lactose intolerance by demonstrating dilatation of the small intestine, dilution of the contrast medium and rapid intestinal transit with barium reaching the colon in under one hour (Laws and Neale, 1966; Bowdler and Walker-Smith, 1969). This is simply a radiological way of establishing diarrhoea after an oral load of lactose.

A blind or stagnant loop syndrome may be diagnosed from a barium follow-through by demonstrating abnormal dilatation and stasis of barium occurring, for example, proximal to an anastomosis after

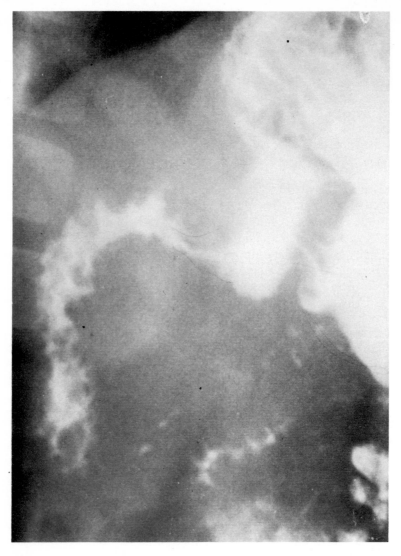

Fig. 3.3. Partial duodenal obstruction due to lymphosarcomatous lymph glands.

surgical resection of the small intestine, or occurring in a child with chronic volvulus, or ileal stenosis (Fig. 3.4).

Radiological investigation is important in diagnosing Crohn's disease in children and when this diagnosis is considered, a barium

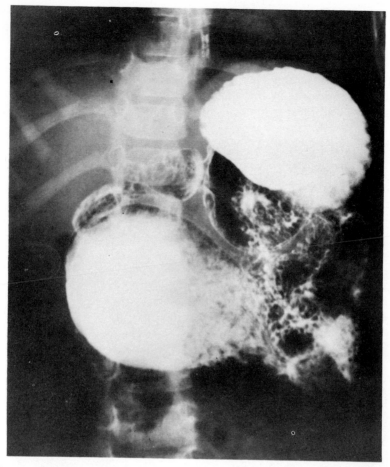

Fig. 3.4. Jejunal stagnant loop occurring postoperatively after resection of atresia.

follow-through should be performed paying particular attention to the ileum. The salient radiological features of this malady are described in chapter 9.

Other Small Intestinal Diseases

Bleeding from the small intestine may be difficult to investigate radiologically but duodenal ulceration, duplication of the ileum, and Meckel's diverticulum may all occasionally be diagnosed from barium studies. However, a negative barium study by no means excludes these disorders.

Haemorrhage into the bowel wall, as may occur in Henoch-Schönlein purpura, may produce deformation in the involved bowel wall and when the terminal ileum is involved may produce an appearance similar to Crohn's disease.

Parasitic infestation may occasionally be diagnosed radiologically. *Ascaris lumbricoides* in the small intestine can be readily recognised (Fig. 3.5) and strongyloidiasis may produce an acute inflammation

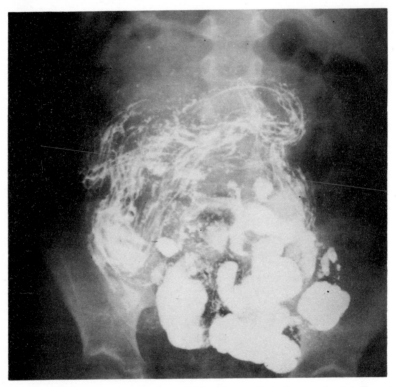

Fig. 3.5. Barium follow-through in a child with ascariasis, barium in the alimentary tract of the worms.

and obstruction in the ileum which may also give an appearance that mimics Crohn's disease.

Lymphangiography may occasionally be useful in the older child in order to demonstrate lymphangiectasia, but in an infant this procedure may be dangerous, severe complications including respiratory failure having been reported.

Endoscopy

Endoscopy is increasingly available in the paediatric age group. It is now often possible, during the course of colonoscopy, for the endoscope to enter the distal ileum and allow an endoscopic ileal biopsy to be taken. In this way a firm diagnosis of Crohn's disease may be made in a child when the appearance of the ileum, on radiology, may be controversial (Campbell, Williams and Walker-Smith, 1978). Endoscopic biopsy of duodenum is also possible at the time of an upper alimentary tract endoscopy.

Technetium Scan

The radionuclide technetium 99M (^{99m} Tc) concentrates in gastric mucosa and appears in gastric juice. When given intravenously as ^{99m} Tc pertechnetate, ectopic gastric mucosa appears as an abnormal localisation on abdominal imaging with a gamma-ray camera, so enabling a Meckel's diverticulum or a duplication of the gut to be diagnosed (Jewett, Duszynoki and Allen, 1970; Leonidas and Germann, 1974) (Fig. 3.6). The technique is simple and non-invasive and the amount of radiation is in the same range as a single abdominal X-ray. It is used to investigate the child with unexplained malaena or rectal bleeding and has a high diagnostic yield although occasional false negatives may occur. Its use should lead to earlier and more accurate diagnosis of Meckel's diverticulum but a negative result in a child with continuing severe symptoms should not deter a surgeon from proceeding with a diagnostic laparotomy.

Laparotomy

Sometimes when all other investigations prove to be negative a laparotomy may be indicated, but this decision should be undertaken only with caution and as a last resort. It may be indicated, for example, in a child who has persistent occult bleeding from the alimentary tract when there is reason to suspect the presence of Meckel's diverticulum. Laparotomy may also be indicated when malrotation with intermittent volvulus is suspected, although there may be no radiological evidence of this, and, again, when the radiological diagnosis is uncertain and lymphoma or Crohn's disease may be suspected.

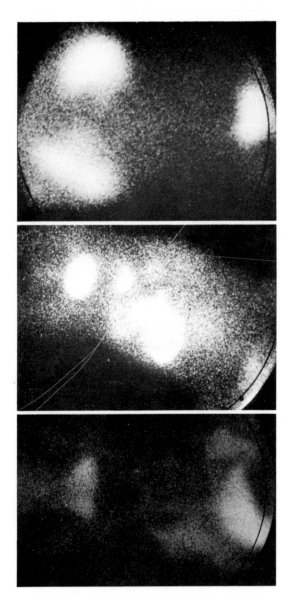

Fig. 3.6. Technetium scan (a) normal appearance, (b) ectopic gastric mucosa in Meckel's diverticulum, (c) ectopic gastric mucosa in a duplication.

MORPHOLOGICAL

Small Intestinal Biopsy

The introduction of small intestinal biopsy to paediatric practice by Shiner in 1957 was a major advance and has led to a great increase in knowledge of small intestinal mucosal pathology. In the same year, Crosby and Kugler in the USA developed for small intestinal biopsy in adults a biopsy capsule that has since been known as the Crosby capsule. In 1962, Read and his colleagues produced a modification of this capsule, and a paediatric version of the modification is now widely used for small intestinal biopsy in children. (Fig. 3.7). This is marketed as the Watson Capsule.

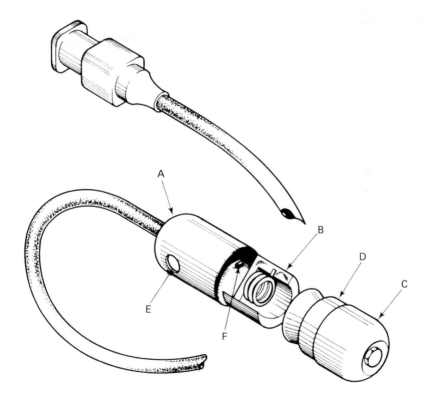

Fig. 3.7. Watson modification of paediatric Crosby Capsule:

A. Body of capsule	C. Cap	E. Port opening
B. Knife blade	D. Expanding skirt	F. Stake

The safety of a capsule in children is related to its porthole size, which in the Watson capsule is 2·5 to 3 mm, compared with 5 mm in the adult capsule. It is dangerous to use the adult capsule in small children as the size of the tissue biopsied may be too large and occasionally lead to perforation. Use of the paediatric capsule, however, is safe in the experience of most observers although there is still a small risk of complications. A modified version of the paediatric Crosby capsule with two port holes, which provides two smaller biopsies at one time, may be useful when the presence of a patchy lesion is suspected, e.g. mucosal damage as a sequel to gastroenteritis. The use of this further modification does not increase the risks of the procedure (Kilby, 1976) (Fig. 3.8).

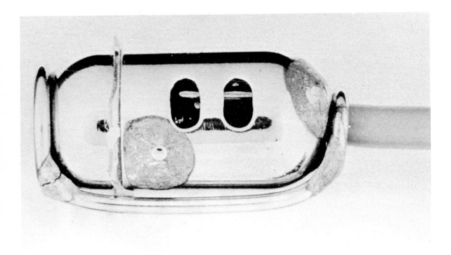

Fig. 3.8. Double port small intestinal biopsy capsule (Kilby, 1976).

The European Society of Paediatric Gastroenterology, in 1969, undertook a review of the safety of small intestinal biopsy in children (Table 3.3).

Table 3.3
Intestinal biopsies and perforations reported by the European Society of Paediatric Gastroenterology

No. of biopsies	4,937
No. of perforations	8 (0·16%)

(Permission of Visakorpi, 1970)

During the author's experience of 704 biopsies in the six-year period 1966–1972 at the Royal Alexandra Hospital, there was only one serious complication; namely, an intraduodenal haematoma which settled spontaneously without any surgical intervention. So, although this is an essentially safe procedure it does still carry some risk. It is vital, therefore, that small intestinal biopsy is performed in children only in special centres where considerable experience and expertise in this technique may be built up and only when there is a valid indication for its performance. Only in this way will safety coupled with minimal disturbance to the child and reliable results, all be appropriately combined. The occasional biopsy performed in inexperienced hands may lead to a disturbed child and, often, inconclusive results.

Technique of Small Intestinal Biopsy

The child is fasted over night but may be given small amounts of water as required. Infants may be given a 10 p.m. and sometimes a 2 a.m. feeding if considered necessary. On the morning of the biopsy the child is sedated. A useful regime of oral sedation is that currently used at the Queen Elizabeth Hospital, namely vallergan and chloral hydrate in appropriate dose for age.

If the child becomes restless or distressed during the procedure intravenous valium may be given with a maximum dosage of 0·5 mg/kg. Once the child is sedated appropriately, the capsule is passed. This is done in the small child by placing a tongue depressor in the mouth and placing the capsule at the back of the tongue. The depressor is withdrawn, the chin held up, and the child swallows. The tubing is then gently advanced till the capsule is in the stomach. A resistance is often felt at the oesophago-cardiac junction. The child is then placed on his right side and the capsule further advanced. It should then fall towards the pylorus.

The next step depends upon whether a flexible tubing is being used or a more rigid tubing, and whether there is to be X-ray screening or progress assessed by plain X-ray of the abdomen. In addition, if a non radio-opaque tube is used, radio-opaque material such as Urografin needs to be injected down the tubing before the position of the capsule can be checked radiologically. Using a flexible tubing and a plain X-ray of the abdomen, as the author outlined in the first edition, is a time-consuming procedure but it does have the virtue of providing an exact record, i.e. an X-ray of the exact site of the biopsy. The author now favours the more rapid technique of using a radio-opaque relatively rigid tube and positioning the capsule under X-ray screening control. The usual speed of this technique makes the procedure preferable from the child's point of view and also permits more than one child to have a biopsy on a particular morning. Care should be taken to monitor the X-ray screening time, which should not exceed two minutes, and is usually far shorter.

Metaclopromide introduced into the tubing or intravenously, in the dosage of 2·5 mg for infants under two, and 5 mg for those over two years, speeds the onward passage of the capsule, and is often used.

Using either procedure, once the capsule is positioned in the fourth part of the duodenum, the duodeno-jejunal flexure, or the first loop of the jejunum, it is 'fired' by rapid suction with a 20 ml syringe and then withdrawn. Ideally, biopsies should be taken from a constant, standard site. A virtue of the screening technique is that it can be done

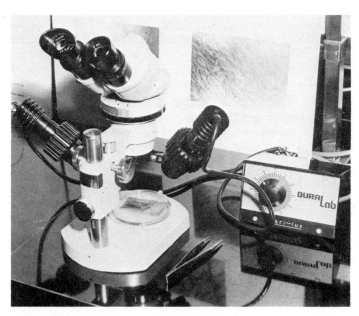

Fig. 3.9. The dissecting or stereo-microscope.

easily and accurately. If Urografin or metaclopromide syrup has been injected down the tube, in order to ensure that it is not blocked it is helpful to inject 2 ml of water followed by 2 ml of air before firing the capsule.

Ideally, some duodenal juice should be obtained either by free drainage before the capsule is fired or at the time of 'firing'. The juice should be examined immediately for the presence of *Giardia lamblia* and sent for culture if bacterial overgrowth is considered as a diagnostic possibility.

Once the capsule has been withdrawn the small intestinal biopsy specimen should be rapidly removed from the capsule. A small portion can be immediately cut off for electron microscope studies. The remainder is placed on a small portion of black paper and then put into formol-saline and examined immediately under the dissecting or stereo-microscope (Fig. 3.9).

It is then possible to study and to photograph the three-dimensional architecture of the mucosal specimen. Once this has been done the mucosa is processed for histological section.

A portion of the small intestinal biopsy may also be removed before fixation for assay of its disaccharidase content; for example to diagnose one of the syndromes of primary disaccharide intolerance.

A number of other observations may also be made on small intestinal biopsy specimens but these are not as yet routine. Some of these are listed in Table 3.4.

Table 3.4
Some possible observations of small intestinal biopsy specimens of clinical and research application

1. Morphology	dissecting microscope
	light microscope
	electron microscope
2. Enzyme assay	disaccharidases
	dipeptidases
3. Histochemistry of enzymes	
4. Transport studies	e.g. sugar transport studies in diagnosis of congenital glucose-galactose malabsorption
5. Metabolic activity	e.g. oxygen consumption, glucose and amino acid uptake, etc.
6. Chemical composition	e.g. increased copper in enterocyte found in Menkes' syndrome
7. Immunofluorescence	immunoglobulin class of plasma cells and their antibody-producing properties
8. Lymphocyte function	e.g. production of lymphokines by cultured biopsies

Morphological Observations of Small Intestinal Biopsy Specimens

Dissecting microscopy: Rubin and his colleagues (1960) were the first to describe the appearance of small intestinal mucosal biopsy specimens when viewed under the dissecting microscope or stereo-microscope. These observations were extended and amplified by Holmes, Hourihane and Booth (1961). The value of this technique of examination has been confirmed by many other workers, both in the field of adult medicine and in paediatrics. Many now consider that examination of a small intestinal biopsy specimen without a dissecting microscopic assessment is an inadequate examination. The value of this method is: firstly, it greatly facilitates orientation of biopsy specimens in readiness for sectioning; secondly, it allows study to be made of the three-dimensional arrangements of mucosal architecture; thirdly, the whole biopsy specimen may be examined which is particularly important in children, where patchy mucosal lesions do often occur; and finally it allows rapid diagnosis of the presence of a flat mucosa.

However, some authors such as Rubin and Dobbins (1965) consider that this method of examination adds little to histology and that its only value lies in the rapid recognition of a flat mucosa. They advocate, instead, serial sectioning for histology of all biopsy specimens. Such a procedure, however, is outside the capacity of most

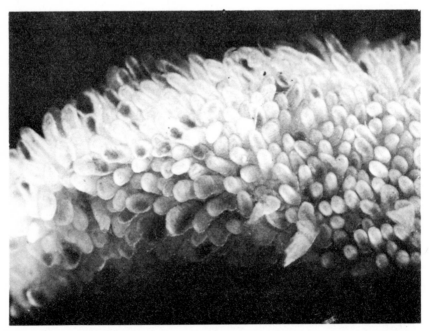

Fig. 3.10. Dissecting microscope appearances: normal small intestinal mucosa in an adult with finger-like villi.

hospitals whereas dissecting microscopy is simple and straightforward and can easily be performed routinely.

When small intestinal biopsies are examined under the dissecting or stereo-microscope the three-dimensional architecture of the mucosal surface may be studied. In normal healthy adults the mucosa is characterised by finger-like villi (Fig. 3.10), but in children the villi tend to be broader (Fig. 3.11). The terms leaf-like and tongue-like are

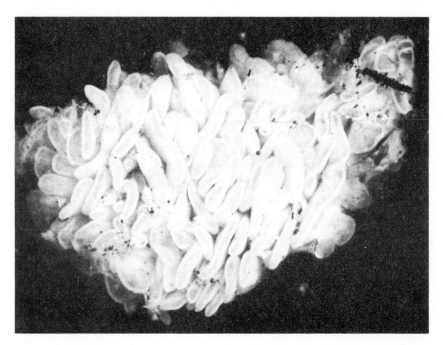

Fig. 3.11. Dissecting microscope appearances: normal small intestinal mucosa in a child with broader villi; long thin ridge-like, tongue-like and leaf-like villi with occasional finger-like villi.

used to describe such villi, and when they are extremely wide the term thin ridge-like villi is used (Fig. 3.12).

When the small intestine is studied at post-mortem by means of a dissecting microscope as described later in this chapter, variation of mucosal morphology with age can be demonstrated. Figure 3.13 indicates the number of children from a group of 85 who had finger-like villous cores as the dominant appearance of the mucosa in the duodenum, the jejunum 50 cm from the duodeno-jejunal flexure and the ileum 50 cm proximal to the ileo-caecal valve at different ages.

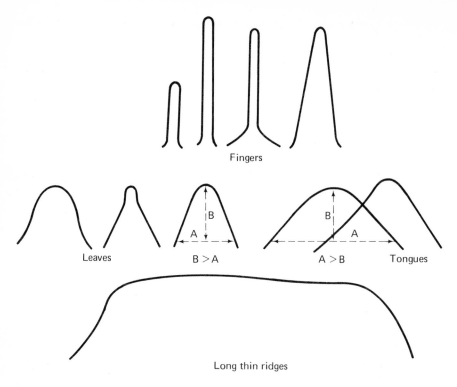

Fig. 3.12. Diagrammatic representation of dissecting microscope terminology based on observations made at autopsy.

It can be seen that throughout childhood up to the age of ten years finger-like villi occurred uncommonly in the duodenum and broader villi were characteristic. This was true, but to a somewhat lesser extent, in the jejunum. In the ileum, finger-like villi were most often found in the neonate, but from one month to four years broader villi were found to be characteristic. Over the age of four years, finger-like villi were again the dominant finding in the ileum, as occurs in adult life. Figure 3.14 demonstrates this by illustrating the distribution of dissecting microscope appearances along the length of the small intestine in a child of five months and shows the transition from broader villi in the proximal small intestine to narrower forms distally.

   Ferguson, Maxwell and Carr (1969) used this technique to study the morphology of 11 stillborn infants and 29 infants dying within 4 days of birth. They found that the jejunal villous pattern was mainly finger-like villi in infants up to 26 weeks gestation, but from 26 weeks onwards they found a preponderance of broader leaf-like and tongue-like villi.

Thus, the observation under the dissecting microscope of broad villi described as leaf-like, tongue-like or thin ridge-like villi on proximal small intestinal biopsy, is accepted as a normal finding in children. The explanation for this observation of broader forms is unknown, but as it is found in infants of 26 or more weeks gestation who have not

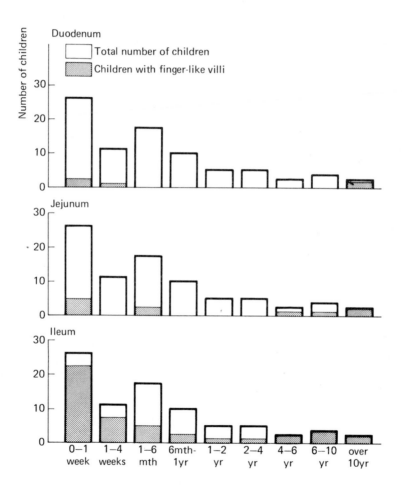

Fig. 3.13. Distribution of finger-like villi in duodenum, jejunum and ileum of children of varying ages.

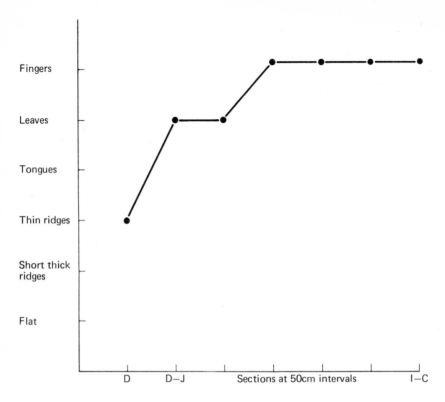

Fig. 3.14. Distribution of dissecting microscope appearances along the length of the small intestine in a child of 5 months without evidence of small intestinal disease.

been fed, it cannot be due to ingestion of food and bacteria after birth, although in-utero ingestion of amniotic fluid or gastric acid secretions *per se*, may play a role.

Abnormal appearances are broadly grouped under two headings: a flat mucosa and a ridged or convoluted mucosa. In both types of mucosae the normal villous architecture is lost.

Table 3.5 indicates a classification of the dissecting microscope appearances of small intestinal biopsy specimens (Fig. 3.15) (Walker-Smith and Reye, 1971).

It is important that a photographic record should be kept of each biopsy examined in order to correlate appearances seen with those observed with the light microscope.

The relationship between dissecting microscopy appearances and histology gradings is illustrated in Fig. 3.16.

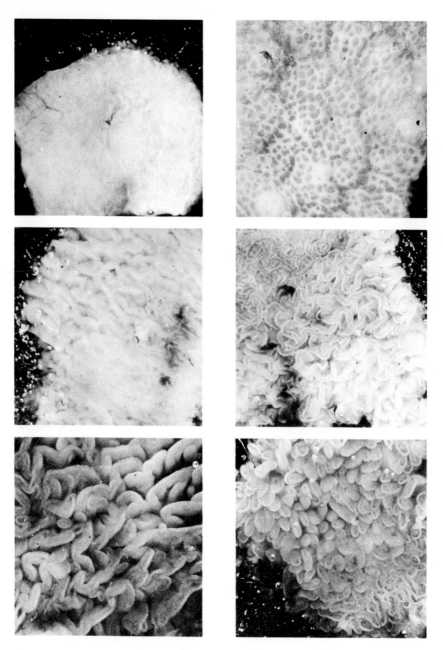

Fig. 3.15. Examples of dissecting microscope appearances in the three groups. From left to right, top row Ia, Ib; middle row IIa, IIb; bottom row IIIa, IIIb.

Table 3.5
Classification of dissecting microscope appearances

GROUP I	Flat Mucosa
	(a) Flat and barren
	(b) Flat mosaic
GROUP II	Thickened Ridges
	(a) short
	(b) taller
GROUP III	Broad Villi
	(a) long thin ridge-like villi and tongue-like villi.
	(b) tongue and leaf-like villi with occasional finger-like villi
	(c) leaf-like and finger-like villi.

Light microscopy: Small intestinal biopsy sections are routinely examined with the light microscope after staining the sections with haematoxylin and eosin. At present an unsatisfactory situation exists in relation to histological terminology. The earliest reports divided pathological small intestinal mucosae into 'sub-total villous atrophy' and 'partial villous atrophy'. The former category was characterised by a flat mucosa with thickening of the glandular layer beneath an atrophic epithelium, and the latter by a less abnormal mucosa. Some authors have further qualified 'partial villous atrophy' with the terms mild and severe, and others have confused the situation further by using the term 'total villous atrophy' to describe a flat mucosa. The fact that the mucosa described as 'subtotal villous atrophy' is in fact not a truly atrophic mucosa, i.e. not thinner than normal (*see* Fig. 4.4), has led to this terminology not being universally adopted (*see* chapter 4). Many authors use the terms flat, abnormal (but not flat) and normal to describe the appearances seen. Others have adopted simple systems of grading, e.g. at the Queen Elizabeth Hospital, since 1960, the following system of grading has been used by Dr N. E. France (Fig. 3.16).

Histological Gradings of Small Intestinal Mucosal Biopsy Specimens

Normal:	Villous height is twice, or more, the length of the crypts. Epithelium is high columnar with basal nuclei and an indented surface. Intra-epithelial lymphocytes number 12 to 35 per 100 enterocytes. There are plasma cells, lymphocytes and a few eosinophils in the lamina propria.

+	Variable picture: Surface epithelium is usually normal but the mucosa shows one or two abnormal features, namely—shortening and occasional widening of villi, increased intra-epithelial lymphocytes, increased round cells in lamina propria and elongation of crypts.
+ +	Villi are replaced by short, usually wide ridges covered by low columnar or pseudostratified epithelium although the epithelium can be normal. Intra-epithelial lymphocytes may be increased, there is a moderate increase of round cells in the lamina propria, and the crypts are elongated.
+ + +	Villi are completely absent, leaving a flat surface covered by pseudostratified, low columnar or, occasionally, normal epithelium frequently vacuolated by fat and often accompanied by considerably increased intra-epithelial lymphocytes. Round cells, mainly plasma cells, in the lamina propria are greatly increased and there is a moderate increase of eosinophils and often some neutrophil polymorphs. The crypts are very elongated and usually show increased mitoses.
±	Used to indicate slight or doubtful mucosal change.
Intermediate Grades: e.g. +–++, ++–+++	are recognised and are particularly useful when used to assess serial biopsies from a single patient.
Patchy Lesions:	show one or more grades of abnormality in a single specimen or different specimens obtained by multiple biopsy, e.g. +/++.
Apparent Abnormality: (+ or ++)	can be present over or in the vicinity of a mucosal lymph follicle or Brunner's gland in an otherwise normal mucosa. This is not significant.
Pathological Lesions:	such as inflammation or changes of cystic fibrosis are not graded.

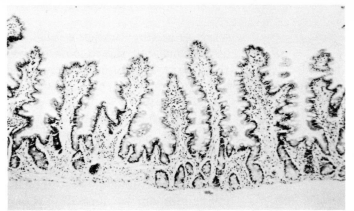

(1)

(2)

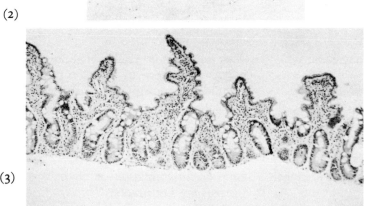

(3)

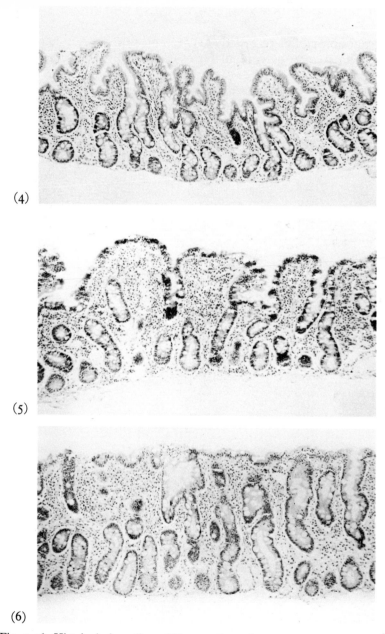

(4)

(5)

(6)

Fig. 3.16. Histological grading of France. Examples (1, 2) are normal, then +(3), + − + +(4), + +(5), + + +(6), same magnification.

Patchy abnormalities recorded as $+/++$ or $++/+++$ indicate that part of a biopsy may be graded; for example, as $+$ abnormality and another part as $+++$, i.e. $+/+++$ (Fig. 3.17). Manuel *et al.* (1979) have divided such patchy lesions into those with a minor degree of patchy abnormality, i.e. a difference of one grade, and those with a major degree where the difference is of two gradings (Fig. 3.17).

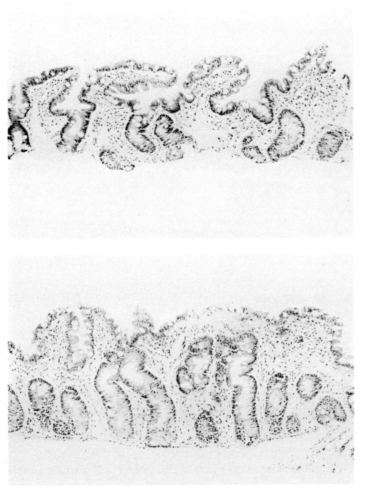

Fig. 3.17. Two parts of a single biopsy specimen showing a patchy enteropathy above $+$, beneath $+++$, whole biopsy is graded as $+/+++$.

Patchiness may be observed within a single biopsy specimen or may be apparent when two specimens are obtained using double port capsule. The dissecting microscope is helpful in diagnosing a patchy enteropathy (Fig. 3.18). Manuel *et al.* (1979) found a significantly increased number of patchy lesions when a double port capsule was used. They found a patchy lesion to be chiefly associated with cow's

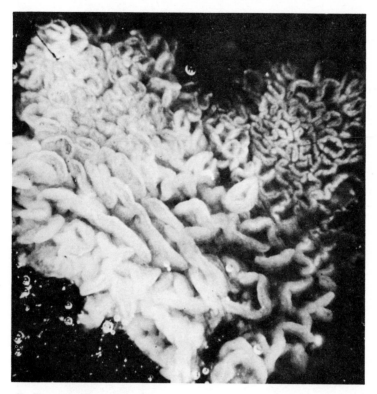

Fig. 3.18. Example of patchy enteropathy viewed with dissecting microscope. Lower part of biopsy is characterised by long thin ridge-like villi; upper portion in each corner by short thick ridges with a convoluted appearance.

milk sensitive enteropathy and post-enteritis syndrome. Table 3.6 relates the finding of patchiness of small intestinal enteropathy to clinical diagnosis in this study.

The wide range in height of villi seen in normal small intestinal mucosae in childhood is illustrated in Fig. 3.16. Normal villi in children are often considerably broader than those found in adult life. Adult pathologists may incorrectly interpret small intestinal biopsies

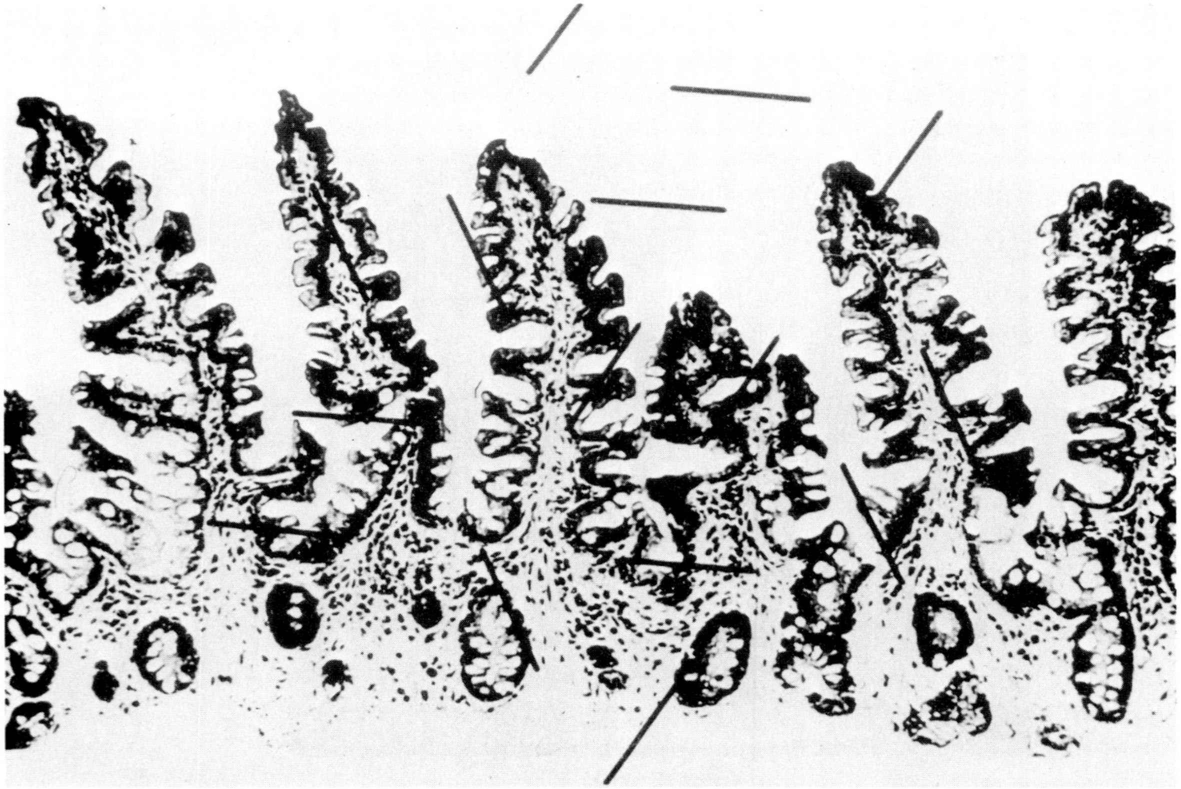

Fig. 3.19. Template superimposed on a biopsy specimen.

Table 3.6
Patchy enteropathy – correlation with disease

Diagnosis	Degree of patchy abnormality		No. of patchy biopsies	No. of uniform biopsies	Total
	minor	major			
Cow's milk protein intolerance	9	13	22	11	33
Post-enteritis syndrome	8	2	10	13	23
Coeliac disease:	0	0	0	14	14
at diagnosis	1	1	2	18	20
on gluten-free diet at challenge	6	1	7	13	20
Others	8	0	8	160	168
	32	17	49	229	278

from children and even diagnose coeliac disease when the mucosa is normal. The author has encountered this on several occasions.

There is clearly an urgent need for an internationally agreed histological terminology to describe the light microscope appearances of small intestinal biopsies. There is a close relationship between dissecting microscopic and light microscopic appearances, but this is not absolute (*see* Fig. 3.22). Nevertheless, examination of small intestinal biopsy specimens with the dissecting microscope is as important as examination with the light microscope and should not be omitted.

Quantitative measurements of villous height and width, mucosal thickness and surface cell height have been reported by many observers in adults and children. Such techniques have wide ranges for both normal and abnormal mucosae. Chapman and his colleagues (1973) have described a technique for measuring changes in the architecture of small intestinal mucosa by using a modification of the technique of television image analysis to measure areas occupied by surface and crypt epithelium and calculation of the ratios of the two areas. This method gives better separation between normal and abnormal compared with the other techniques mentioned above.

Another quantitative technique for evaluating small intestinal morphology i.e. quantitative morphometry has been used (Dunnill and Whitehead, 1972). With this technique, a graticule in a microscope may be used, or histological sections are projected onto a wall on which is applied a template of 15 lines of equal length connecting the vertices of a regular hexagonal point network (Fig. 3.19). The magnification is kept constant. The number of end points of the lines or hits ($\bar{h}$) falling on the tissue between the epithelial cells and the muscularis mucosae is recorded. This value ($\bar{h}$) is proportional to the volume of the mucosa. The number of intersections or cuts ($\bar{c}$) made by the lines with the epithelium is also recorded. This value is proportional to the surface area of the mucosa. The template is superimposed on different fields of sections from each biopsy until a minimum of 200 hits are recorded. The mean number of hits per field, ($\bar{h}$) and the mean number of cuts per field ($\bar{c}$) are recorded.

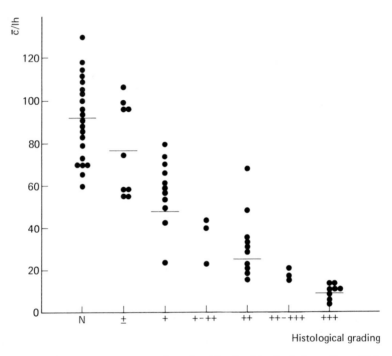

Fig. 3.20. Relationship between $\bar{c}/lh$ and subjective histological grading of biopsies (France.) (Permission de Peyer.)

The ratio $\bar{c}/l\,\bar{h}$ where l is the length of the line is an index of surface to volume. The values of this index and surface area marker $\bar{c}$ may be used as objective markers to compare one biopsy with another, especially serial biopsies from the same patient (de Peyer et al., 1978). This objective technique was used by de Peyer and her colleagues to validate the subjective grading of mucosal biopsies described earlier (Fig. 3.20). Figure 3.20 indicates that although there is some variation around the mean there is a satisfactory agreement between subjective grading and this objective morphometric technique. Furthermore, evaluation of serial biopsies in the same patient with this technique shows a good correlation with subjective assessment. Although this technique of morphometric evaluation is of value as a research tool, especially with serial observations, it is not recommended for routine biopsy assessment.

Another quantitative technique, namely counting the number of lymphocytes within the small intestinal epithelium, is of value for routine use (Ferguson, 1977). It is used to make a differential count of

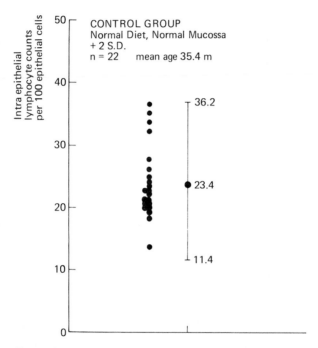

Fig. 3.21. Intraepithelial lymphocyte count in control group of children on a normal diet with a normal mucosa. (Permission of Phillips.)

the lymphocytes within the villous epithelium, i.e. measuring the intra-epithelial lymphocyte count (IEL) per 100 villous epithelial cells. These lymphocytes are intercellular, i.e. they lie between the enterocytes, but are intra-epithelial since they occur within the surface epithelium. Phillips and his colleagues (1977) found a mean of 23·4 IEL per 100 villous epithelial cells in a group of children on a normal diet who had a normal small intestinal mucosa (Fig. 3.21). There was

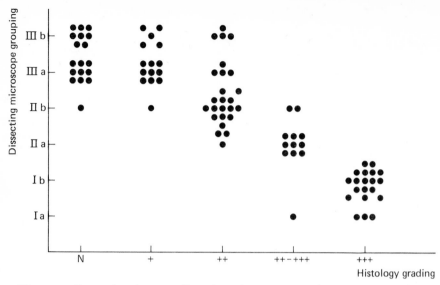

Fig. 3.22. Comparison between dissecting microscope grouping and histology grading of small intestinal biopsies in children.

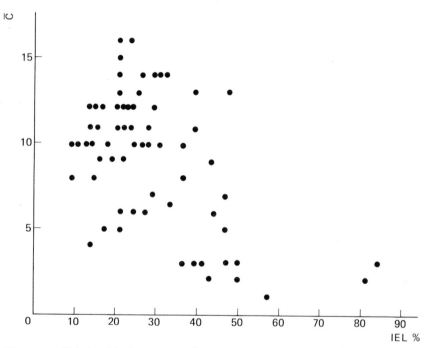

Fig. 3.23. Relationship between surface area measurement $\bar{c}$ and intraepithelial lymphocyte count per cent. (Permission de Peyer.)

no significant variation with age in the children studied and the value is similar to the mean level of 21·1 described by Ferguson and Murray (1971) in 40 adults.

Significantly increased levels of IEL are characteristically found in the small intestinal mucosa of untreated coeliac disease in both children and adults (*see* chapter 4) and also in the mucosa of untreated dermatitis herpetiformis in adults. Increased levels have also been reported in tropical sprue, some children with giardiasis and some with unexplained diarrhoea and failure to thrive (Ferguson, 1977).

The intra-epithelial lymphocyte count falls to within the normal range after introduction of a gluten-free diet in children with coeliac disease. It has been argued that the increase found in the flat mucosa of coeliac disease is merely an effect of the reduction in surface area. However, when intra-epithelial lymphocyte counts are related to surface area ($\bar{c}$) in children with a flat mucosa due to coeliac disease and also those with a non-coeliac enteropathy (Fig. 3.23) it is clear that there is no consistent relationship between the reduction in surface area and the level of intra-epithelial lymphocyte count. Furthermore, there may be localised or patchy areas of increased intra-epithelial lymphocytes, which argues against the level being merely reflection of reduced surface area.

Knowledge of what is normal in children is clearly difficult to determine. It is obviously not ethical to biopsy normal children but observation of morphology of biopsies taken from children suspected of having gastrointestinal disease but who in fact turn out to be normal, observation of control biopsies from children with coeliac disease in remission on a gluten-free diet, as well as post-mortem studies of the small intestine from children dying without evidence of gastroenterological disease (*see* p. 181), do allow some knowledge of 'normal' small intestinal mucosal morphology to be acquired.

It appears that villi broader than those usually observed in normal adults in Britain and Australia occur in children. From autopsy studies this appears to be more apparent proximally (*see* Fig. 3.14). Indeed a greater variation in the range of normal morphology appears to occur in children as compared with adults.

Ultrastructure of the Small Intestinal Mucosa in Childhood

Transmission and scanning electron microscopy have now been used to study the morphology of small intestinal biopsies taken from children as well as adults (Figs 3.24, 3.25). Certain differences in morphology in children have been observed (Phillips, France and

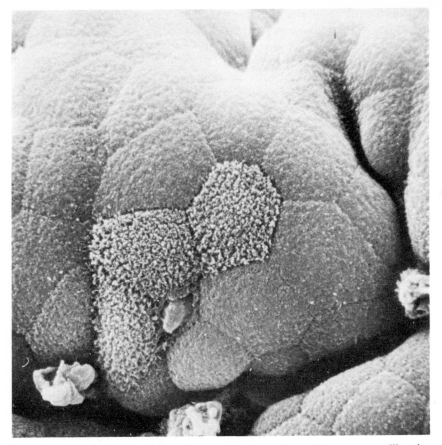

Fig. 3.24 Scanning electron microscope appearance of extrusion zone at a villus tip. Three cells that are about to extrude have lost their glycocalyx. Magnification 14,570. (Permission of Phillips.)

Walker-Smith, 1977). At present such studies are outside the scope of routine assessment of mucosal morphology of biopsy specimens but play an important role in research.

Ultrastructure of the Enterocytes

The small intestine is a dynamic organ. The single-cell-thick layer of epithelial cells covering the mucosa is in a continuous state of turnover. Undifferentiated epithelial cells proliferate in the crypts of

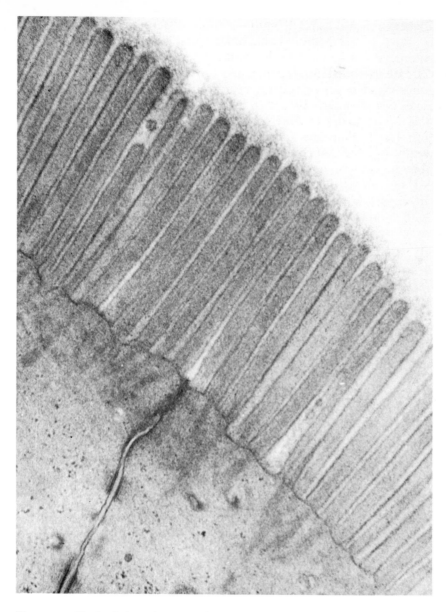

Fig. 3.25. Transmission electron microscope appearances of brush border or microvilli of enterocyte. Magnification 70,000. (Permission of Phillips.)

Lieberkühn and travel up onto the villus, differentiating and maturing as they proceed until functionally mature absorptive cells, the enterocytes, are found on the villus. After a short but active life these cells are extruded into the lumen of the small intestine from extrusion zones which occur principally near the tips of the villi. The extrusion zones may be clearly seen with the scanning electron microscope (Fig. 3.24). The turnover time for normal small intestinal epithelium is from two to four days and it has been calculated that half a pound in weight of epithelial cells is shed into the lumen each day in an adult human (Leblond and Walker, 1956).

If the mucosa is sectioned longitudinally, from crypt base to villous tip, then it is possible to study the ultrastructural appearance of the epithelium in the various stages from immaturity through maturity to extrusion.

Brush Border (Fig. 3.25)

The luminal surface of the enterocyte is a highly specialised region called the brush border. This fraction of the cell may be isolated and its properties investigated. It consists of the microvilli and the terminal web. The microvilli are membrane-bound finger-like extensions of the cell covered by a fuzzy carbohydrate rich layer called the glycocalyx, which is probably produced by the enterocyte itself and may form a barrier against the potentially hostile gut lumen (Walker, 1975). Inside the microvilli are filamentous structures, probably identical with actin, which are attached to the inner aspect of the microvillous membrane and extend down into it to form part of the terminal web.

Some marked differences have been reported between the appearance of the brush border over the villus in childhood and in the adult. In both, the brush border of the crypt region is fairly disorganised, the microvilli few in number and short. In the adult, Brown (1962) has reported that the microvilli become progressively more numerous, longer and thinner as the enterocyte proceeds up the villus until, at the apex of the villus, the microvilli present maximal surface area, being tallest and most numerous in this region. In the child, Phillips *et al.* (1977) found that the microvillous surface area was maximal in the mid-region of the villus in histologically normal small intestinal biopsy specimens, and also, contrasting with the adult finding, there was a reduction in microvillous surface area on the upper third of the villus, the microvilli becoming short and irregular (Fig. 3.26).

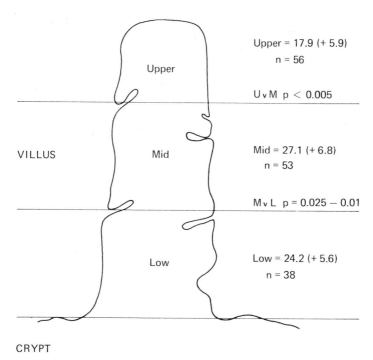

Upper = 17.9 (+ 5.9)

n = 56

U v M p < 0.005

Mid = 27.1 (+ 6.8)

n = 53

M v L p = 0.025 − 0.01

Low = 24.2 (+ 5.6)

n = 38

Fig. 3.26. Surface area mean increase, provided by the microvilli in each of the three villous regions (n = number of observations). (Permission of Phillips.)

Cellular Characteristics

The crypt cell or enteroblast is a flask-shaped cell with a basally located nucleus. Nearly all the cytoplasm is apically located, and there is a preponderance of free ribosomes and polyribosomes with some short lengths of rough endoplasmic reticulum. Mitochondria are few in number. Morphological evidence of secretion by the crypt cells has been reported by Trier (1964) and it is generally accepted that the cells of the crypt region go through a secretory phase.

There is a progressive differentiation and maturation of the crypt cells at the crypt/villus junction. The organelles increase in number, free ribosomes and polyribosomes become less evident, and rough endoplasmic reticulum and smooth endoplasmic reticulum increase. Some cells in the low villus region, described as undifferentiated by Shiner (1974), have dilated rough endoplasmic reticulum and/or swollen mitochondria. Cell extrusion has, in fact, been observed in this low villus region in childhood (Phillips et al., 1977) and this may be a result of immature cells being prematurely exposed to the luminal environment. Thus, the amount of cellular extrusion occurring in this region, the ratio of free ribosomes to rough endoplasm reticulum, and the degree of dilatation and swelling of mitochondria may be taken as indications of immaturity of the epithelial cells. This could be of practical value in assessing morphologically the maturity of the enterocytes in various diseases in which part of the underlying pathophysiology of the disease is attributed to a relative immaturity of cells covering the villi, e.g. in viral gastroenteritis and the post-enteritis syndrome.

The ultrastructure of the mature absorptive enterocyte has been described in several reviews (Trier, 1967; Toner, 1968). Padykula (1962) put forward the theory that, in the adult, the epithelium at the apex of the villus is most active. Some morphological observations (Biempica et al., 1968; Phillips et al., 1977) suggest that in childhood the cells in the mid-region are best adapted for digestion and absorption. Microvilli present maximal surface area in the mid-region (Phillips et al., 1977) and in the tip region, microvilli present the least surface area of the villous enterocytes. Autophagic vacuoles are found in the tip region and residual bodies appear more frequently in the upper part of the villus. Three methods of mitochondrial dissolution have been reported to occur, predominantly near the tip region (Phillips et al., 1977). These organelle changes are indicative either of an ageing phenomenon occurring prior to extrusion, or of an adverse luminal influence on the most exposed enterocytes. It is possible, and perhaps more likely, that there is a combination of the two processes.

Basement Membrane

Although the 'basement membrane' is an inexact term, it is convenient to use it to describe the region separating the epithelium from the underlying lamina propria (Fig. 3.27). It is approximately 1 micron wide, and a single-cell-thick layer of fibrocytes runs along its mid-line. Underneath the epithelium is a lining of homogeneous material 40 nm wide, separated slightly from the basal membrane of the enterocyte by a 50 nm gap which is called the basal lamina and is believed to be produced by the epithelium. Between the basal lamina and the fibrocyte is a region containing some collagen fibrils in a homogeneous, slightly electron dense matrix. On the lamina propria side of the fibrocyte, this is repeated. Capillaries lying next to the basement membrane also have a basal lamina around the endothelium.

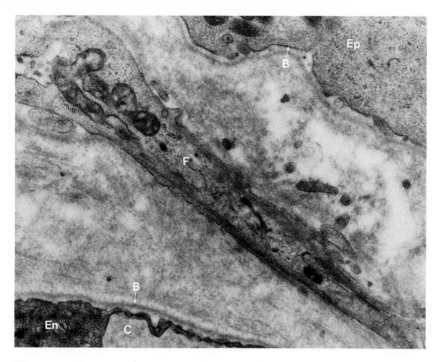

Fig. 3.27. Electron microscope appearance of basement membrane in normal mucosa. Basal lamina (B) of epithelium (Ep) and endothelium (En) of a capillary (C) with a fibrocyte (F) in between.

Lamina Propria Cells

Most of the lamina propria cells can easily be recognised with the electron microscope. Some difficulty may arise when cells are undergoing differentiation from one form to another.

Plasma cells (B cells) have a distinctive pattern of rough endoplasmic reticulum which sometimes expands to form large vesicles, presumably containing antibody, delimited by a single membrane of ribosome-studded endoplasmic reticulum. Lymphocytes are usually small cells with a large nucleus to cytoplasmic ratio. The nucleus often has a cleft in it. Lymphocytes are found not only within the lamina propria but also crossing the basement membrane into the epithelium and within the epithelium (the intra-epithelial lymphocyte).

Mast cells are characterised by their cytoplasmic inclusions. Mast cells contain 0·4 μ wide electron dense bodies which have scroll-like or worm-like patterns in them. Eosinophils are polymorphonuclear leucocytes. They are recognised by their elliptical, electron-dense cytoplasmic granules which have a denser crystalline body in the centre. They are sometimes observed in the epithelial layer.

Neutrophils, polymorphonuclear leucocytes, have a background cytoplasm which is usually slightly more electron dense than that of the eosinophils. There are a variety of cytoplasmic granules present. Normally, they are not seen in the lamina propria but occasionally are observed in capillaries.

Basophils are polymorphonuclear leucocytes that contain similar inclusions to most cells but they are rarely encountered in the lamina propria.

Macrophages are large cells with irregular outlines and large lysosomal inclusions. They are frequently positioned near the basement membrane. Muscle cells, nerve cells and fibrocytes are also an integral part of the lamina propria.

The Role of Small Intestinal Biopsy in Diagnosis

At present, a single small intestinal biopsy has two specific roles that are of value in making a diagnosis in clinical paediatrics. The first is to demonstrate the presence of a proximal small intestinal enteropathy. This may be defined as an abnormality of the upper small intestinal mucosa, which can be demonstrated with the light microscope. The second is to provide a piece of small intestinal mucosa for enzyme assay in order to diagnose a specific enzyme deficiency.

It has recently become clear that two or more biopsies over a period of time, that is, serial small intestinal biopsies related to dietary change (i.e. elimination and challenge), are required before a final diagnosis can be made on, for example, coeliac disease (*see* chapter 4) or cow's milk sensitive enteropathy (*see* chapter 5). The use of biopsy in this way, initially a research procedure, has now become routine. It enables a specific diagnosis to be made that is not at present possible by any other means.

Table 3.7
Disorders in which biopsy is invariably valuable

Abnormal morphology	Normal morphology
Coeliac disease	Congenital alactasia
Abetaliproteinaemia	Sucrase-isomaltase deficiency
Agammaglobulinaemia	

There is a group of disorders in which, to enable a specific diagnosis to be made, biopsy is invariably of value (Table 3.7). These are disorders in which there is a uniform proximal enteropathy or a specific enzyme deficiency.

The demonstration of an enteropathy is an essential prerequisite for diagnosis of coeliac disease, but there is no morphological appearance specific for this disorder. Although a flat, small intestinal mucosa is characteristic of coeliac disease, there are other causes of a flat mucosa in childhood (see chapter 4) and, furthermore, on occasion, lesser degrees of mucosal abnormality may be found in children with coeliac disease.

The enterocyte, in abetalipoproteinaemia, cannot synthesise betalipoprotein and, as a result, chylomicron formation is impaired. Thus, absorbed dietary fat is not properly mobilised from the enterocyte and as a result the cytoplasm of those cells lining the upper half of the villi appear vacuolated in ordinary haematoxylin and eosin sections. By using special stains these cells can be shown to be filled with fat.

Children with agammaglobulinaemia have a complete absence of plasma cells from their lamina propria but the mucosal architecture may range from a flat mucosa to a completely normal one.

Children who have either of the two primary disaccharide intolerances, namely congenital alactasia and sucrase-isomaltase deficiency, have a normal small intestinal morphology but the characteristic enzyme deficiencies may be demonstrated on disaccharidase assay.

When the lesion is non-uniform, i.e. patchy, or when there is penetration of the mucosa by a parasite, biopsy may provide a specific diagnosis, but in this group of disorders, the absence of abnormality (i.e. a normal mucosa) does not exclude the diagnosis (Table 3.8).

Table 3.8
Disorders in which biopsy may or may not be of specific diagnostic value

Giardiasis
Strongyloidiasis
Small intestinal lymphangiectasia
Small intestinal lymphoma
Hypogammaglobulinaemia

The trophozoite of *Giardia lamblia* is often found in the duodenal juice of children with giardiasis, but may also be found on section of small intestinal biopsy specimens. Similarly, in children with strongyloidiasis, larvae of *Strongyloides stercoralis* may be found in the juice and may also be found on section of the mucosal biopsy specimens.

Small intestinal lymphangiectasia may be diagnosed by biopsy of the small intestinal mucosa, but as the lesion is often patchy it may be missed on a single biopsy and multiple biopsies may be indicated. Rarely, small intestinal lymphoma may be diagnosed by biopsy if the lesion has invaded the mucosa.

Children with hypogammaglobulinaemia may be found to have hyperplastic lymphoid follicles on small intestinal biopsy as well as a diminished number of plasma cells and variable morphological abnormalities. *Giardia lamblia* is often found in the duodenal juice of such children.

In another group of disorders in which the lesion may also be patchy, the demonstration of an enteropathy is non-specific (Table 3.9). However, the finding of mucosal abnormality is diagnostically

Table 3.9
Disorders in which biopsy may be abnormal but abnormality is non-specific

Post-enteritis syndrome
Cow's milk protein intolerance
Transient gluten intolerance
Soy protein intolerance
Intractable diarrhoea syndrome
Tropical sprue
Radiation enteritis
Drug induced lesions, e.g. by methotrexate
Protein-energy malnutrition

useful in such patients because it indicates the presence of pathology in the small intestine. Some disorders in this group, e.g. cow's milk protein intolerance, may be diagnosed by serial biopsy related to dietary protein withdrawal and challenge, although there is no specific pathology for this disorder in the small intestinal mucosa.

Finally, for completeness, a group of disorders in which small intestinal biopsy is characteristically normal is listed in Table 3.10.

Table 3.10
Disorders in which biopsy is normal

Cirrhosis
Hepatitis
Exocrine pancreatic insufficiency
Toddler's diarrhoea

Autopsy Studies

It has long been known that rapid autolysis of the surface epithelium of the alimentary tract occurs at death and, indeed, cytology and histology of the small intestinal mucosa at post-mortem is often unsatisfactory and may be misleading. In the past, this knowledge has hindered study of this organ at autopsy and has cast doubts upon the value of any finding observed in the small intestine at post mortem.

However, Creamer and Leppard in 1965 established that dissecting microscopy of autolysed small intestinal mucosa devoid of its surface epithelium gave information of considerable value concerning the three-dimensional morphology of the small intestinal mucosa and, in 1966, Loehry and Creamer reported the findings in 100 adult autopsies. Walker-Smith in 1972 reported observations of 116 childhood autopsies using a modification of the method of Loehry and Creamer.

The small intestinal mucosa consists of the surface epithelium on its basement membrane and the lamina propria. Its lower limit is defined by the muscularis mucosae. The surface epithelium is lost when the method of Loehry and Creamer is used but the lower layers remain intact. The connective tissue cores of the villi are then seen rather than the villi themselves and the overall three-dimensional arrangement of the mucosal architecture can be clearly seen even though the surface epithelium is absent. The appearance then observed may be referred to as the 'skeleton structure' of the mucosa and the surface is now the basement membrane.

Technique of Examination

The small intestine obtained from a child at post mortem is allowed to stand in gently running water for twenty-four hours to dislodge the surface slough of autolysing epithelial cells. The connective tissue cores of villi thus exposed are then stained with ordinary ink and examined under the dissecting microscope. This is best done by taking small sections along the length of the small intestine, but the whole length of the small intestine may be pinned out and scanned with the dissecting microscope. Figures 3.28 to 3.30 illustrate some of the appearances seen with this technique.

The findings in 55 autopsy studies of children dying with evidence of gastroenterological disease has been described by Walker-Smith (1972). An abnormal mucosa chiefly characterised by short thick

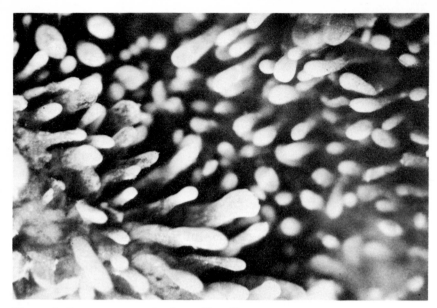

Fig. 3.28. Post-mortem study: finger-like villous cores.

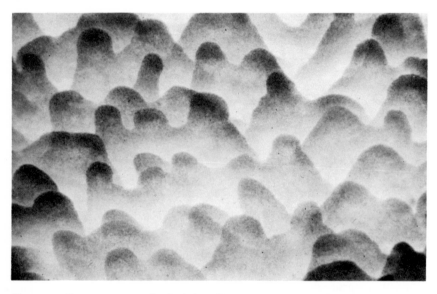

Fig. 3.29. Post-mortem study: broader villous cores (leaves and tongues).

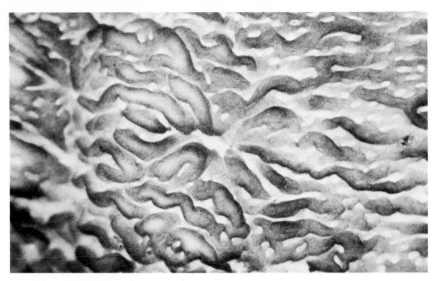

Fig. 3.30 Post-mortem study: short thick ridges with small ulcer.

ridges occurred in 41 per cent (Fig. 3.30). The findings in children dying from gastroenteritis are reported in more detail in chapter 6. An abnormal appearance was also seen in children dying with small intestinal atresia and stenosis, small intestinal lymphangioma, moniliasis, Hirschsprung's disease with enterocolitis and cytomegalovirus infection. No morphological abnormality was found in children dying from liver or pancreatic disease.

The technique was of great value in studying the extent and distribution of the abnormal mucosa along the length of the small intestine. The variations in the pattern of such distribution are illustrated in chapter 6. These studies have made it clear that proximal small intestinal biopsies may not be representative of the mucosa of the proximal small intestine when a patchy lesion is present and certainly give no indication of the extent of the lesion along the small intestine. Fortunately, in coeliac disease most published data suggest that the abnormal proximal small intestinal mucosa characteristic of that disorder is uniformly flat, but in other disorders such as the post-enteritis syndrome more than one biopsy may be necessary to give an accurate assessment of the state of the mucosal morphology in the proximal small intestine.

Examination of autolysed small intestine at post mortem under the dissecting microscope should be employed in all children who die with suspected small intestinal disease.

FUNCTIONAL

Brush-Border Enzymes (Table 3.11)

A number of enzymes have been identified in brush border isolates, and so far all the enzymes identified are hydrolases, degrading substances within the gut lumen. These enzymes hydrolyse their substrates outside the enterocyte. Thus, at least some portion of the protein faces the external surface of the membrane (*see* Fig. 7.3). Non-enzymatic proteins such as the receptor for the intrinsic factor-Vitamin B_{12} complex are also found in brush borders.

Table 3.11
Brush border enzymes

Disaccharidases	maltase
	sucrase
	lactase
	trehalase
Peptidases	oligoaminopeptidase
	γ-glutamyltranspeptidase
	enterokinase
Phosphatases	alkaline
	Ca $++$
	Mg $++$
	ATPase

The microvillus membrane is unique in that it is in contact not only with enzymes in the cystosol and the lysozymes but also with the luminal enzymes and potentially cytotoxic substances in the lumen such as the bile salts. The glycocalyx and intestinal mucus probably play a key role in protecting this membrane.

Brush border enzymes in disease states: A number of diseases in man are associated with a change in the amount of brush border proteins. Alpers and Seetharam (1977) have classified the physiological mechanisms leading to changes in brush-border proteins as follows—

Disease	*Alteration in Protein*
1. *Decreased or altered protein synthesis*	
Sucrase-isomaltase deficiency	Absent sucrase
Enterokinase deficiency	Absent enterokinase
Lactase deficiency	Decreased lactase
Familial vitamin B_{12} malabsorption	Altered receptor

Disease	Alteration in Protein
2. *Increased degradation*	
Stagnant-loop syndrome	Decreased disaccharidases
Gastroenteritis	Decreased lactase
3. *Decreased degradation*	
Cystic fibrosis	Increased disaccharidases

Enzyme Assay of Small Intestinal Biopsies

Disaccharidase assay is now used routinely in paediatric practice. Although assays of other enzymes, such as dipeptidase, have also been investigated extensively in research studies, assay of these enzymes is not performed routinely, hence they are not discussed here.

Disaccharidase Assay

As the small intestinal biopsy specimen that is assayed for disaccharidase activity is so small, and because proximal small intestinal mucosal abnormalities may be patchy and of variable extent, there is often a lack of correlation between disaccharidase activity and other measures of sugar absorption; for example, sugar tolerance tests and stool studies. An example of this is in coeliac disease where there may sometimes be no detectable lactase activity on assay of a biopsy specimen, yet the child has no clinical evidence of lactose intolerance. This is because, although lactase activity is absent in the biopsy specimen, the total amount of small intestinal lactase activity is adequate for the child to absorb lactose further down the small intestine.

Estimation of disaccharidase activity in a single biopsy is of no specific diagnostic importance in the management of disorders where secondary disaccharidase deficiency occurs, such as in coeliac disease and post-gastroenteritis malabsorption. In these circumstances depressed disaccharidase activity merely reflects the state of mucosal damage that is present. Lactase activity appears to be more susceptible to damage than is the activity of the other disaccharidases; depression of lactase levels is usually more severe and takes longer to recover.

The principal indications for disaccharidase assay in clinical practice is in the diagnosis of primary or congenital deficiency syndromes, namely sucrase-isomaltase deficiency and congenital alactasia (*see* chapter 7), and serial estimation as a measure of mucosal damage after challenge, e.g. cow's milk sensitive enteropathy (*see* chapter 5).

Disaccharidase activity may be expressed per gram of protein in the biopsy specimen, or as per gram of wet mucosa (as used at the Queen Elizabeth Hospital) (Tables 3.12 and 3.13).

Table 3.12
Disaccharidase activity in units/g protein in normal jejunal mucosa in children

	Lactase	Sucrase	Iso-maltase	Maltase
Range	14–132	32–338	31–177	83–615
Mean	49	95	89	260

Permission of Burke, Kerry and Anderson, 1965

Table 3.13
Disaccharidase activity in units/g wet mucosa per minute in normal small intestinal mucosa from 112 children

	Lactase	Sucrase	Maltase
Range	2–16	3–20	15–77
Mean	5·6	10·2	31·2

Permission of Burgess, 1974

There is a much wider range of values in the Melbourne series than the series reported from the Queen Elizabeth Hospital. The reason for this is not clear but may be related to differing criteria for 'normality'.

Levels for disaccharidase activity are somewhat lower in the duodenum than the values obtained in the proximal jejunum.

Absorption Studies in Children

As in adults such studies may involve either the administration of an oral load of a particular substance, followed by the serial observation of blood levels as well as stools passed after the oral load, or by investigating the stools while the individual is on a known dietary intake.

Oral Loading Tests

(*a*) *Sugar:* The sugar to be investigated is given by mouth to the fasting child in a dosage of 2 g/kg body weight. Fasting capillary blood is taken and then samples are collected at 30 minute intervals for two hours. An increase of blood glucose of more than 30 mg/100 ml above the fasting level is recognised as normal, a 20–30 mg rise is doubtful, and a rise of less than 20 mg is abnormal (Holzel, 1967).

Rather more important than the rise in blood sugar levels in children is observation of the stools after the load. The demonstration of a 'flat' lactose tolerance test, in the absence of diarrhoea with stool reducing substances, following an oral sugar load is not clinically significant and should not be regarded as an indication that the child should be treated for sugar malabsorption. It could be due to delayed gastric emptying or, on the other hand, indicate some disorder of handling of sugar which is not severe enough to cause symptoms.

(b) *Fat:* A rise in plasma, or serum particulate fat, after an oral load of fat, has been used for some years as a test of fat absorption but without wide acceptance. This was in part due to the unsatisfactory past methods of measuring particulate fat in the plasma or serum. However, Stone and Thorp (1966) have shown that the use of a nephelometer is a reliable and convenient way to make such measurements. This instrument records the light scattering index. Particles in solution scatter light in proportion to their concentration and size, so chylomicrons, as they are large particles, scatter more light than smaller particles. Robbards (1973) has successfully used this instrument in a fat loading test in children and has related the results to the state of small intestinal morphology.

In this test children are given 1 g/kg of fat by mouth after fasting overnight, and a venepuncture of 2 ml of blood. Further blood samples are taken at two and three hours. Robbards found a significantly lower rise in the light scattering index after two hours, in children who had a flat small intestinal mucosa, as compared with those who had a normal small intestinal mucosa on biopsy. Further evaluation of this test continues, its place in paediatric gastroenterology not yet being clear.

Stool Studies

(a) *Sugar:* (i) *Stool reducing substances and stool chromatography for sugar.* When stools are loose the fluid part of the stool may be tested for the presence of reducing substances (Kerry and Anderson, 1964). This may be used as a simple ward test. The fluid portion of the stool is tested by first diluting one part of fluid stool with two parts of water and placing 15 drops of the mixture into a test tube and adding a Clinitest tablet (Ames Company). The amount of reducing substances may then be estimated according to the colour resulting, ranging from 0 to 2 per cent. A value of 0·5 per cent or more is regarded as abnormal. Alternatively, the fluid part of the stool may be diluted with twice its volume of water and then homogenised in the laboratory with a Vortex-genie mixer and then tested as above. This refinement is recommended only when chromatography for sugar is planned. The homogenised suspension is centrifuged and the supernatant used for chromatography. This is only recommended when an excess of reducing substances is present.

It is essential that the fluid stool for testing should be collected in such a way that the fluid does not soak into the infant's napkin and so largely be lost. This may be done by collecting the stool on a non-absorbable material such as plastic or by collecting the stool straight into a container. The effect of allowing the stool to soak into the napkin, in the case of sugar intolerance, is shown in Table 3.14. It is apparent that a significant result turns into a non-significant one.

Table 3.14
Effect of allowing stool to soak into napkin

Time (min)	Nature of stool	Reducing substances (%)
Before soaking	Yellow-green watery	I
0	and curds	
After soaking	Yellow-green curds	0·5–0·75
0	and little fluid	
15	Yellow-green curds	0·25–0·5
30	Yellow-green curds	0·25–0·5
60	Yellow-green curds	0·25–0·5

When chromatography is used, the supernatant should be spotted on to Whatman No. 1 chromatography paper. The technique as described by Soeparto and his colleagues may be used or, alternatively, the technique of Menzies, 1973.

Examples of stool chromatography for sugar are illustrated in Figures 7.4 and 7.5.

(ii) *Stool pH*. A stool pH of less than 6 is regarded as abnormal and has been described as a characteristic finding in children with sugar intolerance (Holzel, 1967). Stool pH is usually tested at the bedside with pH indicator paper with a range of 1–11. Such a method correlates satisfactorily from a clinical point of view with true pH meter readings (Soeparto, Stobo and Walker-Smith, 1972). The value of stool pH estimations in the diagnosis of sugar intolerance is discussed in chapter 7.

(b) *Fat:* Estimation of daily faecal fat levels over 3 to 5 day periods has been used for some time in paediatric practice. The usual method is that used by van de Kamer and his colleagues (1949). The percentage of fat absorbed from dietary fat, i.e. the coefficient of fat absorption, is perhaps a more reliable measure than the absolute value of daily faecal fat estimations, but this depends on precise knowledge of the child's fat intake during the period of study, which may be difficult to obtain. Nonetheless, some attempt should be made to ensure adequate fat intake during the period of stool collection as misleading results may occur when the child is anorexic and his fat intake is low.

Complete stool collections for three or five days are not popular with members of the nursing staff, nor do laboratory technicians like doing faecal fat estimations. Accordingly, it is often difficult to get accurately performed faecal fat estimations outside a metabolic unit.

The need to perform such estimations in children has declined considerably in recent years. Steatorrhoea is no longer regarded as a suitable screening test for coeliac disease (*see* chapter 4). The main indications for this investigation in children in relation to small intestinal disease are massive small intestinal resection, evidence of a stagnant loop syndrome, and chronic diarrhoea of obscure origin, when other investigations have proved negative.

Shmerling, Forrer and Prader (1970) have studied daily faecal fat levels in healthy children and have confirmed earlier observations that higher levels of daily faecal fat are found in infants under one year of age than in toddlers. (Table 3.15).

Table 3.15
Total faecal fatty acids in healthy control children

Age (years)	Fat (g/day)	
	Mean	*Range*
0–1	2·3	1·1–3·6
1–4	1·72	0·2–2·9
4–10	1·79	0·8–3·2
10	2·38	0·9–4·0

Permission of Shmerling *et al.*, 1970

(c) *Protein:* Faecal nitrogen is an investigation not often of much practical help in investigating small intestinal disease. It may be useful, however, in the assessment of children with massive small intestinal resection. Shmerling and his colleagues (1970) have also reported values for healthy children in relation to faecal nitrogen.

Investigation of Deficiency States

Iron Deficiency

Iron deficiency may arise in children with small intestinal disease due, firstly, to poor intake as may occur in association with profound anorexia (for example in Crohn's disease); secondly, due to malabsorption secondary to proximal small intestinal mucosal abnormality as may occur in coeliac disease; and thirdly, due to chronic blood loss as may occur in Meckel's diverticulum.

The diagnosis is usually made on examination of the peripheral blood. The possibility of diagnosing iron deficiency in the absence of anaemia by estimation of serum iron, is uncertain.

Table 3.16
Normal iron values for children, μg/100 ml

Serum iron	50–175
Total iron binding capacity	300–360

Low serum iron values (Table 3.16) may result from inadequate iron intake or absorption, blood loss, or infection. Iron is transported in the blood by transferrin, this protein carrying 30 to 40 per cent of its iron binding capacity. An elevated iron binding capacity occurs in iron deficiency.

Stainable iron on bone marrow aspiration is a useful investigation if there is a need to establish the diagnosis clearly. Recently, serum ferritin estimation has been shown to be a valuable aid to diagnosis.

Folic Acid Deficiency

Folic acid or pteroylglutamic acid is the parent compound of a group of related substances called folates. Naturally occurring folic acid exists chiefly as pteroyl-polyglutamate, which is simple folic acid that has been conjugated in gamma-peptide linkage with up to six additional glutamyl units. Pteroylpolyglutamates are hydrolysed to pteroylmonoglutamate during the process of intestinal absorption. The small intestinal mucosa contains gamma-glutamate carboxypeptidase, a hydrolytic enzyme, usually known as folate conjugase, which releases monoglutamic folate. Folic acid is rapidly absorbed from the proximal small intestine but only poorly from the distal small bowel.

Folic acid is present in cow's milk and in breast milk in approximately equal amounts (54 μg/litre; Ford and Scott, 1968). Goat's milk contains only 6 μg/litre. Folic acid is heat labile and easily destroyed in processing, hence artificial feedings need to be supplemented with folic acid.

The WHO (1972) has laid down recommendations for daily folate intake in childhood (Table 3.17).

Table 3.17

Age	Daily folate requirements (μg)
0–6 months	40–50
7–12 months	120
1–12 years	200
13 years and over	400

It is obvious that much of a child's folate intake will come not only from milk but also from solid foods. Chanarin (1975) has assayed the folate content of a number of foods and has observed that normal cooking can destroy a very high proportion of food folate. He found an important difference between foods freshly bought for assay and those from hospital supply. Examples are shown in Table 3.18.

Table 3.18
Total food folate content μg folate/100 litres
(from Chanarin 1975)

	Fresh	Hospital
Raw tomato	58·0	22·9
Fried tomato	14·8	11·6
Raw brussels sprouts	130·4	
Cooked brussels sprouts	60·0	

It is not only the folate content of food that is important but also its availability. Tamura and Stakstad (1973) found that the polyglutamates in orange juice, lettuce, egg yolk, cabbage, soy bean and wheat germ were only 25 to 47 per cent absorbed, whereas folates in yeast, beans, liver and bananas were well absorbed, 63 to 96 per cent.

Premature infants are at particular risk of developing folic acid deficiency and megaloblastic anaemia (Vanier and Tyas, 1967), but with the use of modern artificial feedings, supplemented with folic acid, megaloblastic anaemia due to folic acid deficiency is now rare in infancy. As has been mentioned above, goat's milk is particularly low in folic acid, and infants fed on this milk alone may develop nutritional folate deficiency, producing megaloblastic anaemia. Davidson and Townley (1976) have described structural abnormalities and disaccharidase deficiency in the duodenal mucosa of four infants with dietary folate deficiency associated with goat's milk. They have attributed these small intestinal abnormalities to folic acid deficiency *per se*, as they were reversed by oral folic acid. Although low blood folate levels may be found later in childhood when there is an inadequate intake of folic acid, megaloblastic anaemia due to dietary folic acid deficiency is almost unknown at that age. Indeed, severe megaloblastic anaemia is rare in infancy and childhood even when there is evidence of folic acid deficiency (Dormandy, Waters and Mollin, 1963).

It has sometimes been assumed as a consequence of this observation that folate deficiency is either trivial or unimportant in children. However, significant folate deficiency may occur in coeliac disease in the absence of megaloblastic anaemia (*see* chapter 4) but folate deficiency has not been recognised as an important feature of other diseases of the small intestinal mucosa in childhood, apart from Crohn's disease in the older child (*see* chapter 9). This probably relates to the fact that in coeliac disease there is a more severe and extensive proximal enteropathy than occurs in the other small intestinal enteropathies of childhood.

In summary, folic acid deficiency in childhood, as in adult life, is most often due to coeliac disease, Crohn's disease, or nutritional deficiency. The criteria for the diagnosis of folate deficiency are shown in Table 3.19.

The diagnosis of folic acid deficiency may first be suspected by detection of macrocytes in the peripheral blood of a child with anaemia, or there may be a dimorphic film, i.e. features of macrocytosis and microcytosis suggesting the presence of both folic acid and iron deficiency. Although such a combination could occur in an infant who has a dietary deficiency, the finding of a dimorphic anaemia is very suggestive of coeliac disease. Bone marrow aspiration classically shows megaloblastic changes but these are difficult to see when iron deficiency is present. Most often, folic acid deficiency is detected by finding low serum and red cell folate levels. Red cell folate reflects the state of the body stores and serum folate reflects more recent changes in folate status. Values normally associated with deficiency are listed in Table 3.20.

Table 3.19
Diagnosis of folate deficiency (Permission of J. Burman)

	Folate deficiency alone	Folate and iron deficiency together
Blood		
MCV	↑	usually reduced
Macrocytes	+	+ but also smaller cells (dimorphic)
Hypersegmented polymorphs	+	+
Marrow		
Erythropoiesis	megaloblastic	megaloblastic change difficult to see
Granulopoiesis	giant metamyelocytes	giant metamyelocytes
Assays	B_{12} normal	B_{12} normal
	Serum folate low	Serum folate low
	Red cell folate low	Red cell folate low
Additional evidence	deoxyuridine suppression test abnormal Figlu excretion raised, response to specific therapy	

Table 3.20
Values associated with deficiency

Serum folate less than 4·0 μg/litre
Red cell folate less than 160 μg/litre
Serum B_{12} less than 160 ng/litre

Table 3.21
Diagnostic approach to child suspected of having small intestinal disease

Initial assessment	Detailed case history
	Physical examination
	Analysis of centile charts for height and weight
Initial investigations	Full blood count and also ESR in older child (?Crohn's disease)
	Serum and red cell folate
	Serum iron and TIBC
	Stool culture for bacteria
	Stool electron microscopy for viruses
	Stool examination for *Giardia lamblia*
	Stool-reducing substances
Next stage	Small intestinal biopsy
	Duodenal juice-examination for *Giardia lamblia* bacterial culture for bacteria anaerobic and aerobic (as indicated)
	Barium follow-through

Rickets

Vitamin D deficiency secondary to small intestinal disease may occasionally be found in children. The diagnosis is based on clinical manifestations plus characteristic X-ray findings and elevated serum alkaline phosphatase levels.

The remaining techniques of investigation listed in Table 3.1, i.e. immunological, bacteriological, parasitic and viral are discussed in later chapters.

Diagnostic Approach

To conclude this chapter on diagnostic techniques it is important briefly to review the diagnostic approach to a child suspected of having small intestinal disease. This is summarised in Table 3.21.

The emphasis nowadays is not so much upon demonstrating malabsorption, e.g. steatorrhoea or xylose malabsorption as formerly was the case, but by pin-pointing a structural abnormality of the small intestinal mucosa, i.e. an enteropathy or a specific aetiological agent. Thus, stool examination and small intestinal biopsy are particularly important investigations. Haematological investigations, such as a full blood count and serum folate, may provide important evidence of a deficiency state that may need to be treated immediately or followed up as a marker of response to treatment. Radiological studies are particularly important for diagnosing Crohn's disease and congenital anatomical lesions of the small intestine.

4

Coeliac Disease

Coeliac disease is a most important disease of the small intestine in children as it has a specific and effective treatment. Failure to diagnose coeliac disease may lead to chronic ill health and arrested development.

TERMINOLOGY

The term coeliac disease originated from a paper by Gee published in 1888, in which he reported a disorder not previously described in any textbook of medicine. He described this 'chronic indigestion which is met with in persons of all ages, yet is especially apt to affect children between one and five years old', as the coeliac affection or coeliac disease. Gee himself did not regard this condition as a newly recognised disorder but rather as a disease that had long ago been mentioned by ancient writers, notably Aretaeus the Cappadocian, who wrote in the first century A.D. (Dowd and Walker-Smith, 1974).

The word 'coeliac' is even more ancient. It was used for example in the second century B.C. by Cato. Aretaeus used the phrase the coeliac diathesis or state, to describe a chronic disorder of adults characterised by the passage of undigested food and accompanied by severe emaciation and weakness. Gee quoted Aretaeus's term in his original paper and he commends its use because the term does not connote anything 'relative to the precise seat or nature of the disorder'.

Some modern authors have preferred the term gluten-sensitive enteropathy but this term does have a precise meaning in relation to the nature of the disorder. As it seems probable that a gluten-sensitive enteropathy may occur in situations other than coeliac disease, for example transient gluten intolerance following gastroenteritis, the term should be avoided as a synonym for coeliac disease. In view of the fact that the fundamental aetiology of coeliac disease remains unknown, it is therefore best to retain the use of this ancient terminology.

DEFINITION

It is, however, vitally important to define precisely what the term coeliac disease does mean at present, because sometimes the phrase 'coeliac syndrome' is used to describe the whole clinical spectrum of malabsorption in children, or to the various conditions that may be associated with a flat small intestinal mucosa.

Coeliac disease may be defined as follows: a disease of the proximal small intestine characterised by an abnormal small intestinal mucosa and associated with a permanent intolerance to gluten. Removal of gluten from the diet leads to a full clinical and pathological remission.

Thus, coeliac disease is a life-long disorder that affects both children and adults and may first present either in childhood or adult life.

This definition makes no specific mention of malabsorption, although malabsorption is usually present in children with coeliac disease. This is because some children with the condition may not have any evidence of malabsorption when simple clinical parameters of absorption, such as daily faecal fat estimation, are used.

INCIDENCE AND GENETIC FACTORS

Environmental factors obviously must influence the incidence of coeliac disease because the disease cannot occur unless gluten is present in the child's diet. It is found, therefore, most often in those countries such as Britain, Australia and North America where wheat is a staple food.

Indeed most children diagnosed as having coeliac disease are children of European origin. There is a genetic explanation for this fact as well as an environmental one, because this disease either does not occur, or is certainly very uncommon, in Negroes living in North America or South Africa and in West Indians living in Britain, nor does the condition appear yet to have been documented in the Chinese or Japanese.

However, Nelson, McNeish and Anderson (1973) in Birmingham,

reported that coeliac disease was present in seventeen Asian children whose parents originated from the Punjab or West Pakistan. Hitherto, there have been few reports of coeliac disease occurring in Asians but interestingly, there have been previous reports in children who came from the northern regions of the Indian subcontinent.

There are now also reports of coeliac disease in Arab children from the middle east. These reports have come from the Lebanon (Bitar, Salem and Nasr, 1970) and from Iraq (al-Hassany, 1975). In addition, Suliman (1978) has described coeliac disease in children from the Northern Sudan, the children being of mixed Arab and African origin. Thus, children with coeliac disease may be encountered over a wide geographical region, but there seems to be a considerable variation in incidence from region to region, with Europe, and Europeans living outside Europe, having the highest prevalence.

There appears also to be a variation in the incidence of coeliac disease in different parts of Europe. Carter, Sheldon and Walker in 1959 estimated that the incidence of coeliac disease in England was between 1 in 2,000 and 1 in 6,000 but by contrast, it has been shown that the incidence of coeliac disease in children in the West of Ireland was 1 in 300. This report used small intestinal biopsy to make the diagnosis whereas the earlier report did not, so the two studies are not exactly comparable. Nevertheless, the order of difference between the two reports appears to be highly significant. Environmental differences in relation to gluten ingestion between the two groups do not appear sufficient to account for this difference in incidence, and so it seems that genetic factors must be the reason for this striking variation.

Other evidence in favour of the importance of genetic factors in the aetiology of coeliac disease includes the observation that coeliac disease may occur in more than one member of the same family, although most children with coeliac disease have no such family history (Gardner and Mutton, 1973). Coeliac disease may occur in twins, but it has now been reported once in adults (Hoffman, Wollalger and Greenberg, 1966) and twice in children (Walker-Smith, 1973; McNeish and Nelson, 1974) that non-discordance for coeliac disease may occur in well-documented monozygotic twins (Fig. 4.1). This provides strong evidence against the hypothesis that coeliac disease is inherited as a dominant gene with incomplete penetrance (Booth, 1970).

At present, the most likely hypothesis to explain the familial occurrence of coeliac disease is that susceptibility to damage by a number of environmental factors is inherited by polygenic variation.

This conception, that there is a genetically determined susceptibility for the acquisition of coeliac disease, was established in 1972 by the independent observations of Stokes and his colleagues in Britain and by Falchuk, Rogentine and Strober in the USA who have found that the histocompatibility antigen HLA-B8 occurred in 80–90 per cent of adults with coeliac disease. A similar pattern has been shown in children with coeliac disease by McNeish and his colleagues in Britain (1974), and Albert and his colleagues in Germany (1973). McNeish and his colleagues have gone on to observe that HLA-B8 individuals are ten times more likely to have coeliac disease than those who do not have this antigen. The highest gene frequencies are found in the countries such as Britain and Australia where coeliac disease occurs most often and where, in addition, the wheat consumption is highest.

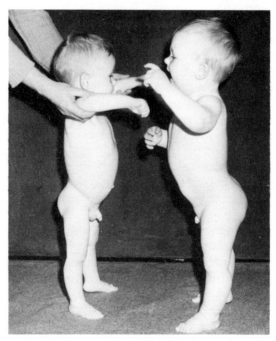

Fig. 4.1. Identical twins: child on left has coeliac disease.

One exception to this is Pakistan, where although wheat intake is lower the HLA-B8 frequency is not; this would account for the frequency of coeliac disease in Pakistani children in Birmingham where the amount of wheat ingested is far higher than in Pakistan.

The frequency of HLA-B8 is higher in the Irish population than in any other country in Europe, paralleling the remarkably high incidence of coeliac disease in Ireland. Thus, the frequency of HL-A8 in a racial group is a good marker for predisposition to coeliac disease.

It is clear that the gene controlling HLA-B8 or a closely linked gene could not be the only gene determining coeliac disease because many people with this histocompatibility gene do not have coeliac disease. Two further genetically controlled antigens have subsequently been associated with coeliac disease. These are the HLA-DW3 antigen (Keunig et al., 1976) and the specific B-lymphocyte associated antigen (Mann et al., 1976). The interrelationships between all these genes and coeliac disease await elucidation.

PATHOGENESIS

Gluten is the germ protein of wheat and some other cereals. Its harmful effect in children with coeliac disease was first established by Dicke in Holland in 1950. Dicke, Weijers and van de Kamer (1953) also established the close relationship between the ingestion of wheat and the degree of steatorrhoea present in children with coeliac disease. The gluten of rye too, has been established to be toxic to such children but there is uncertainty as to whether or not the gluten of barley and of oats is also toxic. Other cereals such as rice and corn are non-toxic to children with coeliac disease.

Wheat gluten is the residue remaining after wheat starch has been extracted from the dough made from wheat flour. It is a large complex molecule that has been divided chemically into four heterogeneous classes of protein: gliadins, glutenins, albumins and globulins. Gliadin is the alcoholic glutamine and proline rich fraction of gluten, but it is itself a very complex protein.

Techniques such as starch-gel electrophoresis have shown that gliadin contains about 40 different components. Most interest has centred around the alpha-fraction. Hekkens, Haex and Willighagen (1970) have produced evidence from in vivo studies that alpha-gliadin is toxic in coeliac disease, whereas Kendal and his colleagues (1972) have shown that pre- and post-alpha-gliadin fractions from an ion exchange separation of gliadin have no toxic effect. Alpha-gliadin is itself still a complex protein and just which fraction of it is toxic remains unknown. Using an in vitro organ culture technique for testing toxicity, Jos and Charbonnier (1976) have found that other fractions of gliadin, namely beta, gamma and omega, are also toxic, although alpha and beta are the most toxic fractions.

As alpha gliadin is present in variable amounts in different wheats, it is possible that some wheats are more toxic than others. High hopes have been raised that a variant of Chinese spring wheat, which lacks alpha gliadin, could be potentially eaten by sufferers from coeliac disease, but evidence that such people can eat this wheat with impunity is awaited (Kasarda *et al.*, 1978).

Another approach to the identification of the toxic fraction of gluten has been the use of enzymatic degradation of gluten or gliadin to determine the size of the toxic portion. When gluten is digested by fresh extracts of small intestinal mucosa from the hog and by crude papain it is rendered non-toxic, although when it is digested by pepsin and trypsin it remains toxic. This observation has been taken as evidence that toxicity is due to a small peptide which is resistant to protein cleavage. Enzymatic degradation studies in one study have suggested that the toxic fraction is an acidic polypeptide having a molecular weight below 1,500 (Kowlessar, 1967). How such a toxic fraction produces its harmful effect remains uncertain.

There are two main theories to account for the toxic effect of ingested gluten in patients with coeliac disease. The first, is a biochemical theory that there is a specific enzyme deficiency, and the second, that the fundamental cause of the disorder is immunological.

EXPERIMENTAL APPROACHES

In order to test these theories experimental approaches have had to be devised, but there are certain limitations to these.

The only way the toxicity of a gliadin or a fraction of gliadin may be determined is by demonstrating damage to the small intestinal mucosa of patients with coeliac disease, which imposes considerable limitations for research in this field. There are, however, two suitable methods now available.

First, there is *in vivo* testing, as described by Hekkens, Haex and Willighagen (1970), where a multiple hydraulic biopsy apparatus is introduced into the jejunum of a gluten-sensitive adult patient in remission, along with a third tube ending about 10 cm above the suction hole in the capsule. Down this tube, a solution of the material being tested may be passed, biopsies being taken sequentially afterwards.

Secondly, there is the technique of *in vitro* small intestinal organ culture (Browning and Trier, 1969; Trier, 1974; Falchuk and Katz, 1978; Jos *et al.*, 1978). This technique enables a small intestinal biopsy to be cultured for 24 to 48 hours. It has proved a useful tool in investigating the pathogenesis of gluten toxicity in coeliac disease. It has been shown that damaged surface absorptive cells from mucosal biopsies of patients with untreated coeliac disease revert towards normal after only 24 hours of culture. This effect is inhibited if the mucosa is cultured in a medium containing gluten peptides. In this way various gluten fractions and sub-fractions have been investigated for their toxicity. The technique has been used with biopsy specimens from both adults and children, and it has the great virtue of permitting *in vitro* evaluation of mucosal function and metabolism. Although it has worked well in the hands of the authors referred to above it has not proved reproducible by all workers.

Whatever experimental approach is used, it must have the following features: (1) specificity, (2) reproducibility, (3) dose-response relationships and, with *in vivo* experiments, reversibility (Hekkens, 1978).

BIOCHEMICAL THEORIES

Several biochemical theories have been put forward to account for the state of gluten toxicity in coeliac disease.

Peptidase Deficiency

The first biochemical theory was enunciated by Frazer in 1956. He proposed that a primary deficiency of an intestinal peptidase resulted in accumulation of a toxic peptide which caused epithelial cell and villous damage. In fact, many mucosal enzymes are deficient in the flat mucosa of active coeliac disease, e.g. several workers have shown that mucosal dipeptidases are deficient. Douglas and Peters (1970) have shown that the activity of these enzymes returns to normal after a clinical response to a gluten-free diet. Thus, such mucosal dipeptidase deficiencies have not so far been shown to be permanent, permanence of such a deficiency being a *sine qua non* for an enzyme deficiency to be regarded as of primary aetiological significance. Furthermore, Douglas and Booth, also in 1970, found no evidence to support this theory when studying the rate of liberation of amino acids from gluten-peptides, using normal mucosa and mucosa from patients treated with a gluten-free diet, i.e. coeliacs in remission.

Cornell and Townley, in 1973, showed that a toxic fraction of gliadin (fraction 9) is defectively hydrolysed by mucosa from treated children, i.e. fraction 9 of a peptide tryptic digest of gluten is digested less by coeliac mucosa in remission than by normal mucosa. Furthermore, this fraction has an effect on organ culture of coeliac biopsies. Controversy has centred on whether the mucosa in these children was completely normal and at present their observation awaits confirmation and the peptidase theory remains unproved.

Deficiency of Intestinal Carbohydrases

A new biochemical theory has been put forward by Phelan and colleagues in Galway (1974). They pointed out that no purified proteolytic enzyme that abolished the toxicity of gliadin in coeliac disease had yet been found, although digestion by fresh extracts of hog small intestinal mucosa and by crude papain render it non-toxic. Conventionally, this has been taken as evidence that toxicity is due to a small peptide, but Phelan *et al.*, believe that this observation may be taken as evidence that toxicity is due to a group of molecules other than a chain of amino acids joined by peptide linkages, i.e. that toxicity is due to a non-protein part of gliadin molecules. They have found that some carbohydrases abolish the toxicity of gliadin, so propose that there is a carbohydrase deficiency in coeliac disease. Again, this observation awaits confirmation. More recently, Phelan *et al.* (1978) have shown some evidence of detoxification of gliadin with enzymes from *Aspergillus niger* and concluded that while this may be due to a carbohydrase but it could be via an enzyme other than a carbohydrase. However, some reservations must exist concerning their studies with this detoxified gliadin *in vivo*. Against this theory, Bernadin *et al.* (1976) were unable to demonstrate the presence of glycoproteins in alpha-gliadin that proved to be toxic in an *in vitro* system. So this theory, too, is still not proven.

Lectin Theory

Lectin is a general term applied to a haemoglutinating substance extracted from plant seeds. Weiser and Douglas, in 1976, also considered the carbohydrate fraction of gliadin and went on to suggest that the underlying defect in coeliac disease is of glycoprotein synthesis or, possibly, of glycolipid synthesis, so that a sugar residue is exposed on the enterocyte surface, i.e. there is an alteration in cell surface membrane. This reacts with wheat gluten in a manner analagous to the interaction of various plant lectins with other cell membranes. Weiser and Douglas (1978) have studied galactosyltransferase activity in coeliac and non-coeliac enterocytes. They found statistically higher values in coeliacs regardless of mucosal lesion, i.e. on or off gluten. This finding, that there were no significant differences in galactosyl-transferase activity between those patients with histologically normal or near-normal mucosa and those with severe histological damage, thus suggests that the abnormality was not of a secondary nature. These findings are consistent with their hypothesis that there may be a difference in the glycoprotein of the enterocyte of coeliac patients. The increase in enzyme could be due to the presence of immature cells in the epithelium of the coeliac mucosa, but against this explanation is: first, that other glycosyltransferases were not increased, and second, that high surface galactosyltransferase activity occurred in coeliac patients regardless of whether they were on or off a gluten-free diet. These preliminary investigations suggest that the underlying defect in coeliac disease involves some aspect of the biosynthesis of carbohydrate-containing macromolecules, but again confirmation is awaited.

Membrane Theory

A third biochemical theory has been put forward by Hekkens (1978). There is increasing evidence that differences in membrane structure exist between coeliacs and non-coeliacs, leading to differences in membrane affinity or permeability. Such alteration in permeability and binding of the cell membrane of the enterocyte may be part of the primary cause of coeliac disease.

IMMUNOLOGICAL ABNORMALITY

A great deal of work has been carried out demonstrating immunological abnormalities in coeliac disease. Among the first of these was demonstration of the presence of circulating antibodies to wheat fractions in the sera of patients with coeliac disease and, later, antibodies to other dietary proteins (Kenrick and Walker-Smith, 1970). Abnormalities of the serum immunoglobulins, namely elevated IgA levels and depressed IgM levels, have also been demonstrated and these appear to be secondary phenomena since they are reversible, return to normal when the child is having a gluten-free diet, and are therefore unlikely to be of primary aetiological significance. In addition, in some children there is a low serum complement (C_3) level at diagnosis, which rises to normal levels on a gluten-free diet.

The number of immunoglobulin containing cells of the various immunoglobulin classes in small intestinal biopsy specimens from children with coeliac disease has been investigated (*see* Figs 6.13, 6.14) by a number of workers, and differences have been observed between childhood and adult coeliac disease. Savilahti (1972) compared the number of IgA and IgM containing cells in the lamina propria of biopsies taken from children with coeliac disease and age-matched controls. He found that in the coeliac group the number of IgA containing cells was twice, and the number of IgM containing cells 2·5 times, the level found in the control group. Falchuk and Strober (1972) have also shown that there is increased synthesis of IgA in coeliac patients after a gluten challenge. It seems that in the early phase of coeliac disease the IgA producing system is stimulated. Because, as in adults with coeliac disease, the number of IgA containing cells has been found to be normal or decreased, it seems possible that the local IgA producing system of the small intestine in the adult patient, which has been previously stimulated for some time, may become exhausted. In some children, IgE cells may be increased (Kilby, Walker-Smith and Wood, 1975, *see* Fig. 6.16). In any event, always in children but less often in adults with coeliac disease, the mucosa returns to normal on a gluten-free diet, both morphologically and in relation to the numbers and distribution of the class of immunoglobulin containing cells.

One immunological abnormality that may be associated with coeliac disease but is not reversed by a gluten-free diet is IgA deficiency. A higher incidence of coeliac disease has been shown to occur in children with this immunological disorder as compared with children without it.

Further information about the pathogenesis of coeliac disease has been provided by morphological and immunological studies of the small intestinal mucosa of coeliac children in remission, following challenge with gluten. Shmerling and Shiner in 1970 demonstrated that the first changes that occurred in the small intestinal mucosa after gluten challenge were not in the epithelial cell itself, but in the lamina propria. They used the electron microscope to study serial biopsies after gluten challenge and they found that the first morphological changes took place in the basement membrane of the epithelial and endothelial cells, the endothelium of the small blood vessels, the connective tissue fibrils, and the infiltrating inflammatory cells. Shiner and Ballard (1972) went on to show that changes involving the deposition of immune complexes occurred parallel with these ultra-structured abnormalities. They found evidence, using immuno-fluorescent techniques, that antibody mainly of the IgA type was formed in the basement membrane following gluten challenge in children previously on a gluten-free diet, and that in some children there was also deposition of complement. Doe, Henry and Booth (1974) have also found evidence of complement deposition in the lamina propria after gluten challenge. These two groups of workers have suggested that an Arthus-type reaction (Gell and Coombs allergic reaction Type III, *see* chapter 5), may be playing an important role in the pathogenesis of coeliac disease. Yet Lancaster-Smith, Kumar and Clark (1974) have not found either immune complexes or complement in the lamina propria of adult patients studied after gluten challenge.

Ezoke, Hekkens and Hobbs (1974) have described lymphocyte dependent antibodies in the sera of patients with coeliac disease which can co-opt lymphocytes known as K or killer cells to attack gluten-labelled targets. Confirmation of this observation is awaited.

The increased numbers of intra-epithelial lymphocytes in the small intestinal mucosa of children and adults with coeliac disease is a characteristic of most patients but the high intra-epithelial lymphocyte count does not always parallel the overall severity of the mucosal lesion. The level falls when the child is placed on a gluten-free diet (Fig. 4.2). Depletion of lamina propria lymphocytes parallels the increase in intra-epithelial lymphocytes. The exact role of the intra-epithelial lymphocytes in the coeliac mucosa remains unknown but their presence is a useful marker for gluten sensitivity. Although they seem to be T-cells they are not markers of local cell mediated immunity (Ferguson, 1976, 1977) but there is an association between intra-epithelial lymphocyte counts and the presence of peripheral blood lymphocytes sensitised to gluten.

Rossipal (1978) has tested cellular immunity in children with coeliac disease using dinitrochlorobenzene (DNCB) and found that 53·8 per cent of the children with untreated coeliac disease had a negative DNCB test compared with 94 per cent of the control group who had a positive DNCB reaction. Only 2·4 per cent of children on a gluten-free diet from 2 months to 4 years had a negative DNCB test.

Thus, from this review it is clear that whatever the basic defect in coeliac disease may prove to be, there can be no doubt that changes in immune status occur, involving both cellular and humoral mechanisms. These may be summarised as follows: when gluten is introduced into the diet of a patient with coeliac disease, he becomes systemically immunised and develops humoral (IgG, IgM) and cell-mediated

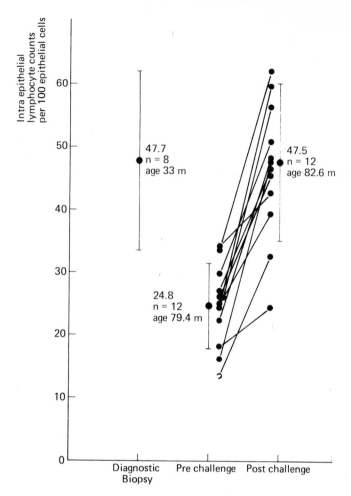

Fig. 4.2. Intra-epithelial lymphocyte count in children with coeliac disease, at diagnosis, pre-challenge on a gluten-free diet and after a relapse following a positive challenge. (Permission of Phillips.)

immunity (gluten sensitised lymphocytes) to gluten antigens in addition to the usual secretory IgA response (Ferguson, 1976), but how central this state of immunisation to gluten is, for the pathogenesis of coeliac disease, is still not clear.

The final end-point of the pathogenetic process, of whatsoever sort, must be the enterocyte. The specificity of the target cell in this disease and the dependence of the disease process upon the presence of gluten suggests that if gluten toxicity operates via an immunological mechanism, then gluten or some fraction of it must bind to the enterocytes and thereby convert them into targets for cytotoxic effector cells or immunoglobulin and complement (Strober, 1976). Rubin and his colleagues (1965) have presented evidence that gluten does bind to the enterocyte in coeliac disease, but so far this observation has not been confirmed by others. On the evidence at present available it does seem possible that an allergic reaction of the Gell and Coombs classification, Types I, II or IV may occur within the lamina propria of the small intestinal mucosa. Such a reaction could be a primary phenomenon or be secondary to a high concentration of a toxic fragment of gluten that has been incompletely digested due to a peptidase deficiency. Thus, the two theories of enzyme deficiency and immunological abnormality are not mutually exclusive (Asquith, 1974). Indeed, Cornell and Rolles (1978) have pursued this point further and have speculated that both an immunological predisposition and a mucosal defect are involved. The mucosal factor may be lack of a mucosal surface protector against gluten's cytotoxic effect.

PERMANENCY OF GLUTEN INTOLERANCE

The full recovery of the small intestinal mucosa to normal in children was first reported by Anderson in 1960, but despite this return to normal on a gluten-free diet, there appears to be no natural recovery in untreated patients, i.e. the intolerance to gluten in children with coeliac disease is permanent (see definition) although clinical manifestations of this may vary widely. Mortimer and her colleagues convincingly demonstrated this in 1968 by showing a persistently abnormal mucosa in untreated patients 18–38 years after the onset of symptoms in childhood.

This observation has recently been challenged by Schmitz, Jos and Rey (1978) in Paris, who have described three children who originally had evidence of a gluten-sensitive enteropathy treated with a gluten-free diet. They all relapsed histologically after return to a gluten-containing diet. They remained well continuing on a normal diet and, later, their mucosa was shown to have spontaneously improved, approaching normality. Whether these children have true coeliac disease, i.e. by definition permanent gluten intolerance, and so will eventually relapse in adult life, or whether, as seems more probable, they have recovered from transient gluten intolerance (see chapter 5) is not yet clear. In any event it was shown, first by Shmerling (1968) and later by many other workers, that when children with coeliac disease, who have fully recovered on a gluten-free diet, are re-challenged with gluten, the mucosa relapses, but it is also clear that although children may have had an histological relapse, they may, for a time, remain symptom free.

The time taken for this relapse to occur is variable. On occasion it takes up to two years, and sometimes even longer (Egan-Mitchell *et al.*, 1978). This may be because of the time it takes to resensitise a potentially sensitive subject.

Much more work is still needed to understand the pathogenesis of this peculiar sensitivity of the small intestine mucosa to gluten in children with coeliac disease and especially in children who have a delayed relapse after returning to a gluten-containing diet.

PATHOPHYSIOLOGY

Increasing attention is being paid to pathophysiological studies of the small intestinal mucosa in children with coeliac disease. Investigation of the level of the enzymes adenyl cyclase and sodium-potassium stimulated adenosine triphosphatase ($Na^+-K^+-ATPase$) by Tripp and his colleagues (1978) have shown that whereas $Na^+-K^+-ATPase$ activity is grossly reduced in the flat mucosa of children with coeliac disease, adenyl cyclase activity is significantly increased in such children when they also have diarrhoea. Those who had no diarrhoea, however, had a basal activity for adenyl cyclase which was not significantly different from the control group. Increased adenyl cyclase activity combined with low Na^+-Ka^+ ATPase activity theoretically would be expected to inhibit sodium coupled glucose absorption, as well as induce active secretion of fluid and electrolytes. In fact, perfusion studies of the proximal jejunum in adults with coeliac disease have been shown, malabsorption of glucose with net secretion of water, sodium and chloride.

PATHOLOGY

Paulley of Ipswich, in 1954, was the first to demonstrate an abnormal small intestinal mucosa in adults with coeliac disease by examining mucosa obtained at laparotomy. Then, in 1957, Sakula and Shiner in London reported, for the first time, observations of a small intestinal biopsy taken from a child with coeliac disease, and they described the characteristic flat mucosa typical of coeliac disease. Earlier reports of an abnormal mucosa in children with coeliac disease had been suggested by some workers and denied by others. Thaysen, in 1932, had asserted that the mucosa was normal in adults with this condition and that any abnormalities previously described as post mortem were artefacts. This was generally accepted as also being true for children with coeliac disease, until 1957.

Since then it has been established that the mucosa of the proximal small intestine is abnormal both in adults and children with coeliac disease. The fact that the most proximal part of the small intestine is the most abnormal accords with the concept of a noxious agent in the diet (namely, gluten) damaging the gut mucosa. Hydrolysed gluten is harmless. By the time any ingested gluten that is not absorbed proximally reaches the ileum it has been completely hydrolysed and so is no longer damaging to the bowel mucosa. Although the distal small intestinal mucosa is usually histologically normal in children with coeliac disease, for this reason Rubin and his colleagues showed, in 1960, that unlike normal mucosa it too becomes abnormal when gluten is directly instilled into the ileum. Thus, the whole length of the small intestinal mucosa is sensitive to gluten.

Characteristically, the proximal small intestinal mucosa is flat, representing a considerable reduction in absorptive surface area. When such a mucosal biopsy is examined under the dissecting or stereo-microscope, it may be completely flat and featureless or it may have a flat mosaic appearance with irregular areas divided by grooves (Fig. 4.3).

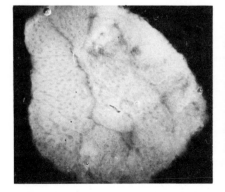 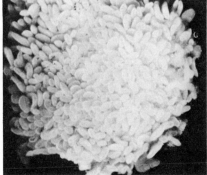

Fig. 4.3. Dissecting microscope appearances. Left: flat mucosa; right: normal mucosa.

Fortunately, from a diagnostic point of view, the proximal small intestinal mucosa in untreated coeliac disease is uniformly flat, so biopsy is a reliable way to obtain a representative section (Table 4.1). However, when biopsies are examined after a gluten challenge, a patchy enteropathy may be seen (Manuel *et al.*, 1979) (Table 4.1), and this may on occasion cause problems in assessment.

Table 4.1
Patchy enteropathy and coeliac disease study of 34 children by Manuel *et al.*, 1979

	Number	*Biopsy*	
Untreated coeliac disease	14	Uniformly flat	14
On gluten-free diet	2	Patchy enteropathy	2
After challenge	20	Patchy enteropathy	7

Histologically, this flat mucosa has an appearance often known as subtotal villous atrophy but sometimes as total villous atrophy (Fig. 4.4). These are unsatisfactory terms because the mucosa is not truly atrophic; indeed, the crypts of Lieberkühn are lengthened. The simple term, a flat mucosa is preferable (*see* chapter 3).

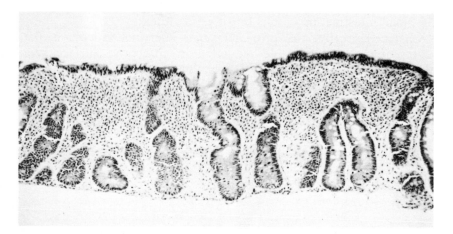

Fig. 4.4. Histological section of a flat mucosa.

There is also a variable cellular infiltration of the lamina propria with round cells. The surface epithelium is low, columnar, pseudo-stratified or cuboidal. Booth (1968) has suggested, using a haematological analogy, that the surface epithelial cells lining the small intestinal mucosa be called enterocytes and the cells in the crypts enteroblasts. He described the surface epithelial cells in coeliac disease as being microcytic enterocytes and the thickening of the enteroblastic layer as enteroblastic hyperplasia with increased mitotic activity occurring in this layer to replace the abnormal enterocytes. Wright (1974) reviewing the morphogenesis of a flat mucosa has observed that this is a most appropriate term. The combined evidence of an elevated mitotic index, decreased cell cycle time, increased cell production rate and increased mucosal cell loss rate, in patients with coeliac disease who have a flat small intestinal mucosa, all supports the concept of enteroblastic hyperplasia to account for this mucosal abnormality.

Polak and her colleagues (1973) reported studies of 16 coeliac children from the Queen Elizabeth Hospital where there was evidence of some degree of hyperplasia of intestinal endocrine cells in the abnormal small intestinal mucosa of 9 of these children. They postulated that this hyperplasia was due to failure to release secretin from the cells.

Polak and Bloom (1978) went on to observe that there is diminished secretion of both bicarbonate and enzymes by the pancreas in coeliac disease in response to a normal meal and to intraluminal acidification which releases secretin. However, the pancreas itself is not diseased, as after intravenous secretin, pancreatic secretion is normal. They also observed in biopsies from seven coeliac children that the secretin cells and CCK cells were increased in number and larger in size, indicating high storage of hormone. These results thus confirm a functional failure of secretin and CCK release. By contrast, it has also been shown that the ileal hormone enteroglucagon is much increased (Bloom and Polak, 1978). This hormone is trophic to the gut and could contribute to increased cell turnover in coeliac disease.

Some children diagnosed as having coeliac disease have a proximal mucosa characterised, under the dissecting microscope, by short thick ridges, sometimes with a convoluted appearance and partial villous atrophy histologically. This appearance is certainly much less common than a flat mucosa in children with coeliac disease and it may occur in a variety of disorders of the small intestine other than coeliac disease. It was found in 4 of 35 children with coeliac disease, the diagnosis being proved by challenge (Table 4.2).

Table 4.2
Initial biopsy appearances in 35 coeliac children proven by challenge

Flat mucosa	31
Partial villous Atrophy	4

The severity of the biopsy findings is less important than the length of the small intestine affected. Figure 4.5 is a diagrammatic approximation of the distribution of the mucosal abnormality along the length of the small intestine in coeliac disease. The precise length of abnormal gut mucosa appears to determine the severity of the clinical state.

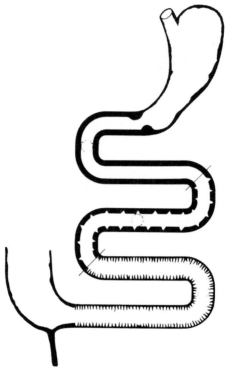

Fig. 4.5. Diagrammatic representation of mucosal abnormality along the small intestine in coeliac disease. (Permission of Gerrard from Gerrard and Lubos, 1967.)

Electron microscope studies of small intestinal biopsies taken from children with coeliac disease reveal abnormality of the enterocytes, which are patchy and of variable severity. Diminution of the size and number of the microvilli with branching is characteristic (Fig. 4.6), as is evidence of epithelial cell damage, but such findings are not constant. There is also, sometimes, an increased deposition of collagen in the region of the basement membrane of the enterocyte, which may be thickened (Fig. 4.7). In the lamina propria there is increased infiltration of plasma cells which Shiner has described as being extremely active.

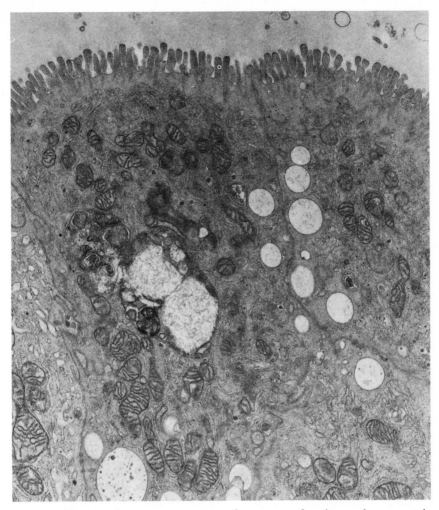

Fig. 4.6. Electron microscope appearances of upper part of an abnormal enterocyte in coeliac disease. Note autophagic vacuoles. (Permission of Phillips.)

Araya and Walker-Smith (1975) at the Royal Alexandra Hospital studied the electron microscopical features of the small intestinal mucosa of 30 consecutive biopsies taken from 14 children with newly diagnosed and untreated coeliac disease, and from 16 children with chronic intermittent diarrhoea due to a variety of causes, 3 having a mild enteropathy and the others a normal mucosa. The most frequent abnormalities of the enterocyte observed were the following: an abnormal brush border, increased numbers of free ribosomes, rich

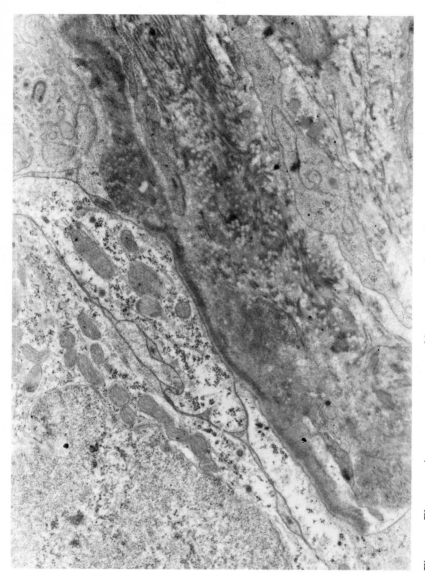

Fig. 4.7. Electron microscope appearance of basement membrane in untreated coeliac disease. Thickening of basal lamina of epithelium and increased collagen deposits in the basement membrane. Compare Fig. 3.25. (Permission of Araya.)

rough endoplasmic reticulum, large Golgi complexes, and thickened basal lamina with poorly developed smooth endoplasmic reticulum. Some of these features, for example the thickened basal lamina, were also found in some of the children who did have coeliac disease. No features were entirely specific for coeliac disease.

CLINICAL FEATURES

There is considerable variation in the age of onset of symptoms in children with coeliac disease. Gee originally described symptoms as presenting most often between the age of one and five years.

However, it is now the trend for most children's symptoms to begin under the age of one year (Table 4.3). In a survey of 110 coeliac children at the Queen Elizabeth Hospital, seen between 1950 and 1969 by Young and Pringle (1971), the onset of symptoms began in most children under the age of a year with a peak between 7 and 12 months, although most were diagnosed in the second year of life (Table 4.3).

Table 4.3
Age of children with coeliac disease at onset of symptoms

Series	Years studied	Number of patients	0–6 months	7–12 months	13–24 months	2–5 years	6 years and over
Young and Pringle, 1971	1950–1969	63	25	29	9	0	0
Hamilton et al., 1969	1964–1968	42	10	11	12	8	1
Walker Smith and Kilby	1972–1975	42	26	9	3	2	2

More recently at the same hospital, in a survey of 42 children diagnosed between 1972 and 1975, the majority had an onset of symptoms under six months and most were diagnosed under a year (Walker-Smith and Kilby, 1977). This trend to earlier diagnosis may be related to increased awareness of the disease but is also clearly related to the earlier age of presentation of symptoms.

The trend towards an earlier introduction of cereals into the diet of infants in Britain has been shown by Anderson, Gracey and Burke (1972) in Birmingham to be associated with a trend to an earlier age of presentation of children with coeliac disease. They compared an eighteen month period in 1950–1952 with a similar period of 1968–1969 and found a dramatic reduction in the age of presentation from 43·6 months to 9·3 months, and a corresponding drop in the mean age of introduction of gluten-containing cereals into the diet from 9·4 to 3·4 months.

If there were an increased incidence of coeliac disease because of this trend to early cereal feeding, it might be expected that children with coeliac disease would have a history of earlier introduction of solids into the diet compared with that of their unaffected siblings. In a study of a group of such children and their unaffected siblings at the Royal Alexandra Hospital, there was no difference in the mean age of introduction of gluten into their respective diets (Table 4.4).

Table 4.4
Age of introduction of gluten into diet

52 coeliac children	mean age 3·2 months
106 non-coeliac siblings	mean age 3·2 months

An opposing view has been put forward by Arneil *et al.* (1973) who believe there has been a significant increase in the prevalence of coeliac disease in Glasgow from 1950 to 1973, associated with very early introduction of solids into the infant's diet.

Since 1975, in Britain, this trend has, in large measure, been reversed. This follows the recommendations of the Department of Health and Social Security in their booklet *Present-day Practice in Infant Feeding*. This booklet states that the introduction of any food to a baby's diet, other than milk, before the age of four to six months should be unnecessary. Furthermore, some products such as Farex, formerly gluten-containing, are now gluten-free and there is an increasing trend to use rice cereal instead of wheat containing products. It seems highly probable, therefore, to predict that in the future the age of presentation of coeliac disease may significantly rise in Britain, and it is even possible that its prevalence may fall.

There is usually a variable 'latent interval' between the introduction of gluten into the diet and the development of clinical manifestations. The explanation for this interval remains unknown. In some children the interval may be months and in others years but some infants may have symptoms immediately gluten is added to their diet. In a study of a group of children at the Royal Alexandra Hospital, 19·6 per cent of the coeliac children had symptoms on their first contact with gluten (Table 4.5) but some workers have not found any children with such a rapid onset of symptoms after gluten ingestion.

The onset of such symptoms following the introduction of gluten

Table 4.5
Adverse reactions to first contact with gluten

Number in group	52
Adverse reactions	10
Nature of reaction:	
Diarrhoea and vomiting	7
Irritability and vomiting	1
Failure to thrive	1
Acute allergic reaction	1

into an infant's diet is not specific for coeliac disease. Often the symptoms may occur transiently after the introduction of solids into the diet without the development of an abnormal small intestinal mucosa. Indeed, 4·3 per cent of 106 unaffected siblings of a group of coeliac children seen at the Royal Alexandra Hospital had such symptoms.

Once symptoms have appeared there may be a delay in diagnosis but with increased awareness of this condition and the ready availability of the technique of small intestinal biopsy in paediatric centres this interval is becoming less. The age at diagnosis in 110 consecutive children with coeliac disease diagnosed at the Royal Alexandra Hospital from 1966–1972 is illustrated in Fig. 4.8. This indicates that

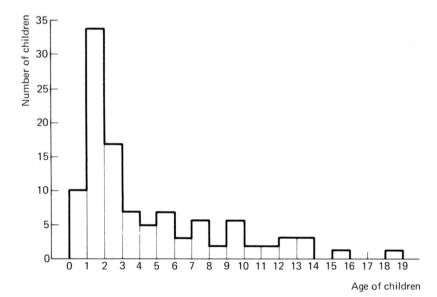

Fig. 4.8. Age at first biopsy of 110 children with coeliac disease seen at the Royal Alexandra Hospital 1966–1972.

most cases are diagnosed in early childhood, but the diagnosis may be made throughout the paediatric age spectrum (Table 4.6).

Table 4.6
Age of children with coeliac disease at time of diagnosis

Series	Years studied	Number of patients	0–6 months	7–12 months	13–24 months	2–5 years	6 years and over
Young and Pringle, 1971	1950–1969	91	–	33	37	18	3
Hamilton *et al.*, 1969	1964–1968	42	0	6	16	15	5
Walker Smith and Kilby	1972–1975	42	8	14	10	4	6

Table 4.7
Mode of presentation of coeliac disease in fifty-two coeliac children at the Royal Alexandra Hospital

Diarrhoea	32
Failure to thrive of no apparent cause	7
Vomiting	6
Weight loss	3
Anorexia	2
Short stature	1
Protuberant abdomen	1

Table 4.8
Symptoms present at the time of diagnosis in fifty-two coeliac children at the Royal Alexandra Hospital

Diarrhoea	45
Abdominal distension	23
Vomiting	32
Lassitude	32
Weight loss	31
Irritability	30
Anorexia	25
Abdominal pain	23
Frequent respiratory infection	14
Failure to thrive	14
Sleep disturbance	9
Appetite increased	8
Acute oedema	7
Muscle wasting	7
Pallor	7
Muscle weakness	4
Constipation	3
Mouth ulceration	2
Rectal prolapse	2
Skin infections	2

The mode of presentation of coeliac disease may be very variable (Table 4.7).

Diarrhoea, which may be acute or insidious in onset, is the commonest presenting symptom and most children with coeliac disease have a history of diarrhoea. The stools are characteristically pale, loose and very offensive and may resemble oatmeal porridge, as Gee described. The child may pass two or three such stools a day but often just one large bulky stool. The child may also have recurrent attacks of more severe diarrhoea, sometimes with the stools becoming watery. However, as has been recognised for some time a few children with coeliac disease may have constipation. These children may have a dilated colon with constipation a clinical pattern that may be confused with that of children who have Hirschsprung's disease, as first described by Bennett, Hunter and Vaughan in 1932 (Fig. 4.9).

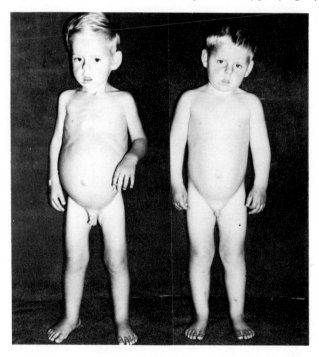

Fig. 4.9. Appearance of a child with megacolon due to coeliac disease, originally mistaken for Hirschsprung's disease, before and one year after treatment.

Failure to thrive is an important way in which coeliac disease may present and coeliac disease needs to be considered in every child with this syndrome. The other modes of presentation listed in Table 4.8

illustrate the broad spectrum of the clinical features of coeliac disease. Sometimes coeliac disease presents as what may best be described as one of its complications, which are discussed later. The symptoms present at the time of diagnosis in a group of children with coeliac disease are indicated in Table 4.8. Their great diversity is readily apparent.

Emotional symptoms are common in children with coeliac disease although they are not often the mode of presentation of this condition. Gibbons, in 1889, drew attention to the fact that the child with coeliac disease 'is extremely irritable, fretful, capricious or peevish. Nothing seems to please him and altogether he is quite unlike himself'.

The coeliac child is often in a state of close dependence on his mother, leading to a pronounced exacerbation of fretfulness and irritability when he is separated from her. This state is best described as 'clingingness'. In addition, the coeliac child is often emotionally withdrawn from his environment and this withdrawal may even resemble autism. Not only may the child have these emotional symptoms but his mother may become depressed, anxious and abnormally pre-occupied with her child (Gardiner, Porteous and Walker-Smith, 1972).

Anorexia is classically said to be present in coeliac children, but only about 50 per cent may have this symptom and some may in fact have an increased appetite. When specifically asked for, there is usually a history of abdominal distension, and some children complain of abdominal pain although this is not usually severe. There is often a past history of respiratory tract infections which may at first suggest cystic fibrosis as a diagnostic possibility.

Although the classical appearance of a miserable child with a distended abdomen and wasted buttocks and shoulder girdles does still occur, abnormalities on physical examination of a child with coeliac disease may be much less obvious (Fig. 4.10). Indeed, some

Table 4.9 Weight percentile at diagnosis in 52 coeliac children, R.A.H.C.	
below 10th	42
10th to 50th	7
50th to 90th	3

Table 4.10 Height percentile at diagnosis in 45 coeliac children, R.A.H.C.	
below 10th	25
10th to 50th	15
50th to 90th	3
above 90th	2

abdominal protuberance may be the only physical sign, but muscle wasting and loss of muscular power with hypotonia may be present and the child may be delayed in his motor milestones. Measurements of height and weight are valuable and the child's height and weight at diagnosis are often found to be below the tenth percentile and sometimes below the third (Tables 4.9 and 4.10).

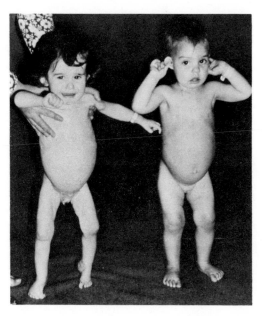

Fig. 4.10. Appearance at time of diagnosis of two children of the same age with coeliac disease: one with and one without classical features.

Nevertheless, single measurements may be within the normal range and so isolated observations may not be useful diagnostically. Knowledge of earlier measurements of height and weight and the plotting of such observations on a percentile chart may prove very helpful diagnostically. Figure 4.11 illustrates a typical percentile chart of a child with coeliac disease. In this case isolated measurements at diagnosis would not have suggested an abnormality, but knowledge of earlier measurements produced the typical percentile chart for weight of a child with coeliac disease; growth was not reduced at the time of diagnosis.

Any child whose rate of weight gain has significantly slowed, especially when this is accompanied by a slowed rate of growth and

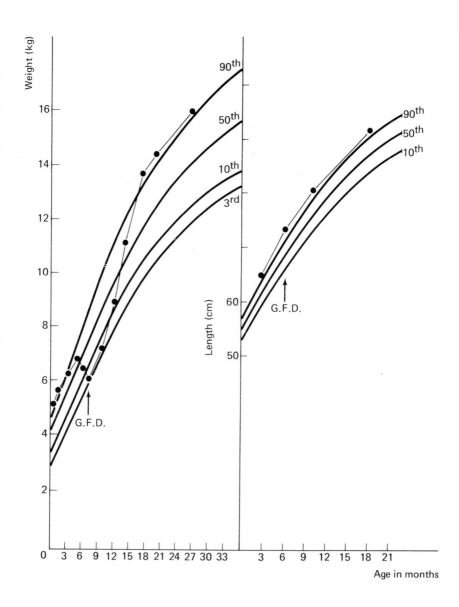

Fig. 4.11. Percentile chart for weight and length of a child with coeliac disease before and after a gluten-free diet (GFD).

gastrointestinal symptoms, merits consideration for the diagnosis of coeliac disease.

In summary, Professor Anderson has divided the commonest modes of presentation of coeliac disease as follows—

1. *Classical Presentation* aged 9–18 months
There is gradual failure to gain weight or loss of weight after introduction of cereals, the child having been previously well. There is also anorexia and alteration in stools which are softer, paler, larger and more frequent than usual. More than half of the 1972–1975 series at Queen Elizabeth Hospital fell into this category.

2. *Presentation in infants before 9 months*
Vomiting is frequent and may be projectable. Diarrhoea may be severe, especially with intercurrent infections, not necessarily gastroenteritis. Abdominal distension may not be marked.

3. *Presentation with constipation*
These children are often very hypotonic with marked abdominal distension.

4. *Presentation at older age*
Short stature, iron resistant anaemia, rickets and personality problems all may occur.

5. *Presentation in Asian children in Britain*
They present later, often with iron-resistant anaemia or rickets and/or short stature. Diarrhoea is not a prominent feature.

6. *Presentation in Asymptomatic siblings*
After a case is positively diagnosed, siblings should have clinical history and growth checked. If a suspicion of coeliac disease arises, full blood count and serum folate and red cell folate should be done. A biopsy should then be performed if there is evidence of a deficiency state.

DIAGNOSIS

The diagnosis of coeliac disease is based initially on the demonstration of an abnormal small intestinal mucosa (usually flat), using the technique of small intestinal biopsy and then upon a clinical response to the withdrawal of gluten from the child's diet. A clinical response is demonstrated when there is significant weight gain and relief of symptoms.

Some paediatricians would then consider that the diagnosis of coeliac disease had been established. The author considers that re-introduction of gluten into the child's diet at a later date, when the small intestinal mucosa has been shown to return to normal, followed by mucosal deterioration with or without a clinical relapse, is necessary before the diagnosis of coeliac disease may be said to have been definitively established. Such a relapse in mucosal appearance may not occur for up to two years after the reintroduction of gluten into the child's diet (Fig. 4.12). These diagnostic criteria for coeliac disease are listed in Table 4.11.

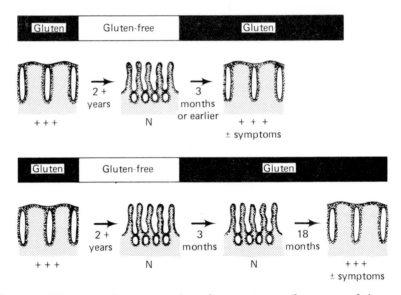

Fig. 4.12. Diagrammatic representation of two patterns of response of the small intestinal mucosa in children with coeliac disease to gluten challenge.

Table 4.11
Diagnostic criteria for coeliac disease

1. Abnormal small intestinal mucosa (usually flat)
2. Clinical response to a gluten-free diet
3. Histological response to a gluten-free diet
4. Histological ± clinical relapse following gluten challenge

A child previously diagnosed as suffering from coeliac disease and having a gluten-free diet should be reinvestigated in order to fulfil these criteria if there is any doubt about the original diagnosis, particularly if the child was started on such a diet without a previous small intestinal biopsy; and also if the child was less than one year of age at the time of diagnosis. It must be appreciated that although a flat small intestinal mucosa is characteristic of coeliac disease, there are other causes of such a mucosa (Table 4.12). Nevertheless, in Western

Table 4.12
Causes of a flat small intestinal mucosa in childhood

Coeliac disease
Gastroenteritis
Giardiasis
Cow's milk protein intolerance
Soy protein intolerance
Tropical sprue
Protein-calorie malnutrition
Acquired hypogammaglobulinaemia

countries the great majority of children with a flat small intestinal mucosa have coeliac disease, but in infants under the age of one year the chances of a flat small intestinal mucosa being due to causes other than coeliac disease are appreciably greater than in the older child, hence the advice to reinvestigate such children. These criteria are sometimes known as the Interlaken Criteria, as they arose from a meeting of the European Society for Paediatric Gastroenterology in Interlaken (Meeuwisse, 1970.) With some modifications, these criteria continue to be a valuable guide to diagnosis. (Harms et al., 1979.)

Such reinvestigation is justified in order to establish clearly the diagnosis of coeliac disease and so to justify the need of a lifetime of dietary restriction. There is evidence that a syndrome of transient gluten intolerance exists (see chapter 5) and this needs to be differentiated from coeliac disease. This reinvestigation may be carried out in the following manner (Fig. 4.13). A small intestinal biopsy is performed while the child is still on a gluten-free diet in order to demonstrate that the mucosa is in fact normal.

If such a preliminary biopsy is abnormal, this suggests either that the child has coeliac disease and is not keeping strictly to a gluten-free diet, or that some other disease is present, so further investigations may be necessary. Usually, such a biopsy is normal when the child has been on a gluten-free diet for two years or more. Earlier reinvestigation in a child with the typical features of coeliac disease is not usually indicated. Once a normal mucosa has been demonstrated the child is given a normal diet containing gluten, or gluten powder is added to his

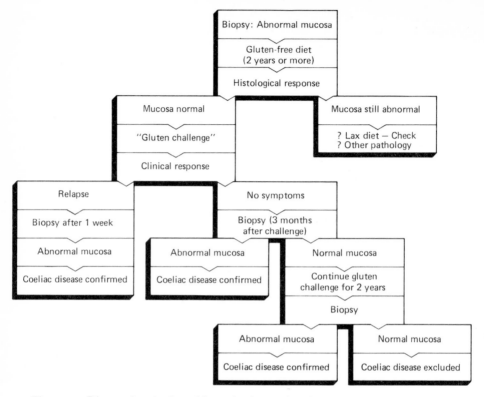

Fig. 4.13. Diagnostic criteria and investigation regime for coeliac disease.

gluten-free diet. Gluten powder may be given to avoid the upset to a child produced by change from a diet already in use for some time. If the child does return to a 'normal' diet, care must be taken to ensure that he does in fact eat gluten-containing foods. A regular check by a dietitian of his daily wheat intake in grams per day is very useful.

Should significant symptoms ensue, a further biopsy is performed after an interval of a week following the return of such symptoms. If the mucosa is then abnormal, the diagnosis of coeliac disease may be said to have been established, i.e. a histological relapse has occurred on reintroduction of gluten to the diet. It is not necessary for the mucosa to be flat to diagnose such a relapse; the presence of significant mucosal abnormalities, for example, increased plasma cells and lymphocytes in the lamina propria and abnormalities of the surface enterocytes, is sufficient.

If symptoms fail to occur, small intestinal biopsy should be performed after three months exposure to gluten since histological relapse may precede clinical relapse. If the mucosa is then still normal, the child is observed and kept on a normal diet, or a diet with added gluten, and another biopsy is performed should symptoms subsequently develop. If symptoms do not develop, a final biopsy is done after two years' exposure to gluten. If the mucosa is then abnormal, coeliac disease is present; but if it is normal, it would be considered that coeliac disease has been excluded. The precise period of two years is somewhat arbitrary and its length may be changed with more experience in the future.

This whole procedure is complex and time-consuming for the child, his parents and his professional attendants, and so should not be undertaken unless really necessary. It is thus particularly important that a child should not be treated with a gluten-free diet unless he has first had a small intestinal biopsy. Failure to do this may lead to the performance some years later of these extensive investigations, only to show that the child did not have coeliac disease and so did not need the diet in the first place. This procedure of reinvestigation should, ideally, be needed only to establish the permanency or otherwise of the state of gluten intolerance in a child previously shown to have an abnormal small intestinal mucosa, and apparently to have responded clinically to the elimination of gluten from his diet.

RE-INVESTIGATION STUDIES

A study of 65 children previously diagnosed as coeliac disease, using the technique outlined in Fig. 4.13 as far as possible, was made at the Queen Elizabeth Hospital (Walker-Smith, Kilby and France, 1978). (Table 4.13). Children were included who had an original diagnosis

Table 4.13
Details of gluten challenges

		Initial abnormal biopsy		No Initial biopsy
Total no. of children challenged	65	44		21
Positive challenges	50	35	⌈31 flat ⌊ 4 PVA	15
Negative challenges	15	9	⌈ 6 flat ⌊ 3 PVA	6

based upon an abnormal biopsy and a clinical response to a gluten-free diet (44 children) and in whom there was no original biopsy but a clinical response to a gluten-free diet (21 children).

Fifty gluten challenges were positive, i.e. there was evidence of histological relapse up to two years on a gluten containing diet. Fifteen were negative, i.e. their mucosa was normal two or more years after a return to a normal gluten containing diet. Looking specifically at the 37 children in this group who had an initial flat mucosa, 6 did not relapse after two years on a normal diet and are clinically well (i.e. 16

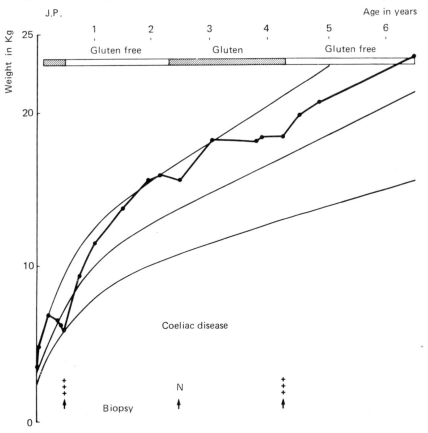

Fig. 4.14. Serial biopsies and weight gain related to centile chart and to dietary gluten in a child with coeliac disease.

per cent). This is a higher figure than the 3·6 per cent reported by Shmerling (1978) to the members of the European Society for Paediatric Gastroenterology but is in closer accord with findings of colleagues in Sweden, 8 of 35, or 22 per cent (Lindberg), and in Finland 8 of 83, or 9 per cent (Kuitunen *et al*., 1977).

Figures 4.14 and 4.15 illustrate serial biopsies and weight gain with dietary gluten in a child with coeliac disease and non-coeliac enteropathy.

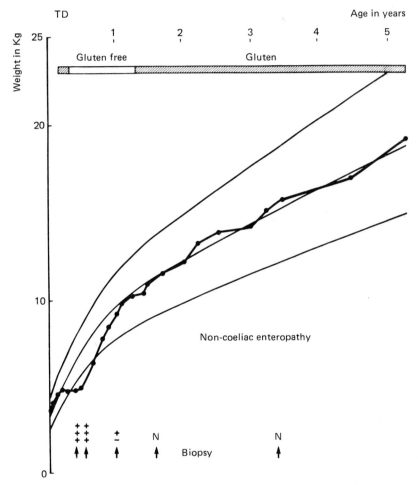

Fig. 4.15. Serial biopsies and weight gain related to centile chart and to dietary gluten in a child with non-coeliac enteropathy.

The serum immunoglobulins were compared in a group of children at the time of initial diagnosis, i.e. untreated, and also at the time of a positive challenge, i.e. in relapse (Table 4.14).

Table 4.14
Serum immunoglobulins in coeliac disease (from Walker Smith, 1977)

	Untreated		Positive challenge	
	No.	Total	No.	Total
Elevated IgA	7	20	I	14
Depressed IgM	3	20	I	14
Depressed IgG	6	20	I	14

It is clear that abnormalities of serum immunoglobulins occurred less frequently in the children who have relapsed after a challenge compared to the untreated group. This may be related to clinical severity since all children reinvestigated after gluten challenge had relatively minor symptoms when these were present at all.

Duration of Diet and Time to Relapse

Of these 35 children who had an histological relapse, 27 were studied for the relationship between the duration of their gluten-free diet and the time to histological relapse. Six of this group were asymptomatic at the time of histological relapse (Fig. 4.16), the remainder had

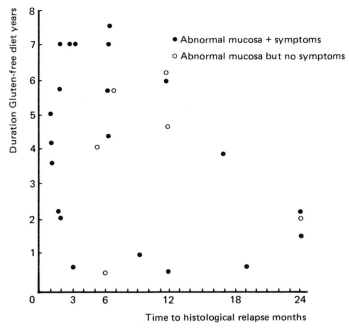

Fig. 4.16. Relation between duration of a gluten-free diet and time to relapse, after gluten challenge in 27 children.

symptoms. There was no correlation whatever between the duration of their gluten-free diet and the time to histological relapse, nor indeed with those who had clinical symptoms as well.

Delayed Relapse

Of the children who had a positive challenge, 45 had definite evidence of mucosal relapse at the time of their first post-challenge biopsy, but 5 did not. Table 4.15 indicates that these five children's first

Table 4.15
Data concerning five children whose first post-challenge biopsy was not diagnostic

Patient	Sex	Age challenge started	Post-challenge biopsy	Time interval on gluten	Final biopsy	Time interval on gluten
B.H.	F.	2 yr. 2 mo.	N.	14 mo.	++/+++	2 yr.
R.J.	M.	3 yr.	N.	5 wks.	+++	2 yr.
J.J.	M.	1½ yr.	N.	5 wks.	+++	2 yr.
S.L.	M.	2 yr.	+	4 mo.	++	9 mo.
J.P.	M.	2 yr. 3 mo.	N.	5 wks.	+++	2 yr.

post-challenge biopsy was taken at intervals ranging from 5 weeks to 14 months on a gluten-containing diet. Only one child subsequently became symptomatic and he had a biopsy after 9 months gluten which was more abnormal than the earlier biopsy. The remainder, despite a grossly abnormal mucosa were symptom-free and were having a routine two-year post-challenge biopsy.

Packer *et al.* (1978) have stated that a normal biopsy, three months after a gluten challenge, for practical purposes excludes coeliac disease provided gluten intake is adequate. The author has seen two children, B.H. above, 14 months on gluten and another 6 months on gluten (Walker-Smith, 1972), who had unequivocally normal biopsies at those times, yet who finally had an abnormal biopsy at a later date. It is essential to have a normal biopsy after two years on a gluten-containing diet before coeliac disease can be said to have been excluded, and even then Egan-Mitchell *et al.* (1978) believe it may take longer.

Short-Term Gluten Challenges

Sinaasappel and Hekkens (1978) have endeavoured to find a satisfactory way to find a short-term challenge in view of the time-consuming procedure discussed above. In a preliminary study of four children they found a rapid depression of disaccharidase activities in biopsy specimens taken under 12 hours after an oral load of gluten fractions. Interestingly, at this early time intraepithelial lymphocytes counts did not rise.

INVESTIGATION OF A CHILD WITH COELIAC DISEASE

Investigation of a child with coeliac disease at initial diagnosis may reveal evidence of multiple deficiencies in absorption, e.g. steatorrhoea, hypoprothrombinaemia, iron and folic acid deficiency anaemia, low serum iron, low serum folate and low red cell folate levels, a flat glucose tolerance test and abnormal xylose absorption. Doubt has been cast upon the reliability of the xylose absorption test in adults; neither urine excretion rates nor serum concentrations alone were found by Sladen and Kumar (1973) to distinguish patients with or without an abnormal small intestinal mucosa. Rolles and his colleagues (1973) have commended as a useful investigation the estimation of a one-hour blood xylose level in children.

In centres where small intestinal biopsy is available a xylose test appears, however, to be of little use because it may occasionally be misleading. Its remaining place may be as a screening test for referral elsewhere in centres where small intestinal biopsy is not available and also as an indication of mucosal relapse after gluten challenge. Perfusion studies of the jejunum in adults, reported by Holdsworth and Dawson (1965), measuring absorption of glucose and water, are a more sensitive measure of jejunal function. Glucose absorption can be shown in this way to be severely depressed despite normal xylose absorption. This research technique has also shown that in some of these patients there is a net secretory state with respect to water and electrolytes. This is reversed by a gluten-free diet.

Gluten antibodies and other dietary protein antibodies may be found in some children with coeliac disease. The percentage that have such antibodies varies in different reports and with the methods of investigation used. Reticulin antibodies may be present, e.g. 85 per cent of one group of 22 children with coeliac disease reported from the Queen Elizabeth Hospital (Seah et al., 1973).

None of these investigations is abnormal in 100 per cent of children who have coeliac disease and so none of them is of value as a screening procedure, but some may be useful to document as a baseline for future observations.

The diagnosis of coeliac disease can only be made using small intestinal biopsy. The indication for biopsy is when any of the clinical features as described above are present and the diagnosis of coeliac disease appears to be a possibility. There is at present no other screening test.

COMPLICATIONS

Most of the complications of coeliac disease are due to malabsorption. While malabsorption of many different substances may occur in coeliac disease, in some children there may be no clinical evidence of malabsorption. In other children there may be evidence of a defect of absorption of only one substance, or there may be malabsorption of a number of different factors.

RICKETS AND OSTEOPOROSIS

In the days before any treatment was available, rickets was a frequent complication of childhood coeliac disease. Photographs in old text-books reveal the horrible deformities that rickets used to produce in such children, but in recent years rickets has been reported relatively infrequently in children who have this disorder. Young and Pringle (1971) in their report of 110 children followed at the Queen Elizabeth Hospital from 1950–1969, found only 2 children with clinical rickets and in a series of a similar number of children seen at the Royal Alexandra Hospital from 1966–1972, none were seen. However, rickets still does occur as a complication of coeliac disease and 3 children from a total of 46 new cases of coeliac disease seen at the Queen Elizabeth Hospital from 1971–1973 had rickets. In two of the children, additional factors, namely anticonvulsant therapy and dietary deficiency (in a Pakistani child), played a role in the development of rickets.

When rickets complicates coeliac disease it is believed to be due to malabsorption of fat soluble vitamin D. The hypocalcaemia that may accompany rickets in coeliac disease, producing tetany and paraesthesiae, is related to the impairment of absorption of dietary calcium and endogenous calcium of the digestive juices due to the binding of calcium to fatty acids to form soaps (Fink and Laszlo, 1957). Thus, calcium and vitamin D deficiency in children with coeliac disease may lead to secondary hyperparathyroidism.

Some children with coeliac disease may have osteoporosis but this is not as severe or as important a complication of coeliac disease in children as it is in adults.

GROWTH AND DEVELOPMENTAL RETARDATION

Severe growth retardation and delayed development, sometimes with delayed onset of puberty, were well known to the early observers of coeliac disease. Gee, in 1888, remarked 'while the disease is active children cease to grow; even when it tends slowly to recovery, they are left frail and stunted'. Growth retardation and delayed puberty continue to be important complications of coeliac disease, albeit less common now, owing to earlier diagnosis and treatment. Prader and his colleagues (1963 and 1969) have shown that 'catch-up growth' occurs once there has been a response to a gluten-free diet.

Day, Evans and Wharton (1973) have studied the effect of intravenous tolbutamide and oral Bovril on growth hormone levels in ten children with coeliac disease at the Queen Elizabeth Hospital. They found that the response of growth hormone levels to tolbutamide was less in children with coeliac disease than in control children. Three children out of the ten had a poor response to Bovril stimulation.

Vanderschueren-Lodeweyckx and her colleagues (1973) went on to compare insulin tolerance tests in 13 children with untreated coeliac disease and 60 normal pre-pubertal children. The fall of blood glucose after insulin was comparable in both groups but the subsequent response of blood glucose levels to the induced hypoglycaemia in the children with coeliac disease was significantly reduced. This was restored to normal after treatment with a gluten-free diet. Out of the 13 children with coeliac disease, 9 had a diminished rise in the level of plasma growth hormone (Fig. 4.17). These authors considered that some degree of hypothalamic hypofunction might account for these observations. It is clear that coeliac disease needs to be considered whenever a child with short stature has evidence of impairment of release of growth hormone.

ANAEMIA IN COELIAC DISEASE

The incidence of anaemia in children with coeliac disease is variable. The most common type is a hypochromic microcytic anaemia due to iron deficiency.

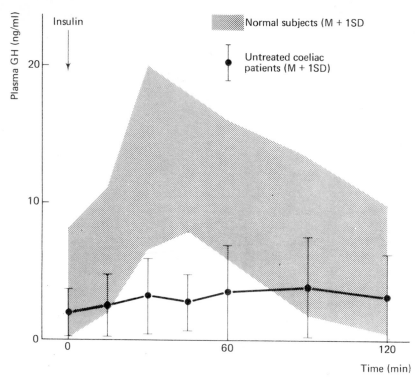

Fig. 4.17. Plasma growth hormone after intravenous administration of insulin in 13 untreated coeliac patients.

Shaded area represents the mean ± 1SD of the values observed in 60 normal pre-pubertal subjects. (Permission of Eggermont from Vanderschueren-Lodeweyckx *et al.*, 1973.)

In a detailed study of 12 patients with untreated coeliac disease (Burman *et al.*, 1978) found a third had haemoglobin concentrations less than 10·0 g/dl, 80 per cent had MCV less than 80 fl, all were iron deficient and two-thirds also folate deficient. Serum iron concentration was reduced in all, but despite iron deficiency TIBC was raised in less than half. If iron deficiency is accompanied by folate deficiency serum iron concentration may be misleadingly high. Six of the patients were looked at more fully, and bone marrow was examined for morphology and tested using the deoxyuridine suppression test (Killmann, 1964). Of the six, four were folate deficient and had abnormal deoxyuridine suppression tests. Two were not folate deficient and had normal deoxyuridine suppression tests. All of the six had absence of iron stores in the bone marrow. Anaemia was prominent in three of the patients and although both iron deficiency and folate deficiency were found, the factor responsible for most of the anaemia was iron deficiency.

Following treatment with a gluten-free diet, serum folate rose from an average of 4·0 (range 1·1 to 12·6) to 8·0 (range 3·0 to 14·8) and red cell folate from an average of 141 (50 to 227) to 256 (range 135 to 426) (period of treatment from 1 to 14 months). In most children values had begun to improve within a month of beginning treatment. Conversely, these values fell when gluten was reintroduced to patients who were in remission on a diet free of gluten when they relapsed histologically.

Only rarely does megaloblastic anaemia occur in children with coeliac disease (Dormandy, Waters and Mollin, 1963). Despite this, serum folate and red cell folate levels are usually reduced in children with untreated coeliac disease. Not surprisingly, a red cell folate level has, therefore, been claimed to be useful as a screening test for coeliac disease in childhood, but although a low level is usually found in children with coeliac disease it cannot be relied upon as a screening test as an occasional child may have normal levels at the time of diagnosis. Folate levels rapidly rise on a gluten-free diet and tend to fall, albeit not always to a pathological level after a gluten challenge. Estimation of folate levels is thus a useful way to evaluate progress on a gluten-free diet of a child with coeliac disease. The cause of these low levels is folic acid malabsorption, and folic acid malabsorption has been well documented in adult studies. Malabsorption of dietary folate (pteroylpolyglutamate) has also been demonstrated (Hoffrand *et al.*, 1970). Perfusion with (^{3}H) pteroylomonoglutamate and pteroyl u (^{14}C) glutamylmonoglutamate, i.e. conjugated folate, have also shown, in adults, marked impairment of luminal disappearance, which improved after gluten withdrawal but did not return to normal values (Halsted *et al.*, 1977). This appeared to result from impaired hydrolysis and also from decreased mucosal uptake of the hydrolytic product. Curiously, *in vitro* analysis of mucosal biopsies in adults with coeliac disease has shown that folate conjugase is increased, whereas disaccharidase is decreased, suggesting that measurement in whole mucosal homogenates overestimates its significant digestive activity. It is likely that the two enzymes are concentrated in different cell types, i.e. the enterocyte and the crypt cell. Halstead *et al.* suggest that increased folate conjugase activity in coeliac disease may be due to predominance of this enzyme in hyperplastic crypt epithelium.

HYPOPROTEINAEMIA

Hypoproteinaemia is a common complication of coeliac disease; for example, Hamilton, Lynch and Reilly (1969) found hypoalbuminaemia to be present in 12 out of 37 children. There is good evidence from radioisotope studies, that the hypoprotinaemia found in children with coeliac disease, is due to protein-losing enteropathy.

When there is severe hypoproteinaemia the child may present with generalised oedema mimicking the nephrotic syndrome. The oedema is relieved by therapy with a gluten-free diet.

HYPOGAMMAGLOBULINAEMIA

Low levels of serum IgA and IgM have been described in children with coeliac disease. The IgA deficiency is not reversible with a gluten-free diet whereas IgM levels rise to normal. It is possible that IgA deficiency predisposes to coeliac disease, as there is an increased incidence of coeliac disease in children with IgA deficiency.

HYPOPROTHROMBINAEMIA

An abnormal prothrombin time due to malabsorption of vitamin K may occur in coeliac disease. Some authorities recommend the estimation of prothrombin time and other parameters of coagulation before small intestinal biopsy is performed. Hypoprothrombinaemia is rapidly corrected by intramuscular vitamin K_1.

LIVER DAMAGE

Lindberg *et al*. (1978) have described liver damage as judged by raised aminotransferase levels in children with coeliac disease, and also cow's milk protein intolerance with severely damaged mucosa. They consider this is connected to the damaged mucosa and could be caused by 'toxic substances' absorbed from gut. This hepatic dysfunction improves on dietary therapy and they suggest that it is another reason for lifelong treatment with a gluten-free diet.

MALIGNANT DISEASE

The most serious complication of long-standing coeliac disease is the development of malignancy. It appears however, to occur only in adult life and so should not ordinarily be discussed with parents of children with coeliac disease.

Gough, Read and Naish in 1962 described three adults with coeliac disease who developed lymphoma of the small bowel, apparently as a complication of coeliac disease. Since then, there has been a number of reports of malignant disease occurring as a sequel to coeliac disease. Harris and his colleagues in Birmingham, in 1967, clearly demonstrated this association in a group of 202 adult patients. The Birmingham group went on to review the incidence of malignant disease in 250 coeliac patients diagnosed between 1941 and 1969 and found lymphoma in 20 cases, gastrointestinal cancer in 16 and some other malignancy in 4.

Cooper, Holmes and Cook (1978) have described 17 lymphomas in long-diagnosed adult patients with coeliac disease. They also report an adult, presenting at age of 39 years with lymphoma, who had been diagnosed as coeliac disease in childhood before days of biopsy but who had been well through adolescence up to the time of presentation.

A further review of this subject in Birmingham (Holmes *et al.*, 1976) failed to show any protection against this risk of malignancy in adults by the use of a gluten-free diet. It would have been unreasonable perhaps to expect such a benefit when an oncogenic stimulus may have existed so long. Only long-term studies of individuals managed from childhood will reveal whether a gluten-free diet provides such protection.

TREATMENT

Elimination of gluten from the child's diet usually leads to a dramatic and rapid clinical response (Fig. 4.18), but this may sometimes be delayed. Weight gain (*see* Fig. 4.11), and relief of emotional symptoms in the mother as well as the child usually occur first, before cessation of diarrhoea and other signs of improvement. There is, however, some disagreement as to precisely what constitutes a gluten-free diet. All authorities are agreed that wheat and rye should be eliminated from the diet, but some also recommend elimination of barley and oats, although it is still uncertain whether these two cereals are also toxic to children with coeliac disease.

Dissanayake, Truelove and Whitehead (1974) have provided some evidence that oats are not toxic in adults, but their period of observation following challenge with oats was far too short to draw firm conclusions. A survey of coeliac children in Britain showed that 12 per cent were upset by oats (Segall, 1974). Thus, the evidence that

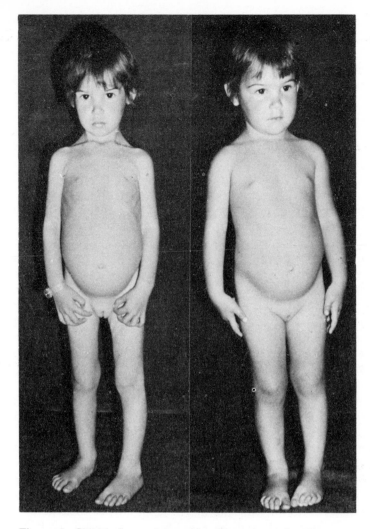

Fig. 4.18. Child before and 6 months after a gluten-free diet.

oats and/or barley are toxic in coeliac disease remains controversial, and further studies are required to clarify the situation. Rice and maize (corn) are certainly not toxic to children with coeliac disease.

Although secondary disaccharidase deficiency has clearly been demonstrated, by assay of small intestinal biopsies, to be present in virtually all children with coeliac disease at the time of diagnosis, in only 5 per cent of infants is lactose intolerance present. Only when there is evidence of such intolerance, i.e. an abnormal amount of reducing substances in the stool, diarrhoea after a lactose load, etc. is elimination of lactose from the diet indicated.

When malnutrition with a severe degree of steatorrhoea is present, a feeding formula based on medium chain triglycerides, such as Pregestemil, may be used for the first weeks after starting treatment, in order to hasten recovery.

In addition, some infants appear to be intolerant of cow's milk protein. This is suggested if symptoms first occurred with the introduction of milk to the child's diet before the child was exposed to gluten. When this happens temporary avoidance of cow's milk may speed recovery.

The need for the restriction of lactose, long chain triglycerides and cow's milk protein is temporary, in contrast to the need for gluten restriction, which is permanent in individuals with coeliac disease.

The need for such permanent dietary restriction is based on three principal premises. First, there is the fact that eventually the small intestinal mucosa will always become abnormal again when it is exposed to gluten, despite years of normality while on a gluten-free diet. Secondly, although such a mucosal relapse may not be followed at once by a clinical relapse, it may lead to slowing of growth and a failure to achieve full growth potential, or it may produce general malaise and lack of energy, often not appreciated by the patient himself, except retrospectively when his gluten-free diet is reintroduced. Thirdly, it is possible that long-term gluten restriction diminishes the risks of developing malignant disease as a complication of coeliac disease. This has yet to be established.

The patient with coeliac disease and his parents should be advised that there is a permanent need for him to adhere strictly to his gluten-free diet. He should only depart from it, on medical advice, as part of a gluten challenge to reinvestigate his state of gluten tolerance, or to establish definitively the diagnosis of coeliac disease.

The child with coeliac disease and his parents need careful support to provide them with up-to-date facts about a gluten-free diet. This may in part be given in Britain by the Coeliac Society, but regular attendance at a coeliac clinic is the ideal. There, a specially trained dietitian is available to advise about a gluten-free diet and to discuss with the parents and child any problems they may have encountered with such a diet. At such a clinic the child's progress and general development can also be observed by the paediatrician, and, if unsatisfactory, investigated appropriately. However, such attendance once or twice a year should not undermine the general advice to the child that he is in every way a normal child as long as he continues on his gluten-free diet.

Finally, we should mention briefly the management of the so-called 'coeliac crisis'. This now very uncommon diagnosis, typically occurring in children under two years of age, is made only when a child with coeliac disease presents with severe diarrhoea, dehydration and weight loss, often accompanied by acidosis, hypokalaemia, hypomagnesaemia and hypoprothrombinaemia. While immediate intravenous replacement therapy is indicated and fluid and electrolyte balance restored, recovery may be delayed even though the child has no gluten in his diet.

Lloyd-Still and his colleagues (1972) have reviewed the use of corticosteroids for such children. They have concluded that there is a rapid reversal of symptoms when steroids are used during the acute stage of therapy as a temporary expedient. The theoretical justification for this therapy is based on the observation of Wall and his colleagues (1970) who found that oral prednisolone in adults with coeliac disease led to a prompt histological recovery of the small intestinal mucosa despite continued ingestion of gluten.

ASSOCIATIONS OF COELIAC DISEASE

IgA deficiency has already been mentioned as an association of coeliac disease.

Diabetes mellitus has been reported more commonly in patients with coeliac disease than in the general population. In a series of 110 new cases of coeliac disease at the Royal Alexandra Hospital from 1966–1972, there were two children with diabetes mellitus.

A possible explanation for the association between diabetes mellitus and coeliac disease may be a common genetic predisposition. It is now clear that approximately 80 per cent of patients with coeliac disease have the histocompatibility antigen HLA-8. Cudworth and Woodrow (1974) have also found that 54 per cent of patients with juvenile onset diabetes have the HLA-8 antigen. It has been suggested that one or more immune-response genes are in linkage disequilibrium with HLA-8 and this may be the basis for the predisposition to both coeliac disease and diabetes mellitus that possession of the HLA-8 antigen appears to endow.

In adult patients there is an association between dermatitis herpetiformis and coeliac disease (Marks et al., 1966). This association does not appear to occur in childhood, when dermatitis herpetiformis is uncommon, although children with coeliac disease may have parents or relatives who appear to have both coeliac disease and dermatitis herpetiformis. Whether the enteropathy that occurs in most adults who have dermatitis herpetiformis is identical with that of adult coeliac disease is still uncertain. Both are sensitive to gluten but the mucosa of the proximal small intestine of the former group was noted to be patchily abnormal in 21 out of 22 patients investigated by Brow and his colleagues (1971). However, Kumar and her colleagues at St Bartholomew's Hospital (1973) found no evidence of a patchy lesion in five patients, but they did not perform as many multiple biopsies as Brow and his colleagues. They studied the effect of a gluten-free diet on jejunal morphology and function in six adults with dermatitis herpetiformis and found a significant improvement comparable to that found in coeliac disease.

5

Dietary Protein Intolerance

Clinical food 'intolerance' has many causes and many manifestations, which include psychological aversion to the sight, smell or taste of food as well as intolerance to one or more of the many constituents of food.

Intolerance to various food proteins in childhood, especially the protein of cow's milk, has been recognised for many years. Such food intolerance may result from a variety of causes; for example, specific enzyme deficiencies, and small intestinal mucosal damage, which may be the result of a food allergy. Indeed, food may contain a number of substances that are potentially harmful to infants and children. Bleumink (1974) has classified adverse reactions after food ingestion as follows—

1. Toxic effects, including those due to bacterial contamination and food additions.
2. Intolerance phenomena due to enzyme deficiencies, e.g. lactose intolerance as a sequel to lactase deficiency.
3. Allergic reactions.
4. Symptoms resembling allergic reactions but not elicited by immunological phenomena. To this category belong symptoms caused by histamine releasers, e.g. strawberries, where the histamine release is not the consequence of an immunological reaction.

There is increasing evidence that dietary protein intolerance may be mediated via an allergic reaction. In this chapter, the varieties of food protein intolerance in which there is some evidence for such an allergic reaction or reactions will be discussed.

When the term allergy is used, it implies a heterogeneous group of conditions which have in common a state of altered reactivity to foreign proteins, i.e. antigens (Gell and Coombs, 1968). These antigens are called allergens when they produce symptoms in an allergic person. A child who has an allergy is distinguished from other children by an abnormal response to contact with an allergen or allergens, a response that does not occur when a non-allergenic child is exposed to the same potential allergen. The typical features of an allergic reaction are: first, the lack of any untoward reaction to the child's first exposure to the allergen, and second, that subsequent exposure to the allergen produces a hypersensitivity reaction. Indeed, Ferguson (1976) regards the term 'hypersensitivity' as preferable to the term "allergy' when used to describe tissue damage resulting from the immune reaction to a further dose of antigen occurring in a previously immunised host.

Gell and Coombs (1968) have classified the allergic or hypersensitivity reactions that may produce tissue damage of some kind into four types, as follows—

Type I Anaphylactic or Immediate Hypersensitivity

This is initiated by an allergen reacting with mast cells that have been passively sensitised by IgE (reaginic) antibody with release of vasoactive agents such as histamine. The reaction occurs within minutes of exposure.

Type II Cytotoxic

This reaction is initiated by antibody reacting with an antigenic component of a cell or tissue element or one that is intimately associated with these. Complement is usually necessary to effect cellular damage.

Type III Toxic or Immune Complexes (Arthus-type)

In this type of reaction, antigen and antibody (IgG or IgM) react in the presence of antigen excess with subsequent complement fixation to form complexes, with consequent local inflammatory response. This reaction is maximal a few hours after exposure to antigen.

Type IV Delayed Hypersensitivity (Cell-Mediated Immunity)

This reaction is mediated by T-lymphocytes and macrophages and manifests by infiltration of lymphocytes and macrophages at the site where antigen is present, due to release of lymphokines. These are soluble factors secreted by lymphocytes on contact with antigen. This reaction takes 1 to 2 days after antigen exposure.

Evidence of such an allergic reaction, with tissue damage, in children who show clinical intolerance to dietary protein is not always available. Therefore, in clinical practice, the descriptive term 'food protein intolerance' is preferred to the more precise term 'food allergy', until more is known about the pathogenesis of the disorder, or what is likely to prove more probable, this group of disorders.

The first case report of food allergy was made by Finkelstein in 1905, who described cow's milk as a cause of acute death in an infant.

Schloss, in 1911, related gastrointestinal symptoms to food allergy. He made the diagnosis of egg allergy on the basis of a positive skin test with a protein fractionated from ovomucoid. Although many subsequent observers have clearly established that skin tests are only of limited value in the diagnosis of gastrointestinal allergy, food protein intolerance has come to be recognised as an important cause of gastrointestinal symptoms in infancy.

Many paediatricians in the past, however, have been sceptical about this diagnosis because of the absence of precise and objective diagnostic criteria, nevertheless most paediatricians now accept the existence of the condition. There is still debate, however, concerning its frequency and importance in different parts of the world.

Gastrointestinal symptoms may be the only manifestation of clinical intolerance to food protein but there may also be respiratory symptoms and signs as well as atopic eczema. Only gastrointestinal effects will be discussed in any detail here.

DEFINITION

Dietary protein intolerance is the clinical syndrome resulting from the sensitisation of an individual to one or more dietary proteins that have been absorbed via a permeable small intestinal mucosa. Clinically, it appears to be a transient phenomenon of variable duration in children.

Lippard et al. (1936) showed that at whatever age a child first begins to drink cow's milk, cow's milk antigen and then cow's milk antibody can be detected in his blood. More recently, Delire et al. (1978) have found that neonates fed on cow's milk have in their blood circulatory immune complexes containing cow's milk protein antigens, and IgG antibodies of maternal origin. Despite these findings, only a few children go on to develop cow's milk protein intolerance. How such a state of clinical intolerance comes about is unknown.

Even the presence of a high level of antibodies is not necessarily damaging, e.g. there is a high incidence of elevated titres of cow's milk antibodies in children with both coeliac disease and kwashiorkor (Chandra, 1976) yet, as a rule, these children improve clinically on cow's milk diet. Presumably, although antigen exclusion was defective, elimination was adequate.

The definition above makes it clear that food protein intolerance is a transient phenomenon in childhood, at least in its clinical manifestations, although there are adults who give a history of apparent intolerance to dietary proteins. The relationship of such adult syndromes to those of childhood remains unknown. The one exception to the transient nature of food protein intolerance in childhood is coeliac disease which, by definition, as described in chapter 4, is characterised by a permanent state of gluten intolerance and so is excluded from discussion here.

INCIDENCE OF FOOD PROTEIN INTOLERANCE

The reported incidence of food allergy in childhood has ranged widely from a low 0·3 per cent in one series to a high 38 per cent in another. Part of this apparent disparity is related to differing diagnostic criteria, but this is not the whole explanation.

In Finland, there has for some time been a particular interest in this subject as it seems to be a relatively frequent problem there; 7·8 per cent of children had this condition in a recent survey. Peltonen, Kassanen and Peltonen, in 1955, observed that there were more allergies among people born in Finland in the 1940s than among those born in the 1930s. Koivikko (1973) believes that it is relevant to this observation that in the 1940s breast feeding began to decline in Finland, and he has recently reviewed the evidence that breast feeding per se could reduce the incidence of allergies in children and suggests that the increase in allergies from the 1940s onwards in Finland was related to less breast feeding. A basis for such an explanation is provided by the high level of secretory IgA in breast milk which could act as an immunological barrier against foreign food antigens such as those found in mixed cereals. Taylor and his colleagues in London (1973) have demonstrated that transient IgA deficiency in infancy may be associated with the subsequent development of allergic symptoms. Breast feeding in such infants with its high secretory IgA level could play a role in preventing the development of allergy, and breast feeding, of course, also results in avoidance of early contact with cow's milk protein antigens at a time when IgA levels may be low.

The early introduction of mixed feeding into an 'at risk' infant's diet, e.g. the child of atopic parents, may also be associated with an increased incidence of food protein intolerance, particularly when such an infant is not breast fed. Thus, the incidence of breast feeding, the age at which mixed solids are introduced into the infant's diet, and the type of artificial feeding used in a community, as well as variable diagnostic criteria, may all influence the incidence of cow's milk protein and other types of dietary protein intolerance.

VARIETIES OF FOOD PROTEIN INTOLERANCE

Intolerance to many food proteins, including those of egg, shell-fish, etc. has been described, but only in the cases of cow's milk protein, soy protein and the wheat protein, gluten, have alterations in small intestinal structure and function been documented in children. Only these varieties of food protein intolerance will be discussed here.

Clinical intolerance to a variety of food proteins has been described. The most common are cow's milk, eggs and fish, but intolerance to tomatoes, oranges, bananas, meat, nuts, chocolates and cereals, including soy protein, have been described (Bleumink, 1974).

Chemically, allergens are usually glycoproteins with a molecular weight of between 20,000 and 40,000.

COW'S MILK PROTEIN INTOLERANCE

Intolerance to cow's milk protein may occur as an isolated phenomenon causing gastrointestinal symptoms or it may be associated with other manifestations of allergic disease such as eczema and asthma. It may also occur as a secondary phenomenon in children with coeliac disease, and disappear as the child responds to a gluten-free diet.

Cow's milk and human breast milk have different protein compositions, as Table 5.1 illustrates.

Human milk does not contain beta-lactoglobulin, which represents the major protein in cow's milk whey proteins, and most observers, including Visakorpi and Immonen (1967) and Freier and his colleagues (1969), have noticed that this protein is often the responsible factor for cow's milk allergy, although the other proteins may also be allergenic in children. Cow's milk contains three times more protein

Table 5.1
Protein content in g/100 ml mature milk

	Cow's milk	Human milk
Total proteins	3·5	1·1
Casein	2·8	0·4
Proteins in lactoserum (whey protein)	0·6–0·8	0·7
Beta-lactoglobulin	0·37	—
Alpha-lactalbumin	0·18	0·35
Immunoglobulins, total*	0·05	0·1–0·15
Other proteins	0·13	0·2

* Pahud, J. J. Thesis, University of Lausanne (1971).
Permission of Montreuil, 1971.

than human milk (due to its higher content of casein), but the same content of soluble proteins (Table 5.1). In so-called 'humanised milks' the total protein content is lowered to about the level of human milk and the proportion of soluble proteins to casein is corrected by the addition of whey proteins (i.e. all the soluble proteins in milk after precipitation of casein either by the action of rennin or by acidification to the iso-electric point pH 4·6).

The immunoglobulins present in breast milk are chiefly of the IgA class. Table 5.2 indicates the difference in the immunoglobulin composition of breast and cow's milk.

Table 5.2
Immunoglobulin content in mg/100 ml

	Cow's milk	Breast milk
IgA	100	1,735
IgG	4	150
IgM	–	43

Permission of Silverman, Roy and Cozzeto, 1971.
St. Louis: The C.V. Mosby Co.

PATHOGENESIS

At present, the pathogenesis of the cow's milk sensitive enteropathy of cow's milk protein intolerance is not clear, but a number of observations that do shed some light on this subject are known, and give rise to interesting speculations.

Clinically there seem to be two syndromes of cow's milk protein intolerance, a primary and a secondary. In the primary there appear to be no predisposing factors, but in the secondary it follows acute gastroenteritis. Two factors may be important in both: first, the permeability of the small intestinal mucosa to antigen, and secondly, the control of the antigen once it has been absorbed. The primary syndrome may be due to a primary disturbance of the local immune system for antigen control, particularly exclusion. The secondary syndrome, may be a sequel to primary gut damage due to gastroenteritis permitting excess antigen entry, perhaps coupled with a defect of local antigen control. An immunodeficiency state, such as transient IgA deficiency, may be an important predisposing factor for both syndromes. Table 5.3 outlines this hypothesis for secondary cow's milk protein intolerance, and suggests a relationship between gastroenteritis and lactose intolerance with cow's milk sensitive enteropathy.

Table 5.3
Hypothesis
Relationship between gastroenteritis and lactose intolerance with cow's milk sensitive enteropathy

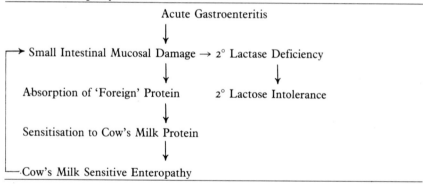

It has been shown by Barnes and Townley (1973) that acute gastroenteritis causes small intestinal mucosal damage. As a result, there may be excess absorption of foreign protein, as was shown by Gruskay and Cook (1955). They studied 21 children with acute gastroenteritis severe enough to warrant intravenous fluids. They gave them an oral egg albumin load and found a greater concentration in the serum than in controls. It is also known from Barnes and Townley's observations that the small gut mucosa usually heals rapidly, and it is also known from Gruskay and Cook that 1 to 2 weeks after that acute episode, egg albumin levels, after a further load, had significantly fallen in most cases. It is hypothesised then that, in some children with acute gastroenteritis, sensitisation occurs to cow's milk protein and that the mucosal damages does not heal but persists with associated lactase deficiency. This may be due to excess antigen entry, defective antigen control by the mucosa, possibly due to temporary immunodeficiency, or immaturity of the immune system of the small intestinal mucosa.

In both syndromes the net result is that the small intestinal mucosa is sensitised to a cow's milk protein or proteins. The resulting local reaction in the small intestine may be mediated via one of the allergic reactions as classified by Gell and Coombs (1968), namely type I, type III, and type IV, although it must be pointed out that these mechanisms have only been established systemically and not in the small intestine. Evidence that these three types of reaction may occur in children with cow's milk protein intolerance include the following observations.

First, in relation to Type I reaction, elevated titres of IgE antibodies to cow's milk protein, using the RAST technique, have been observed. However, such elevated titres can be found in milk tolerant children and the IgE milk antibody titre does not correlate with symptoms, although in early infancy there is a better correlation with the height of the titre. Positive skin prick tests may be found in milk intolerant children but, again, correlation with symptoms is variable. The involvement of IgE in the immunological response of the lamina propria to milk challenge in children with cow's milk protein intolerance has been described by Shiner and her colleagues (1975), also by Kilby, Walker-Smith and Wood (1976), who showed an increase in IgE cell numbers in the small intestinal mucosa after a milk challenge in a child with cow's milk sensitive enteropathy. However, whether IgE mediated small intestinal disease due to sensitised mast cells releasing mediators at the site of reaction between cow's milk protein, and reaginic IgE antibody fixing to mast cells really occurs, has not yet been proved. If this does happen, disodium cromoglycate may help.

Second, in relation to Type 3 reaction, elevated titres of IgG and IgM milk antibodies have been described, but again with a poor clinical correlation. Increased numbers of IgA cells, but not in general IgM plasma cells after a positive milk challenge, may occur. Matthews and Soothill (1970) have observed the effect of milk feeding on complement activation, and reports of circulating immune complexes in children fed with cow's milk has already been referred to. Whether such complexes are associated with cow's milk protein intolerance is unclear.

Third, abnormalities of cell mediated immunity leading to abnormal lymphocyte transformation tests (Fontaine and Navarro, 1975) have been reported.

Any or all of these mechanisms are possible and may be variously involved in individual children. With this background it is possible to speculate further concerning the involvement of these mechanisms. First, the local immune system of the small intestine has no memory. Presumably, after a few weeks of a milk-free diet, i.e. antigen withdrawal, the small intestinal mucosa would lose its immunity to milk. Thus, on rechallenge, there would be neither protective immunity nor damaging hypersensitivity possible for a few days (3 to 4 days) if local immunity were solely involved.

On the other hand, systemic immunity *does* have memory. It is possible that in the mucosa there may be systemic anti-milk IgE antibody fixed to mast cells allowing a type I reaction in the gut to occur. The gut would also be washed by systemic IgG and IgM cells with some anti-milk specificity which would cause intermediate but, probably mild, damage. Within 2 or 3 days secondary immunisation would occur with greatly increased reaction to the antigen.

The importance of the type I reaction in the gut, and the mild intermediate reaction, would be in allowing increased amounts of antigen to cross a damaged mucosa, and by causing capillary dilatation and increased permeability, allowing large amounts of antigen into the systemic circulation to set up secondary immunisation. If this antigen meets tissue fixed IgE then type I reaction would occur, e.g. in the skin (rash), in the gut (mucosal damage), in bronchial mucosa (wheeze), generally (anaphylaxis). This would depend on just where the antibody was, which would explain the very variable reactions encountered.

The involvement of systemic immunity, and the local immune system, would also explain the transient nature of the illness. The illness could disappear after a period on a milk-free diet when, (1) the systemic immune system lost its memory (which would probably take months), and (2) the small intestinal mucosa local immune system was mature enough to prevent much antigen getting through. The role of cell-mediated immunity in all this is not clear but its possible importance should not be underestimated.

GENETIC FACTORS

Boys and girls appear to be equally affected (*see* Table 5.4). Although an atopic family history is very common, no definite genetic factor has been identified. Kuitunen *et al.* (1976) have shown an HLA status identical to that of the community. However, Swarbrick, Stokes and Soothill (1979) have shown, in animals, a genetic variation in the control of antigen by the gut, which suggests certain individuals may be predisposed to develop dietary protein intolerance.

PATHOLOGY

Most children with cow's milk protein intolerance who produce gastrointestinal symptoms appear on biopsy to have an abnormal small intestinal mucosa at the time of initial diagnosis (Kuitunen *et al.*, 1975; Fontaine and Navarro, 1975; Harrison *et al.*, 1976). However, unlike coeliac disease, this enteropathy does not appear to be an invariable finding on a single proximal biopsy from all such children. When present, the enteropathy can be shown to be cow's milk sensitive by serial biopsies related to withdrawal and challenge with cow's milk (Fig. 5.1). Unlike the gluten sensitive enteropathy of

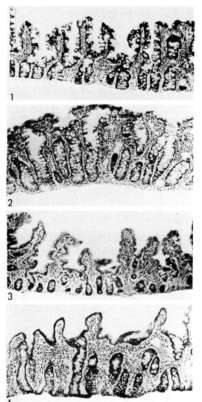

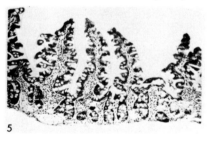

Fig. 5.1. Serial small intestinal biopsies in an infant with cow's milk protein intolerance.

(1) Aged $3\frac{1}{2}$ months at time of first biopsy on a cow's milk-free diet. (2) Biopsy appearances aged 4 months after return of diarrhoea on milk containing diet. (3) Biopsy appearances aged 1 year on a cow's milk-free diet. (4) Biopsy appearances $3\frac{1}{2}$ days later after a further positive milk challenge. (5) Biopsy appearances aged 21 months on a cow's milk free diet. This was followed by an uneventful return to a normal cow's milk containing diet.

untreated coeliac disease, this cow's milk sensitive enteropathy is of variable severity on proximal mucosal biopsy, and is patchy in distribution, while a flat mucosa, indistinguishable from the mucosal appearances found in coeliac disease, may occur (Fig. 5.1).

More often, lesser degrees of mucosal abnormality may be found. After a positive milk challenge, alteration in microvilli of the enterocyte may be seen (Fig. 5.2) in parallel with a fall in disaccharidase activity (Fig. 5.3). Although the numbers of intra-epithelial lymphocytes may rise after a positive milk challenge (Fig. 5.4), the level reached is usually within the normal range.

Figure 5·5 indicates the relationship between lactose intolerance and cow's milk challenge.

Some observers have claimed that eosinophilic infiltration of the mucosa is characteristic in children who are intolerant to cow's milk protein but others have found it to be an inconstant finding. It has been reported to be present as a characteristic finding by Silverberg and Davidson (1974) in children who have 'allergic gastroenteropathy'. In these children, apart from the increase of eosinophils in the lamina propria, the mucosa is otherwise normal.

Eosinophilic or allergic gastroenteritis is a disorder of unknown aetiology, described in the American literature but which has not been recognised by the author either in Britain or Australia (Waldmann et al., 1967). It is characterised by protein-losing enteropathy, peripheral eosinophilia and iron-deficiency anaemia secondary to gastrointestinal blood loss. Some patients respond to a cow's milk free diet but others are apparently resistant to dietary management and have been treated with steroids. Katz, Goldman and Grand (1977) have described the presence of a gastric mucosal lesion in six children aged 6 months to 15 years with eosinophilic gastroenteritis. They suggest that the gastric lesion may contribute to the protein loss and gastrointestinal lesion found in this disorder, and go on to recommend gastric mucosal biopsy as an aid to diagnosis.

CLINICAL FEATURES

Most children with cow's milk protein intolerance have symptoms within the first six months of life. The symptoms fall into two principal categories, namely, those that are predominantly gastrointestinal and those related to organs outside the alimentary tract; for example urticaria and wheezing.

Children with chiefly gastrointestinal manifestations may present with acute symptoms or with a chronic syndrome, sometimes with evidence of malabsorption, producing a clinical picture resembling

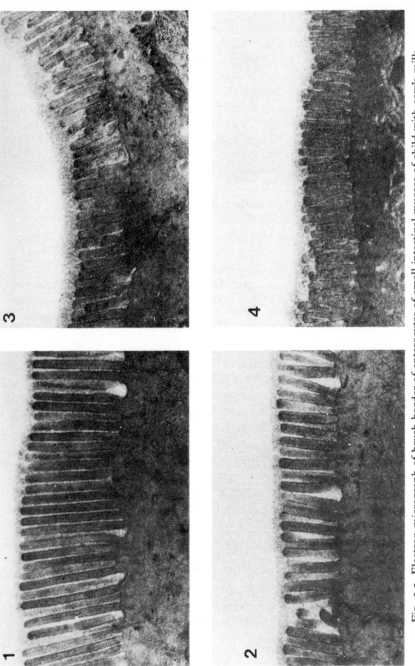

Fig. 5.2. Electron micrograph of brush border of enterocytes of small intestinal mucosa of child with cow's milk protein intolerance.
(1) and (2) on a cow's-milk-free diet, (1) mid-villus region, (2) villus-tip region, (3) and (4) after a positive cow's milk challenge, (3) mid-villus region, (4) villus-tip. (Permission of Phillips.)

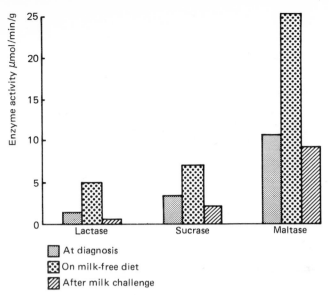

Fig. 5.3. Mean disaccharidase activity related to cow's milk intake in 5 infants with cow's milk sensitive enteropathy.

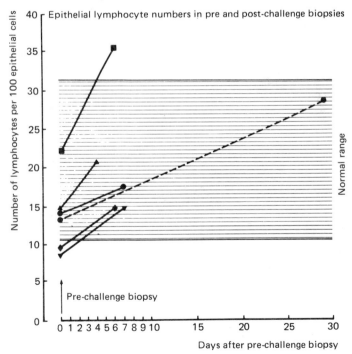

Fig. 5.4. Intraepithelial lymphocyte counts in relation to a cow's milk challenge, pre- and post-challenge levels indicated.

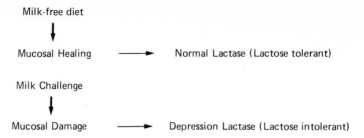

Fig. 5.5. Relationship between milk challenge and lactose tolerance.

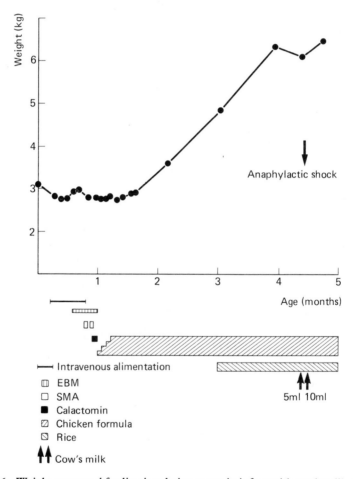

Fig. 5.6. Weight curve and feeding in relation to age in infant with cow's milk protein intolerance.

coeliac disease. In some of these children there may be a family history of atopy but in others no such history is present.

The acute syndrome is usually characterised by the sudden onset of vomiting, occasionally followed by pallor and a shock-like state, but acute anaphylaxis is rare. When it occurs, acute anaphylaxis is a dramatic syndrome (Fig. 5.6) (de Peyer and Walker-Smith, 1977) and can be fatal. The role of cow's milk hypersensitivity in the genesis of sudden unexpected death or 'cot death' was raised by Parish et al. (1960). The postulated mode of death was an acute anaphylactic reaction to cow's milk. Devey et al. (1976) in Cambridge, went on to report that guinea-pigs given cow's milk to drink, instead of water, soon became anaphylactically sensitised to the proteins of cow's milk. After 14 days, all the guinea-pigs could be fatally shocked, following either intravenous injection or intratracheal inhalation of cow's milk. Coombs, Devey and Anderson (1978) then found that when the drinking of cow's milk was continued by the guinea-pigs for more than 70 days they became refractory to the effect. Anderson et al. (1979) have now shown that there are differences in the anaphylactic sensitising capacities of different milks in their animal model. Evaporated whole cow's milk was practically without sensitising capacity to beta lactoglobulin, and a formula in a liquid concentrate form had an extremely low sensitising capacity to both casein and beta lactoglobulin. In both cases this only occurred when given to the guinea-pigs by mouth, sensitising capacity being retained when given parenterally. This suggests that these formula are handled differently in the small intestine from other milk feeds, i.e. they may be more digestible. These observations have far-reaching implications if they are true for human infants, because they suggest that modification of artificial feeding formulae may profoundly influence their allergenic or sensitising capacity.

Often the onset of vomiting in the acute syndrome is followed by diarrhoea, and the clinical syndrome may be identical with the features of acute gastroenteritis. Since cow's milk protein intolerance may occur as a complication of infective gastroenteritis, and especially as it may also be accompanied by secondary lactose intolerance, it may be impossible, at the time of the initial illness, to make an accurate differential diagnosis between cow's milk allergy and acute gastroenteritis. This is particularly difficult as it is not possible at present to identify routinely a stool pathogen in most cases of acute gastroenteritis unless electron microscopy is available to identify the stool viruses. This acute presentation is the commonest mode in the author's experience (Table 5.4).

Table 5.4
Mode of presentation of cow's milk protein intolerance in 30 children at Queen Elizabeth Hospital for Children – Permission Harrison

Males 21		Females 19

5 children. Chronic diarrhoea, vomiting and failure to thrive.

25 children. Acute onset of diarrhoea and vomiting ?gastroenteritis.

Evidence for gastroenteritis
8 – stool pathogen identified
6 – contact with infective diarrhoea and vomiting.

Iyngkaran *et al.* (1978) have followed up the role of cow's milk protein intolerance in prolonging diarrhoea after acute gastroenteritis in Malaysia. Based on biopsy studies before and after cow's milk challenge, they found a high incidence of cow's milk protein intolerance after gastroenteritis, especially in infants under two years of age.

The chronic syndrome is characterised by the gradual onset of vomiting and diarrhoea with failure to thrive. Some children may pass the typical fatty stools of steatorrhoea. Visakorpi (1970) indeed states that most children with cow's milk protein intolerance have laboratory evidence of malabsorption, but others such as Freier and his colleagues (1969) do not agree.

Some children may pass watery stools containing blood. Gryboski (1967) has described sigmoidoscopic findings in such children which are typical of colitis but which respond to elimination of milk from the diet.

Buisseret (1978) using Goldman's criteria to diagnose cow's milk allergy in children found in a study of 79 children aged between 11 months and 17 years a wide variety of clinical manifestations. These included constipation as well as diarrhoea, vomiting, intestinal colic, eczema and asthma, all being reversed by milk withdrawal.

DIAGNOSIS

Until recently, the only satisfactory way to make the diagnosis of cow's milk protein intolerance has been based purely on clinical observations of repeated withdrawal of milk and challenge with milk, associated with clinical remission and relapse as formulated by Goldman and colleagues in 1963, and since spoken of as the Goldman criteria (Table 5.5).

Table 5.5
Goldman criteria

1. Symptoms subside following dietary elimination of milk.
2. Symptoms recur within forty-eight hours after milk challenge.
3. Reactions to three such challenges must be positive and have similar onset, duration and clinical features.

These criteria have obvious drawbacks. Most mothers are reluctant to submit their infants to three potentially hazardous challenges, especially after one positive challenge. Diagnosis of clinical relapse can be misleading, e.g. intercurrent illness may cause vomiting and diarrhoea and lead to error in interpretation. It is also now clear that children may take longer than 48 hours to relapse after a milk challenge. Finally, such positive challenges do not always have a similar onset, duration and clinical features. The use of these criteria has led to under-diagnosis of this syndrome.

Serial small intestinal biopsies at the time of initial presentation, after a clinical response to milk withdrawal and, finally, after the return of symptoms following a milk challenge, now permit a firm diagnosis to be made; on the basis of one diagnostic milk challenge.

The first stage in making the diagnosis is the suspicion that the child's symptoms relate to milk ingestion. If the small intestinal mucosa is shown to be abnormal on biopsy at the time and there is a clinical response to withdrawal of cow's milk from the diet a provisional diagnosis of cow's milk protein intolerance can be made. The final diagnosis of cow's milk protein intolerance depends upon the response to a milk challenge after the period of milk withdrawal.

Technique of Cow's Milk Challenge

It is important that a challenge with cow's milk should be carried out in hospital so that it may be critically evaluated and because of the occasional risk of an acute anaphylactic reaction. The infant who is having a milk-free diet (almost the same as a lactose-free diet) is admitted to hospital. First, he has a control pre-challenge small intestinal biopsy to show that his mucosa has returned to normal or near normal. If it is still abnormal, challenge should be deferred and the diagnosis reconsidered, the diet being carefully checked. In these circumstances if the child is truly on a milk-free diet but continues to have gluten in his diet coeliac disease must be considered.

When the mucosa has been shown on biopsy to have healed, the following day an oral lactose load of 2 g lactose/kg is given. This is followed by a lactose mixture containing 7 per cent lactose for 24 hours. During this period the infant should be observed carefully and any loose stools tested for reducing substances. If watery diarrhoea with excess reducing substances occurs, the infant is clearly lactose intolerant and goes back to his milk-free diet, and milk challenge is deferred. If there is no diarrhoea the milk challenge takes place the next day. The amount given in the challenge will depend upon the previous severity of symptoms. If the history suggests the possibility of a previous anaphylactic reaction an intravenous infusion should be set-up before the challenge and the initial amount of milk given should be small; for example 0·2 ml. In most children 5 ml of milk should be given, followed after an hour by a further 10 ml when no symptoms occur. If this is tolerated the child is then regraded in quarters back onto cow's milk or his normal milk feeding. Should symptoms recur, such as vomiting and diarrhoea, milk is withdrawn and he goes back to his milk-free diet, and a further small intestinal biopsy is done as soon as possible. If the previously normal mucosa is now abnormal, then this is regarded as a positive challenge, i.e. a cow's milk sensitive enteropathy has been shown and a firm diagnosis of cow's milk protein intolerance is made. If the mucosa is still normal, he continues on milk, and other causes for the symptoms are sought, such as an intercurrent hospital acquired illness. It is only a biopsy that can distinguish this from relapse. An occasional child may clinically relapse after a milk challenge despite a normal biopsy. This poses a difficult problem in diagnosis and may be due to patchiness of the cow's milk sensitive enteropathy.

Table 5.6
Clinical features of a positive milk challenge in 30 children at the Queen Elizabeth Hospital for Children, Permission of Harrison

Feature	No. tested	No. positive
Diarrhoea	30	30
Vomiting	30	29
Occult blood in stools	25	24
Weight loss >300 g in 24 hours	30	27
Rise in T.° to >38° C.	29	21
Rise in eosinophils >450 × 10/dl	28	19
Reducing substances in stools 0·5–2%	30	28
Rash/urticaria	30	9
Wheezing	30	3
Anaphylaxis	30	3

The symptoms that occur after challenge vary considerably and range from an alarming anaphylactic reaction that comes on rapidly after the child has ingested cow's milk, to the development of diarrhoea, with stools obviously blood-stained twenty-four or more hours after exposure to milk protein (Table 5.6). Vomiting is usually a striking symptom and is often the first to appear.

However there is still no unanimity concerning the diagnostic criteria for cow's milk protein intolerance; for example, there is no consensus as to how a milk challenge should be performed; some use whole milk for the challenge and others use milk protein fractions such as lactoglobulin.

Goldman and his colleagues in 1963 reported investigations of 89 children with cow's milk protein intolerance and found the following frequencies of reactions to challenge with various milk protein fractions: beta-lactoglobulin 66 per cent, casein 57 per cent, alpha-lactalbumin 54 per cent, bovine serum albumin 51 per cent.

In addition to the above challenge procedure, various laboratory tests have been studied to help to diagnose cow's milk protein intolerance. Anderson and Schloss in the USA in 1923, found antibodies to cow's milk protein in the serum of infants exposed to cow's milk. Since then the occurrence of circulating milk precipitins in the serum of children has been reported in a wide variety of disorders, including chronic respiratory disease and IgA deficiency. However, most authorities believe that the presence of circulating milk antibodies cannot be correlated with clinical intolerance to this protein. A good example of this is provided by some children with coeliac disease who still have cow's milk antibodies in their sera while on a gluten-free diet and yet have no symptoms with milk ingestion.

Skin tests have been advocated as being of diagnostic value in children suspected of being intolerant to cow's milk protein. Matthews and Soothill (1970) found positive skin tests to cow's milk protein in all eight children they reported with this disorder, but previously, Goldman and his colleagues (1963) found positive skin tests in only 59 per cent of a group of children who were intolerant to cow's milk. Of 16 children with cow's milk protein intolerance at Queen Elizabeth Hospital for Children who were tested, by no means all had positive prick tests (see Table 5.7).

Some observers, e.g. Matthews and Soothill (1970), have studied complement activation after milk challenge. Five children with gastrointestinal symptoms due to milk protein intolerance had evidence of complement activation after milk challenge with 5 ml of milk. Further studies of complement activity after milk challenge may

Table 5.7
Immunological investigations in children with cow's milk protein intolerance at Queen Hospital Hospital for Children. From Harrison *et. al.*, 1976

| | Skin Prick Tests | | | Serum Antibody Tests | |
	Milk	Casein	Lactalbumin	Cow's milk precipitins	Serum IgA below normal
Number tested	16	16	16	23	20
Number positive	13	9	10	12	8

provide a useful laboratory confirmation of the diagnosis of cow's milk allergy in addition to observation of the clinical response to milk challenge and the response of the small intestinal mucosa.

DIFFERENTIAL DIAGNOSIS

The most important differential diagnosis for cow's milk protein intolerance is to distinguish this condition from lactose malabsorption. Usually this is impossible at the time of initial presentation as both cow's milk protein intolerance and lactose intolerance may co-exist. In a classic paper, Liu, Tsao and Moore, in 1967, showed that challenge with cow's milk protein could produce intestinal malabsorption of lactose and fat in children who were intolerant to cow's milk protein. It is now clear that lactase deficiency with secondary lactose intolerance may be produced by cow's milk challenge in children who have cow's milk protein intolerance, particularly when this has occurred as a sequel to acute gastroenteritis. The secondary lactase deficiency is a consequence of mucosal damage produced by cow's milk protein, see figure 5.1 (Harrison, 1974; Harrison *et al.*, 1976).

While it may be impossible at the time of initial presentation to make the differential diagnosis, at the time of milk challenge it is practicable and important that the distinction should be made.

Visakorpi (1970) has described cow's milk protein intolerance as a transient accompaniment of coeliac disease, sometimes with intolerance symptoms preceding those of gluten intolerance. He and his co-workers have also described transient gluten intolerance accompanying temporary cow's milk intolerance. It is clear that cow's milk protein intolerance may also accompany other forms of dietary protein intolerance.

Treatment

The obvious treatment for this condition is to eliminate cow's milk from the child's diet and also all foods based on cow's milk. This latter point is most important as therapeutic failure is sometimes related to neglect of a restriction of foods such as ice-cream, which are based on cow's milk, despite strict adherence to avoidance of cow's milk itself.

Various milk substitutes such as soy protein based feedings and goat's milk have been recommended for these children. Goat's milk may not be suitable as often there is cross-reactivity between some goat's milk proteins and cow's milk protein fractions. Soy formulae such as Pro-Sobee or Velactin are usually satisfactory milk substitutes but some children are also intolerant to soy protein.

The need for such dietary restriction of milk ingestion is nearly always temporary, although there is little documentation concerning the precise duration of this intolerance. On clinical grounds, most children over two years of age, are apparently able to to tolerate milk without any untoward sequelae. The timing of a re-challenge with cow's milk is arbitrary and varies from paediatrician to paediatrician.

Cow's milk protein intolerance does occur in adult life. The best evidence for this is the observation by Gerrard *et al.* (1967) that 17 per cent of mothers of infants with milk allergy still had adverse reactions on challenge with milk. The relationship of this adult intolerance to the childhood malady described in this chapter is not clear. Equally, the presence or absence of a small intestinal enteropathy in such people is unknown.

SOY PROTEIN INTOLERANCE

A soy bean food prepared to resemble milk has been used in many countries since its first recommendation by Hill and Stuart in 1929 for infants with milk allergy. Glaser and Johnstone in 1953 suggested that soy bean milk when used as a substitute for cow's milk could play an important role in the prevention of allergy to cow's milk in those who were at risk.

Although it has been shown that soy bean has low antigenicity, over the past ten years there has been an increasing number of reports of intolerance to soy protein. Such reactions have varied from a dramatic anaphylactic response, to the onset of respiratory symptoms and to the appearance of gastrointestinal symptoms.

In 1972, Ament and Rubin clearly documented soy protein intolerance in an infant using challenge with soy protein and monitoring the clinical and small intestinal mucosal response to such challenges. Their report was unusual, as unlike other reports of a gastrointestinal reaction to soy milk, the reaction in their child occurred at the time of the first exposure to soy, not after multiple exposures. Challenge with soy protein in their infant, however, produced a flat small intestinal mucosa indistinguishable from that found in untreated coeliac disease. The lesion was reversible and serial biopsies revealed that it disappeared within four days of withdrawal of soy protein, only to recur on further challenge with soy protein. Varying degrees of small intestinal mucosal abnormality have been recognised by other workers in children with such intolerance.

TRANSIENT GLUTEN INTOLERANCE

Definition

Transient gluten intolerance may be defined as the syndrome seen when a child with gastrointestinal symptoms and an abnormal small intestinal mucosa responds to a gluten-free diet, but subsequently thrives on a normal gluten-containing diet and after two years on such a diet is found to have a normal mucosa.

Dicke in Holland, in 1952, described a transient wheat sensitivity in pre-school children after enteritis. Visakorpi and Immonen in Finland, in 1967, described a state of transient gluten intolerance in 28 children associated in some cases with temporary cow's milk protein intolerance, but their reports did not include serial small intestinal biopsies. In 1970, a child with transient gluten intolerance was described in Australia and this report included such biopsies (Walker-Smith, 1970). This child had an abnormal mucosa (a severe degree of partial villous atrophy) and he responded clinically to a gluten-free diet. After one year, while he was still having a gluten-free diet, a further biopsy revealed a normal mucosa. He was put back on a normal diet and 16 months later a further biopsy demonstrated a persistently normal mucosa. He has subsequently remained in excellent health.

Although a diagnosis of transient gluten intolerance was made in this child, retrospectively, more recent criteria lay down stricter requirements for this diagnosis. These are first, the need to provide evidence that gluten toxicity was in fact present and that the apparent response to gluten restriction was not fortuitous (McNeish, 1974), and second, the need to demonstrate the presence of a normal small intestinal mucosa two years or more after the return to a normal diet, as laid down by the European Society for Paediatric Gastroenterology in Interlaken in 1970 (Meeuwisse, 1970).

The precise criteria necessary to establish the existence of any form of transient intolerance to a dietary substance associated with small bowel mucosal abnormality have been outlined by McNeish (1974) and are indicated in diagrammatic form in Fig. 5.7.

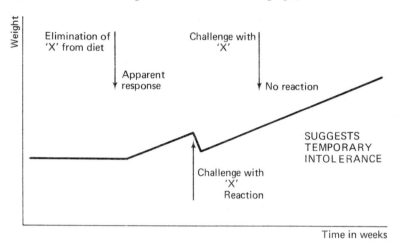

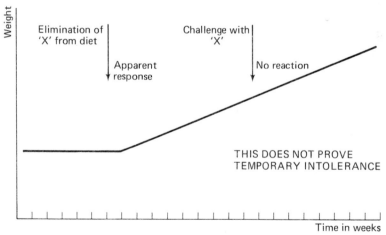

Fig. 5.7. Diagrammatic representation of diagnostic criteria for transient gluten intolerance. (Permission of McNeish, 1974.)

The McNeish criteria for the diagnosis of transient gluten intolerance thus requires objective evidence of gluten toxicity, which later disappears. McNeish et al. (1978), in fact, have demonstrated such early evidence of gluten toxicity by serial xylose absorption studies at the time of an early gluten challenge in an infant with an enteropathy who had previously responded to a gluten-free diet. Serial biopsies were not used to establish gluten toxicity at that time in their infant, but the mucosa has been shown to be normal two years after return to a normal gluten-containing diet. Now, at the Queen Elizabeth Hospital, a child has been observed who completely fulfils both the Interlaken and McNeish criteria for the diagnosis of transient gluten intolerance (Table 5.8). This child had an early gluten challenge at age

Table 5.8
Features of child with transient gluten intolerance

Age	Small intestinal biopsy grading	Diet	Intraepithelial lymphocyte count	Symptoms
6 mo.	+++	Gluten started 2½ mo. of age	51·8	Severe diarrhoea and vomiting
1 yr 2 mo.	N	Gluten-free	16·8	Symptom-free
1 yr 5 mo.	+++	Gluten 10 g powder daily for 3 mo.	48·2	Anorexia Irritability
4 yr 7 mo.	±	Gluten-free 3 years 2 mo.	21·7	Symptom-free
4 yr 10 mo.	±	Gluten 5 g in diet, daily for 3 mo.	35·0	Symptom-free
6 yr 9 mo.	N	Gluten 5–10 g in diet, daily for 2 years 2 mo.	25·9	Symptom-free

of 1 year 2 months, having previously had a flat mucosa and a clinical response to a gluten-free diet. She relapsed clinically and histologically with gluten. Subsequently, after a second challenge with gluten, she has remained clinically well and her mucosa two years three months after return to a normal gluten-containing diet has remained normal. It thus seems very probable that this child had transient gluten intolerance from which she has now recovered.

The time interval of two years to exclude coeliac disease after a return to a gluten-containing diet has been a matter of controversy since McNicholl *et al.* (1974) described two children who took more than two years to relapse after return to a normal gluten-containing diet. A survey by the European Society of Paediatric Gastroenterology and Nutrition suggested that others had a similar experience (Shmerling, 1978) but only one case has yet had clinical details published (Egan-Mitchell, Fottrell and McNicholl, 1978). In that case the intraepithelial lymphocyte count rose and disaccharidases fell before frank mucosal relapse. No case yet described, in which intra-epithelial lymphocyte counts and disaccharidase levels, as well as morphology, have remained normal two or more years after return to a normal gluten-containing diet, has relapsed. The author has never seen a child whose mucosa has been normal after this interval relapse, and is convinced that the child illustrated in Table 5.8 will not subsequently do so, but only time will tell.

Pathogenesis

Two explanations have been proposed to explain the development of this syndrome. Firstly, it has been suggested that there may be a temporary depression of dipeptidase activity occurring in the small intestinal mucosa, secondary to non-specific mucosal damage, such as may occur as a sequel to gastroenteritis. Such a suggestion at present is only speculative and is based on reports of this syndrome following clinical episodes of gastroenteritis where there has been the demonstration of an abnormal small intestinal mucosa on biopsy. Secondly, it is possible that a transient 'allergy' to gluten may occur in a similar and equally unknown manner to that suggested earlier in this chapter in relation to cow's milk protein, possibly secondary to mucosal damage. There is little evidence available so far to support either theory.

Pathology

The small intestinal mucosa is by definition abnormal, i.e. thickened ridged mucosa characterised by partial villous atrophy histologically or, sometimes, a flat mucosa. The demonstration of a flat mucosa should not ordinarily suggest this diagnosis, a flat mucosa being characteristic of coeliac disease. It seems probable that the mucosal abnormality may be less severe than that found in coeliac disease. Only long-term follow up with subsequent reinvestigation would allow the retrospective diagnosis of transient gluten intolerance to be made in a child with a flat mucosa who earlier has responded clinically to gluten withdrawal, but who is now thriving on a gluten-containing diet.

In the child referred to in Table 5.8 it is notable that there was an increase in the intra-epithelial lymphocyte count in the initial diagnostic biopsy, a fall in the count after a gluten-free diet, followed by a rise on mucosal relapse following a gluten challenge and, finally, a return to normal level which has remained normal on a gluten-containing diet. Thus, the intra-epithelial lymphocyte count in the mucosa of this child at the time when the child was gluten sensitive, appeared to be as responsive to gluten in the diet as does the mucosa of children with coeliac disease (i.e. permanent gluten intolerance).

Clinical Features

Transient gluten intolerance should be considered as part of the differential diagnosis of the infant who develops gastrointestinal symptoms when he first encounters wheat protein, especially when he appears to be intolerant to other food proteins such as milk and egg. It should also be considered as a possibility in a child who fails to thrive following gastroenteritis in the presence of an abnormal small intestinal mucosa and the absence of other explanations, such as secondary lactose intolerance, particularly when such an infant has not responded to several other dietary measures.

There appear to be two clinical syndromes associated with transient gluten intolerance; first, when gluten intolerance accompanies other forms of food intolerance, and secondly, when there is gluten intolerance alone (Walker-Smith, Kilby, and France, 1978; Nusslé *et al.*, 1978).

Diagnosis

As explained earlier, this is difficult to establish definitively. Once a child who has an abnormal small intestinal mucosa is started on a gluten-free diet and apparently responds clinically to such dietary restriction, the differential diagnosis lies between coeliac disease and transient gluten intolerance. All such children should be reinvestigated at a later interval in the manner outlined for the reinvestigation of children diagnosed as suffering from coeliac disease, by means of a gluten challenge and further small intestinal biopsies. If a child is shown subsequently to have a normal small intestinal mucosa two years after resumption of a normal diet containing gluten, and has earlier had a clinical response to gluten withdrawal, then the presumptive diagnosis, retrospectively, is transient gluten intolerance.

The biggest difficulty in making the diagnosis of transient gluten intolerance, however, and a factor of importance in making the diagnosis of coeliac disease itself, is the critical evaluation of a clinical response to a gluten-free diet. In some children it may be difficult to know whether an apparent clinical response, e.g. weight gain and relief of diarrhoea following dietary restriction of gluten, was directly attributable to gluten withdrawal. As an example of this difficulty, Fig. 5.8 illustrates the weight response of six aboriginal children seen at the Royal Alexandra Hospital and treated with a gluten-free diet.

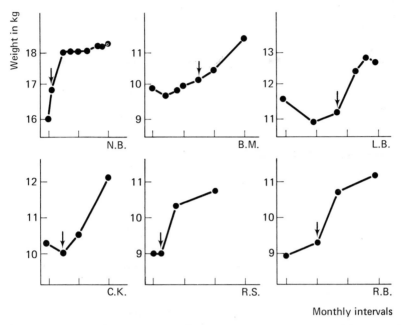

Fig. 5.8. Response of weight gain of six Australian aboriginal children to the withdrawal of gluten ($\downarrow$) from their diet.

Such a response could be due either to the response of a child previously having a low calorie diet, now being given an adequate diet, a spontaneous recovery, or a direct response to gluten withdrawal (Walker-Smith and Reye, 1971). Three of these children have subsequently thrived on a normal diet. Whether they were ever intolerant to gluten remains uncertain.

The timing of such reinvestigation and re-challenge with gluten is problematical and will vary from clinician to clinician. Early reinvestigation, a month or so after beginning treatment, may reveal evidence of persisting gluten intolerance and so does not necessarily indicate the diagnosis of coeliac disease. It is quite unknown how long transient gluten intolerance may last in these children. However, early reinvestigation and the demonstration of a relapse with gluten and the later demonstration of normal gluten tolerance as outlined in Fig. 5.7

is the only way to diagnose this condition definitively. Many clinicians may not feel that such early reinvestigation is justified. Indeed, the child referred to in Table 5.8 was exceptional, and it is not the author's ordinary custom to reinvestigate such children early, i.e. the diagnosis in clinical practice is usually presumptive, rather than definitive.

Reinvestigation Studies in Children with Probable Transient Gluten Intolerance

In a study of 65 children, originally diagnosed as having coeliac disease, at the Queen Elizabeth Hospital (*see* chapter 4), 15 proved on reinvestigation not to have coeliac disease (Walker-Smith, Kilby and France, 1978). Of these, 9 had a documented abnormal initial biopsy at the time of the original presentation on a normal gluten-containing diet.

These 9 children had an initial abnormal biopsy and responded clinically to a gluten-free diet, but despite this, they had a final biopsy which was normal or near normal, after two or more years on a gluten-containing diet, i.e. they do not appear on present evidence to have had coeliac disease. Figure 5.9 demonstrates the histological findings in one of these children.

Seven of these children had serial disaccharidase assay after start of challenge. On two occasions, disaccharidase activity fell despite normal morphology as reported in such children by McNicholl, Egan-Mitchel and Fottrell (1974).

In only one child has there tended to be a rise in intra-epithelial counts (IEL), which is shown in Table 5.9 related to disaccharidase activity; in view of the rise in IEL his last biopsy was graded as ±. At present he is absolutely well after 3 years 10 months on a normal gluten-containing diet. What is going to happen to this child and the others with a negative challenge? Will the two who had falling disaccharidases, and especially the one who also had a rise in his intraepithelial lymphocyte count after return to a normal diet, eventually relapse? Only time will tell, but it would seem highly unlikely that children with normal IEL and disaccharidases will relapse. Table 5.10 indicates the time over which these children have now been followed up and their present condition.

What was wrong with these 9 children originally? (Table 5.10). Their ages ranged from 8 weeks to 1 year 5 months at the time of the initial biopsy, i.e. all were less than two years of age at that time. A critical review of the early history in three children reveals evidence of

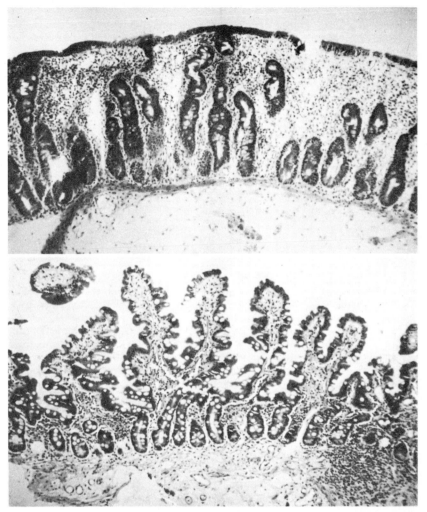

Fig. 5.9. Original diagnostic biopsy in a child aged 3 months. (Above) with non-coeliac enteropathy and presumed transient gluten intolerance. (Below) Mucosa two years two months after return to a normal gluten containing diet, aged 5 years 3 months.

a preceding episode of acute enteritis and evidence of other food intolerances, e.g. cow's milk protein intolerance, but in the remainder there was no such evidence and this group have been designated as non-coeliac enteropathy.

Within this group there were some children who met all the classical criteria for the initial diagnosis of coeliac disease as they had flat

Table 5.9
**Histological grading, lactase activity and intra-epithelial lymphocyte counts/100
epithelial cells (IEL) in serial biopsies from a child S.S. related to age and
gluten-containing (G) or gluten-free diet (GF)**

Patient	Age	Diet	Histology	Lactase	IEL
S.S.					
	3 mths.	G	++	0·5	81
	3 yr. 1 mo.	GF	N	—	31
	4½ yr.	G	N	8·1	32
	5 yr. 3 mo.	G	N	2·6	29
	7 yr. 4 mo.	G	±	3·3	48

Table 5.10
Nine children with negative gluten challenges

Patient	Age at initial biopsy	Sex	Histology	Duration of follow-up on normal diet	Final diagnosis
D.B.	8 wks.	M.	PVA	5 yr	Post-enteritis enteropathy
M.M.	10 wks.	M.	Flat	5 yr	Non-coeliac enteropathy
S.S.	3 mo.	M.	Flat	6 yr	Non-coeliac enteropathy
T.D.	4 mo.	F.	Flat	5 yr	Non-coeliac enteropathy
L.S.	4 mo.	F.	PVA	6 yr	Post-enteritis enteropathy
T.J.	5 mo.	M.	Flat	5 yr	Post-enteritis enteropathy
T.C.	10 mo.	F.	PVA	5 yr	Non-coeliac enteropathy
A.K.	1 yr.	M.	Flat	6 yr	Non-coeliac enteropathy
P.M.	1 yr. 5 mo.	F.	Flat	6 yr	Non-coeliac enteropathy

PVA = Partial Villous Atrophy

mucosa and evidence of malabsorption, and responded dramatically to
a gluten-free diet alone without any evidence of other food intolerances.
It is impossible now to convince the mothers of these children that a
gluten-free diet at that time did not account for their clinical
improvement. Figure 5.10 shows the weight progress over the years of
one of these children. What was wrong with this boy originally? It is
probable that he had transient gluten intolerance from which he has
recovered. Although McNeish's strict criteria for transient gluten
intolerance in this boy, or in the other eight children in this study,
have not been fulfilled; nonetheless, the original diagnosis of transient
gluten intolerance is presumptive.

Nusslé et al. (1978) have described a similar group of 6 children,
initially diagnosed as having coeliac disease, who have had a normal
small intestinal mucosa 2½ to 4½ years after reintroduction of gluten to

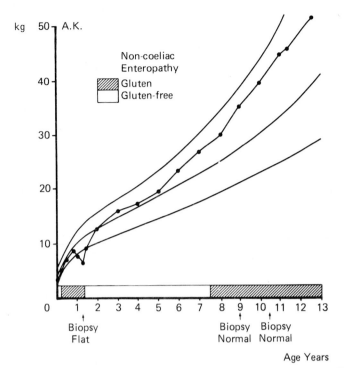

Fig. 5.10. Serial weight measurements related to dietary gluten and small intestinal biopsies in a child with non-coeliac enteropathy and presumed transient gluten intolerance.

their diet. All had normal IEL, and all except one normal disaccharidases. Thus, again, these children appear to have had transient gluten intolerance from which they have recovered. Schmitz, Jos and Rey (1978), from Paris, in a very important paper have described three children who had earlier responded to a gluten-free diet but who then developed flat mucosae on a gluten-containing diet at the ages of 10 years, $6\frac{1}{2}$ years and 4 years 8 months respectively. However, they did not return to a gluten-free diet but continued on a gluten-containing diet. Further biopsies after more than 9 years, 12 years and 5 years respectively on a normal gluten containing diet, showed surprisingly normal or near normal mucosae. The third case was having a low gluten intake but had relapsed earlier on a similar low gluten diet. Thus, these three children appear to have recovered spontaneously on a gluten-containing diet. The author would regard this as good evidence that all three had had transient gluten intolerance from which they had recovered, but Schmitz, Jos and Rey raise the possibility that the mucosal lesion of coeliac disease may disappear during adolescence only to reappear in adulthood. Further prospective studies will establish whether this is so. There is thus a particular need for detailed and long-term follow-up into adult life of these children with apparent non-coeliac enteropathy.

Thus, at the most, a clinical response to a gluten-free diet, may be taken as indirect evidence only of gluten intolerance.

Management

The dietary management is identical with that prescribed for children with coeliac disease but the need for such dietary restriction is, of course, by definition, a temporary one. The duration of the need for such dietary restriction will vary from child to child.

It is clear that at present this is a confusing field and in need of much clarification. It has been discussed here at some length, not because of the intrinsic importance of transient gluten intolerance itself, but rather because of the importance of distinguishing the condition from coeliac disease.

Finally, it is most important that those children diagnosed as non-coeliac enteropathy, who were also, in all probability, transiently gluten intolerant, but who have completely recovered, should have long-term follow-up. It is possible that these children could eventually relapse. It is the author's practice to follow-up such children throughout their childhood and then refer them to adult gastroenterologists for indefinite follow-up.

6

Gastroenteritis

Acute gastroenteritis is a common diagnosis in paediatric practice. It is a clinical diagnosis and in many cases in Western countries at the present time no aetiological agent is identified. Its commonest symptoms are acute vomiting and diarrhoea, which are such frequent symptoms in infancy that children having them may incorrectly be labelled as suffering from acute gastroenteritis without any real justification. It is thus important to define what is meant by acute gastroenteritis, although it must be appreciated that in the clinical situation it may be difficult at times to be certain of the diagnosis.

DEFINITION

Acute gastroenteritis is the clinical syndrome of diarrhoea and/or vomiting of acute onset, often accompanied by fever and constitutional disturbance which is of infective origin and not secondary to some primary disease process outside the alimentary tract.

AETIOLOGY

No bacterial pathogen can be isolated from the stools of the majority of children with gastroenteritis who are admitted to hospital in a developed country, but in developing countries over 50 per cent of children may have bacterial isolations.

Table 6.1 indicates the percentage bacterial isolation from the stools of children with gastroenteritis admitted to children's hospitals in Britain, Australia and Indonesia.

The percentage isolation of enteropathogenic *Escherichia coli* is far higher in the Indonesian series than the British or Australian reports,

Table 6.1
Bacterial isolation in gastroenteritis

	Britain (London)	Australia (Sydney)	Indonesia (Bandung)	Britain (London)
Author	Gribbin et al. (1975)	Dorman (1968)	Suprapti et al. (1968)	Walker-Smith (1977)
No. of children	472	828	466	530
% isolation				
Salmonella	1·9	12	2·4	2·2
Shigella	1·5	6	11·2	3·4
Enteropathogenic E. coli	11·6	7·5	32·2	6·4
Cholera El Tor	—	—	0·9	—

while the percentage isolation of salmonella is higher in the Australian series than in the British or Indonesian reports.

The high percentage of bacterial isolation in the Indonesian series is related to the prevalence of malnutrition and poor hygiene in the community. This is well illustrated by the observations of Gracey (1973) in young malnourished aboriginals with acute diarrhoea in Australia, where there is a similar prevalence of malnutrition and poor hygiene. He found that from a group of 251 such patients, 47 excreted a serotype of enteropathogenic *E. coli*, 17 a species of salmonella and 25 a shigella. A similar high isolated rate of bacterial pathogens in another developing community, was reported by Maiya et al. (1976) who found recognised bacterial pathogens in the stools of 66 per cent of a group of children under two years of age with acute gastroenteritis in Southern India, who were observed over a twelve-month period.

Infection with individual bacterial pathogens will be discussed in more detail later, but the mere isolation of a known bacterial pathogen from the stool of a child with acute gastroenteritis does not establish that it is the causative agent of the syndrome. Feldman, Bhat and Kamath (1970) in South India have shown a dissociation between the pattern of clinical illness and the pattern of isolation of bacterial pathogens in an impressive epidemiological survey of pre-school Indian children. However, such isolation does provide good presumptive evidence of a cause and effect relationship at the time of an outbreak of infective diarrhoea when other children are found to excrete the same pathogen, but care has to be taken when interpreting the significance of the results of stool culture taken from an individual child with acute diarrhoea and vomiting.

There are important differences in the manner in which these bacterial pathogens may produce their toxic effects. Salmonellae penetrate the mucosa relatively deeply but do not produce an enterotoxin whereas *Shigella shiga* produces a powerful enterotoxin which may cause ileal hypersecretion, almost to the same degree as that which occurs in cholera. It is believed that it is this penetration or invasion of the mucosa by salmonellae, and some strains of enteropathogenic *E. coli* and most shigellae, that permits the endotoxin they produce to exert its toxic effect.

Thus, salmonellae, shigellae and some strains of *E. coli* may invade the intestinal epithelial cell and multiply within the mucosa. Animal studies have greatly helped our understanding of the pathogenetic mechanisms involved. Formal *et al.* (1976) have shown that in both salmonellosis and shigellosis bacterial invasion of the colonic mucosa does occur. This is associated with acute inflammatory reaction and mucosal damage and, in turn, there is abnormal colonic salt and water transport. In the animals studied they have also found that the jejunum is in a net secretory state despite the absence of bacterial invasion or morphological abnormalities in the jejunum. They suggest, therefore, that in these circumstances the diarrhoea produced by invasive organisms results from the inability of the colon to reabsorb the increased volume of fluid entering the colon from the small intestine.

Enterotoxins are synthesised within the bacterial cell body and are elaborated into broth cultures containing intact bacteria, whereas endotoxins are associated with the bacterial cell wall and so are not found in broths unless there is damage or destruction of the bacteria. Enterotoxins have classically been shown to be produced by *Vibrio cholerae* but also by some strains of *E. coli* and food poisoning strains of *Staphylococcus aureus* and *Clostridium perfringens* as well as *Shigella shiga*.

One of the most fascinating observations in this field in recent years has been the demonstration that cholera enterotoxin produces its hypersecretory effect via 3′–5′ adenosine monophosphate (cyclic AMP). Field (1971) and others have shown that cholera enterotoxin increases intestinal levels of cyclic AMP. It also has been shown to activate adenyl cyclase, the enzyme that converts adenosine triphosphate (ATP) into cyclic AMP. It is this activation of adenyl cyclase which is believed to account for the fluid hypersecretion by the gut.

Invasive enteropathogens such as salmonellae as well as enterotoxin-producing bacteria like *Vibrio cholerae* can produce elevated levels of adenylate cyclase activity. This could result from stimulation by prostaglandins synthesised locally. Indomethacin, a potent inhibitor of prostaglandin synthesis, has been shown in the experimental animal to abolish adenylate cyclase activation and fluid secretion induced by *Sal. typhimurium* (Gianella *et al.*, 1975).

So, to summarise, two mechanisms have been recognised whereby bacterial pathogens may produce the syndromes of acute gastroenteritis. These are toxin production and mucosal invasion. The particular organisms may thus be designated toxigenic or invasive.

Sometimes bacteria not ordinarily regarded as pathogens may be associated with outbreaks of diarrhoea. These include *Pseudomonas aeruginosa*, especially in premature infants, and some strains of klebsiella. Two bacterial pathogens, not previously known to be aetiological agents for acute gastroenteritis have now been identified. These are *Yersinia enterocolitica* and *Campylobacter* (Vantrappen *et al.*, 1977; Tauwers, De Boeck and Butzler, 1978).

The role of viruses in the remaining children with acute gastroenteritis who did not have a bacterial pathogen in their stool had until 1973 been uncertain. Several epidemiological studies were made in the USA and Canada where echoviruses were found more often in infants with diarrhoea than in controls. Similarly, culture of adenoviruses were reported both from North America and Europe but other workers considered that adenoviruses and enteroviruses were unlikely to be significant causes of uncomplicated diarrhoeal disease. In support of this view a virological survey of stools and throat swabs from 639 children admitted to the gastroenteritis unit at the Royal Alexandra Hospital in 1970 produced a positive viral culture in only 21 children. The positive cultures revealed no consistent pattern, Echo, Coxsackie, adeno and influenza viruses being randomly isolated. Thus, it seemed unlikely that any of these viruses played a major role in the causation of gastroenteritis of unknown aetiology.

However, exciting new work was reported from the United States by Blacklow and his colleagues (1972) who studied an outbreak of winter vomiting disease among adults in Norwalk, Ohio. They found that bacteria-free stool filtrates derived from infected people during this outbreak led to acute vomiting and diarrhoea when administered to human volunteers. The infectious agent in this outbreak has come to be known as the Norwalk agent. Its general properties suggest that it may belong to the parvovirus group. Paver and his colleagues (1973) in Bristol have also found a small virus resembling parvoviruses in the stools of adults with gastroenteritis using an immunological electron microscope technique.

Bishop and her colleagues (1973) from Melbourne using the

electron microscope found virus particles in the epithelial cells of duodenal mucosa obtained on small intestinal biopsy from 6 out of 9 children with gastroenteritis. The morphology of the virus bore a resemblance to an orbivirus rather than a parvovirus and, interestingly, had a pronounced morphological similarity to the viruses causing epizootic diarrhoea of infant mice. The virus particles were found more readily in small intestinal biopsies obtained early after the onset of symptoms in these infants and less readily in those who had a longer history at the time of biopsy.

Bishop and her colleagues in Melbourne (1974) went on to use electron microscopy of negatively-stained faecal extracts to reveal particles that resemble orbiviruses in 11 out of 14 children aged less than three years who had acute non-bacterial gastroenteritis. Independently, in Birmingham, Flewett and his colleagues (1973) using diagnostic electron microscopy of the faeces described identical virus particles, which they called rotavirus. Reports of similar particles in the stools of children came rapidly from the United States, Canada, Singapore, Rhodesia and India.

This technique for examining stools with the electron microscope for the presence of virus particles has now been widely applied in the investigation of diarrhoeal states in children with gastroenteritis, and a number of viruses have been recognised by their morphological appearance. These are listed in Table 6.2.

Table 6.2
Viruses identifiable in stools by electron microscopy in acute gastroenteritis in children and adults

	Diameter nanometres (nm)
Rotavirus (family Reoviridae)	65–70
Adenovirus (family Adenoviridae)	70
Coronavirus (family Coronaviridae)	c. 150
Small viral particles	
Calici virus (family Picornaviridae)	30
Astro virus (unclassified)	30
Enterovirus (family Picornaviridae)	28
includes poliomyelitis, Coxsackie, ECHO	
Norwalk agent	28*
Hawaii agent	28*
Montgomery County agent	28*

* Morphologically identical.

Most interest has centred on the demonstration of the virus particle originally described as the orbi virus (Fig. 6.1). It has subsequently been described not only as the rotavirus but as the duovirus, the reovirus-like agent (RLA) the human reovirus-like agent (HRVLA) and the infantile gastroenteritis virus (IGV). It seems probable that the term rotavirus will become generally accepted.

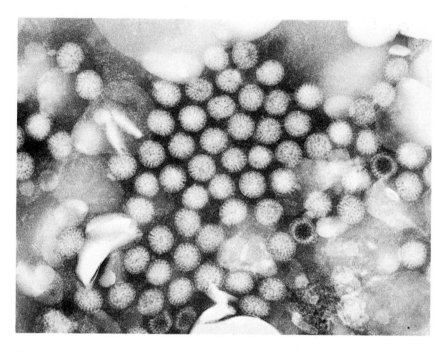

Fig. 6.1. Rotavirus particles in stool demonstrated by electron-microscopy × 198,000. (Permission of Phillips.)

These viruses have been detected in about 60 per cent of some series of children with acute gastroenteritis. At the Queen Elizabeth Hospital, in two studies, rotavirus was found in 30 and 28 per cent respectively of stools examined from children with non-bacterial gastroenteritis (Shepherd et al., 1975; Walker-Smith, 1978).

This human virus has been very difficult to isolate in tissue culture but Banatvala and colleagues, in 1975, showed that the virus would infect cells if the inoculum and cell monolayer were centrifuged together at 2,000 to 4,000 rev/minute. Until viruses identified in the stools can be conveniently cultured there will be some element of doubt concerning their aetiological significance, but the observation that rotavirus is found in small intestinal mucosa, duodenal juice and stools provides firm evidence for regarding it as a pathogen. Flewett (1976) remarked 'their guilt by association makes the identification of these virus particles in the stool a highly significant finding', and this represents a major breakthrough in our understanding of the aetiology of acute gastroenteritis in infancy and childhood. The precise criteria for the pathogenicity of rotavirus are discussed later (page 202).

An enzyme-linked immunosorbent assay (ELISA) has been developed for the detection of rotavirus in human stools. Yolken *et al.* (1977) found this technique to be as sensitive as electron microscopy or radioimmunoassay. They recommend its use as being simpler and requiring less sophisticated equipment. However, the technique is specific for rotavirus. Stool electron microscopy has the virtue of allowing the presence of other virus particles to be detected. Some of these will be discussed briefly.

Adenoviruses may be found in the stools of children with acute diarrhoea (Fig. 6.2) and may be present in large numbers even though

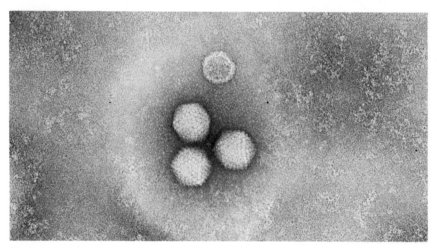

Fig. 6.2. Adenovirus particles in stool demonstrated by electron-microscopy × 626,000. (Permission of Bird.)

the adenovirus is not often cultured from tissue culture of these stools. The evidence that these adenoviruses are in fact pathogenic in these circumstances is again based on 'guilt by association' (Flewett 1976), but as earlier workers in this field established, adenoviruses may be found in the stools of apparently well controls, whereas in children outside the neonatal period rotaviruses may be found only in the stools of children with gastroenteritis.

Coronaviruses, which are known to be causes of acute gastroenteritis in piglets and calves, have also been found in stools from young adults (Caul *et al.*, 1975) as well as from children with acute diarrhoea (Fig. 6.3).

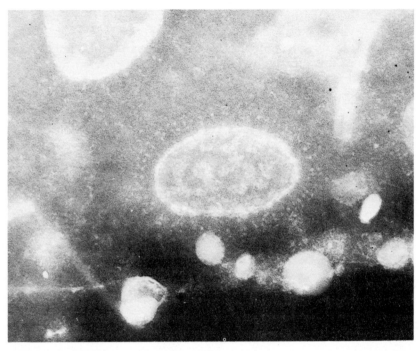

Fig. 6.3. Coronavirus particle in stool demonstrated by electron-microscopy × 203,200. (Permission of Phillips.)

Another small virus particle found on electron microscopy of stools of children with gastroenteritis (Fig. 6.4) has been designated the astrovirus because of its star-like appearance (Madeley and Cosgrove, 1975); it is 30 nm in diameter. Kurtz, Lee and Pickering (1977) have described an outbreak of gastroenteritis in a paediatric ward in which 17 of 27 symptomatic children, and 4 of 14 members of the staff with diarrhoea had this virus particle in the stool. In 7 excretors, other viral or bacterial pathogens were found.

Another small virus particle that has been identified is the calici virus, as well as several small-sized enteroviruses ranging from

20–30 nm, variously classified as parvo-like, picorna or picodna viruses.

In 142 consecutive stool electron-microscopy examinations, Phillips (1978) found the viruses listed in Table 6.3.

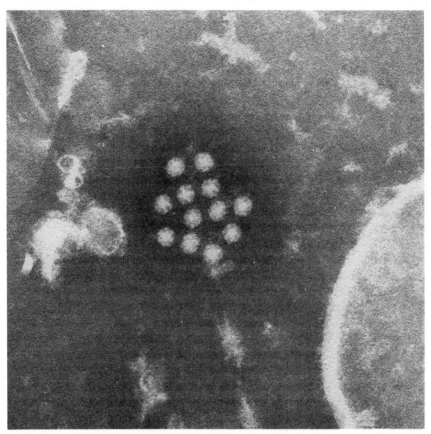

Fig. 6.4. Astrovirus particles in stool demonstrated by electron-microscopy × 175,000. (Permission of Phillips.)

Two other agents similar to the Norwalk agent have now also been implicated aetiologically and have been named the Hawaii and Montgomery County (MC) agents after the locations of epidemics of gastroenteritis where they were first identified. Infectious filtrates containing the Norwalk, Hawaii and MC agents all contain morphologically indistinguishable viral particles which are 26 to 29 nm in diameter. Despite this morphological similarity, these agents seem to be distinct, since infection with one agent does not appear to confer immunity against infection from another of them. These parvovirus-like agents appear to be primarily responsible for disease in adults and older children rather than infants, although parvo-like virus particles have sometimes been found in enormous numbers in the stools of children with acute gastroenteritis, often at the same time as adenoviruses.

Table 6.3
Results of electron microscopy of stools for viruses in children with acute gastroenteritis at Queen Elizabeth Hospital—permission Phillips

1st February–1st June, 1978			
No virus	92	64·8%	
Rotavirus	31	21·9%	
Rotavirus + Astrovirus	3	2·1%	26·1%
Rotavirus + Adenovirus	3	2·1%	
Adenovirus	6	4·2%	
Corona virus	1	0·7%	
Astrovirus	1	0·7%	
Parvovirus	2	1·4%	
Calici virus	1	0·7%	4·2%
Picorna virus	2	1·4%	
Total	142		

Indeed, it is now clear that several different viruses may be found at the same time in the stools of children with gastroenteritis. Furthermore, a bacterial pathogen may also be present, and there is some evidence that when viruses and bacterial pathogens appear together, clinically more severe disease results. It is often difficult to determine which potential aetiological agent is of pathogenetic significance, just as in the past it has been shown in the developing world that the mere identification of a stool bacterial pathogen does not establish it as a cause of the child's clinical symptoms (see page 172).

While discussing the possible viral aetiology of gastroenteritis, it is important to recall that acute diarrhoea may accompany a number of viral illnesses. In developing communities, where measles is often a severe illness and a common problem, acute diarrhoea is a frequent manifestation of the malady. In developed communities, diarrhoea is usually a less important manifestation of measles but there are occasional children in whom severe diarrhoea accompanies measles.

Gilles, Monif and Hood (1970) reported post-mortem findings in a child who developed severe diarrhoea with measles, followed by sudden death. The ileocolitis diagnosed on histopathological section was attributed to the measles virus.

In adults, Sheehy, Artenstein and Green (1964) have studied small intestinal mucosal morphology using biopsy in a variety of viral illnesses and they have found a significant incidence of abnormal findings in a number of viral illnesses including infectious hepatitis and measles.

PATHOLOGY

The small intestine is the organ principally affected in most children by gastroenteritis but the stomach and colon may also be involved to a varying extent. Barnes (1973), in a study of 21 children with non-bacterial gastroenteritis, found evidence of inflammation in stomach, duodenum and rectum of some children, indicating that the disease may affect the whole gastrointestinal tract. In particular, in 15 of 21 biopsies there was some inflammation of the stomach.

This variable distribution of the site of pathology along the gastrointestinal tract has important functional significance. The area of bowel principally affected may influence the composition of diarrhoeal fluid, e.g. the considerable bicarbonate losses resulting from small intestinal damage will be reduced if there is no colonic involvement and the reabsorptive capacity of the colon remains intact. Indeed acute infectious diarrhoeas may produce, in the rectal mucosa, changes that are virtually indistinguishable from the appearance of colitis found in chronic inflammatory bowel disease. Granulomata with giant cells have been described in some adults with salmonellosis (McClelland and Gilmour, 1976).

In the past, based on autopsy studies, the pathological findings in children with gastroenteritis have been regarded as non-specific and inconsistent. Giles, Sangster and Smith (1949) described, at post mortem, the pathological features in 49 fatal cases in a childhood epidemic of gastroenteritis. There was mild hyperaemia of the small intestine in 28, submucosal haemorrhages in 13, ulceration of the mucosa in 4, and the small bowel was normal in 4 children.

The rapid autolysis of the surface epithelium of the small intestine, which occurs very soon after death, has in the past greatly hindered critical evaluation of the state of the small intestinal mucosa in children dying from gastroenteritis. In fact, much may be learned from post-mortem studies of the small intestine taken from children who have died following acute gastroenteritis. This is because of the discovery by Creamer and Leppard in 1965 that, although autolysis of the surface epithelium at death is rapid, autolysis of the basement membrane and lamina propria is delayed. By taking advantage of this fact they were able to study the three-dimensional morphology of the small intestine closely along its whole length with a dissecting microscope, once the surface epithelium had sloughed off.

Details of this technique are discussed in chapter 3. Ten children who died as a consequence of what proved at autopsy to be enteritis or enterocolitis were studied in this way at the Royal Alexandra Hospital. Death in each case followed the clinical syndrome of acute gastroenteritis after varying intervals. In some children this syndrome accompanied other disease processes, e.g. acute leukaemia, but in others, it was the only disease present. Table 6.4 lists the age at death of these 10 children, the diagnosis and the appearances seen under the dissecting microscope in the duodenum, the jejunum, 50 cm distal to the duodeno-jejunal flexure, and the ileum, 50 cm proximal to the ileo-caecal valve. The dominant appearance is listed first and any other morphological variant also observed is listed below, roughly quantitated + to +++.

The presence of short thick ridges (*see* Fig. 3.28) or a flat mucosa was considered abnormal, as these appearances have been shown to correspond histologically to partial villous atrophy or subtotal villous atrophy, respectively. Long thin ridges, tongues, leaves and fingers were regarded as normal variants.

This study showed that the dissecting microscope appearances within the area surveyed, particularly proximally, showed a variable morphology. When mucosal abnormality was present this was also of variable severity, i.e. the lesion was patchy. In addition, there was a variable pattern of distribution of the mucosal abnormality along the small intestine. In the majority of children the mucosa was most abnormal in the proximal small intestine but in two children the whole length of the small intestine was equally abnormal and in one child the ileum was chiefly affected. The mucosal abnormality occurred more commonly in the children under six months of age and the most extensive lesions observed, i.e. involving the whole length of the small intestine, occurred in two of the infants under six months.

Figures 6.5, 6.6 and 6.7, illustrate diagrammatically the distribution of the dominant mucosal appearances along the length of the

Table 6.4
Findings in children with enteritis

Child	Sex	Age	Diagnosis	Duodenum	Jejunum	Ileum	Ulcers
E.M.	M	3 wk	Enteritis Bronchopneumonia	STR TR++	STR TR++	STR	Whole small intestine
F.O.	F	3 wk	Enteritis Adrenal haemorrhage	TR T++	T	F	—
K.F.	F	6 wk	Enterocolitis Chronic pancreatitis Septicaemia Sugar malabsorption	STR Flat+	STR Flat+	STR T+	Chiefly terminal ileum
B.W.	M	2 m	Enterocolitis Pseudomonas and Candida albicans	TR STR++	T TR++	STR	Terminal ileum
R.S.	M	7 m	Congenital heart disease Enterocolitis	NE	STR	T STR+	—
J.P.	F	9 m	Enteritis	STR+++ TR+++	T STR++ TR+	T L++	—
R.O.	M	1 y 4 m	Enteritis Pulmonary haemorrhage	STR	STR	L	—
J.C.	M	1 y 5 m	Enteritis Pulmonary oedema	STR TR++	TR	T	—
R.C.	M	5 y	Acute leukaemia Enteritis probably due to Cl. welchii	F L++	F	F	—
M.R.	F	10 y 4 m	Mongolism Diabetes Pancreatic atrophy Enteritis	T	F	F	—

STR = Short Thick Ridges. TR = Thin Ridges. T = Tongues. L = Leaves.
NE = Not Examined. F = Fingers.

small intestine, showing the three patterns, and contrasting them with the morphological findings in a child dying from a nongastro-enterological cause (*see* Fig. 3.14). Histologically, all children had enteritis with an infiltration of inflammatory cells in the lamina propria, but the three-dimensional morphology ranged in appearance from fingers to a flat mucosa. The flat mucosa when sectioned

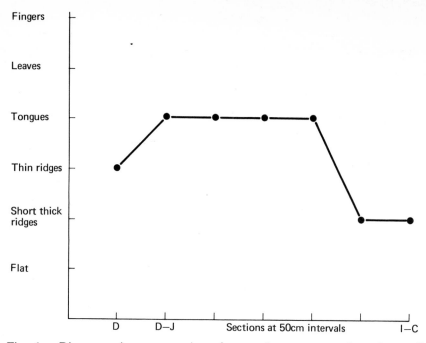

Fig. 6.5. Diagrammatic representation of mucosal appearances along the small intestine in a child dying from gastroenteritis.

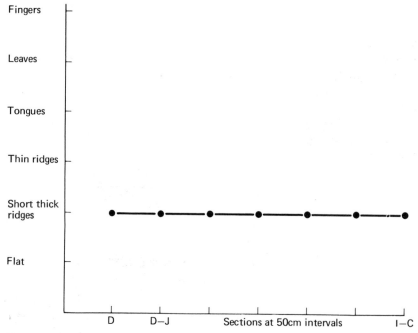

Fig. 6.6. Diagrammatic representation of mucosal appearances along the small intestine in a child dying from gastroenteritis.

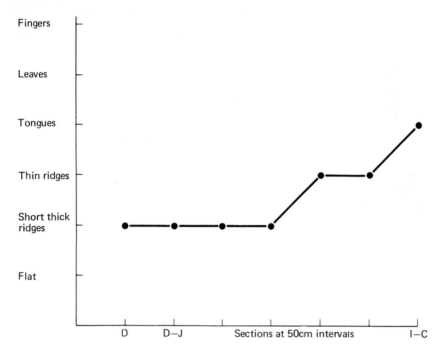

Fig. 6.7. Diagrammatic representation of mucosal appearances along the small intestine in a child dying from gastroenteritis.

histologically (Fig. 6.8) had an appearance identical with that seen in children with coeliac disease.

In these children the most abnormal appearances tended to occur on the tops of the mucosal folds (plicae circulares) or on the edges of mucosal ulcers. In between the mucosal folds the mucosa was less severely abnormal and this difference in morphology between the top of the folds and the valleys between, is shown in Fig. 6.9.

In some children inflammatory ulcers were seen with varying patterns of distribution along the small intestine.

From this study it may be concluded: first, that the mucosal damage that occurs as a consequence of gastroenteritis is of variable severity in the proximal small intestine, i.e. it is a patchy lesion; second, that the pattern of distribution of this mucosal abnormality along the small intestine is very variable, and thirdly, that ulceration of the small intestine is relatively common.

It may be inferred that a single proximal small intestinal mucosal biopsy could not be interpreted as reflecting the state of the whole small intestinal mucosa along its length, nor may it reflect accurately

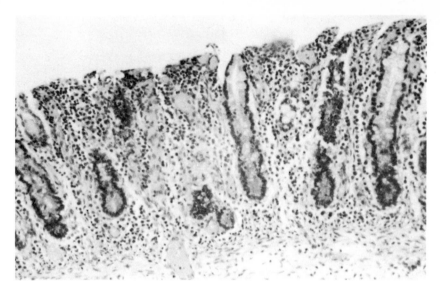

Fig. 6.8. Flat mucosa from a child dying from gastroenteritis.

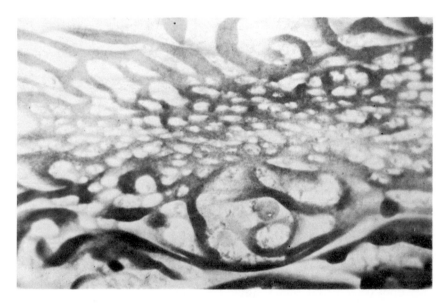

Fig. 6.9. Dissecting microscope appearances showing flat mucosa on top of mucosal folds with ridges on the side of the folds.

even the overall state of the mucosa in the region of the small intestine biopsied in these children.

These observations raise difficulties in interpretation of both single and serial biopsies. It is possible, however, that proximal biopsies are taken most often from the more accessible exposed tops of mucosal folds rather than the more inaccessible valleys in between. Serial biopsies may thus tend to be taken from roughly the same area, but this is pure speculation. This study does suggest that multiple biopsies would reflect more accurately than single biopsies the true state of the small intestinal mucosa.

Barnes and Townley (1973) used single small intestinal biopsies to investigate the state of the duodenal mucosa in 31 infants with acute gastroenteritis. Their study confirmed the observations that a mucosal lesion similar to that seen in coeliac disease may occur in children who have gastroenteritis, as 5 of these infants had such a lesion on biopsy. Only 5 infants had normal small intestinal biopsies, and in the remaining infants mild (11) or moderate, (10) mucosal abnormality was present. In 3 patients, serial biopsies after three days, eight days and seven weeks showed significant improvement.

Schrieber, Blacklow and Trier (1973) in the USA have studied the effect of oral administration of a stool filtrate containing the Norwalk agent upon the small intestinal mucosa in 15 adult volunteers. All the volunteers had normal baseline small intestinal biopsies; 12 developed clinical gastroenteritis and an abnormal small intestinal mucosa with villous shortening, crypt hypertrophy and mucosal inflammation. One of the three asymptomatic volunteers also developed mucosal abnormality. Biopsies six to eight weeks later were normal. These authors used a multiple biopsy technique. In some cases, when two simultaneous biopsies were taken, the severity of the mucosal abnormality varied and it was concluded that the mucosal lesion involving the proximal small intestine could be patchy, thus supporting the observations made in the above childhood autopsy study.

They postulated that the Norwalk agent initially damages the villous absorptive cell, causing acute inflammation. Then, probably as a compensation, the crypt hypertrophy and epithelial cell proliferation occurs to replace the damaged enterocytes.

MORTALITY

Before the development of modern methods of preventive medicine and of intravenous therapy, gastroenteritis had a high mortality in the

Western world (Fig. 6.10). This has been substantially reduced, but in developing countries, as Kretchmer (1969) has pointed out, a child under the age of seven years still has a 50 per cent chance of dying from a diarrhoeal disease.

It has been estimated that during 1975, there were between 5 and 18 million deaths attributed to diarrhoea. Gastroenteritis thus remains a factor of the greatest importance in the continuance of a high death rate in infancy and early childhood in many developing communities (Rohde and Northrup, 1976).

Spencer and Coster in Johannesburg (1969) have shown a striking fall in mortality rate from gastroenteritis in African children, in the age group 0–11 months, during the ten year period 1956–1966. They attributed this improvement more to betterment of socio-economic and environmental circumstances than to improved medical services and therapeutic techniques. However, such improvements do not lead to a disappearance of gastroenteritis from the community but may in fact alter its aetiology and, also, its clinical severity.

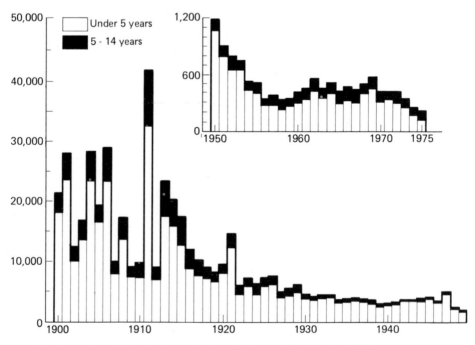

Fig. 6.10. Annual deaths from diarrhoeal disease in England and Wales 1900–1975.

In Sydney, in 1970, at the Royal Alexandra Hospital, there were six deaths from gastroenteritis out of 610 public admissions to the gastroenteritis unit, i.e. a mortality of 0·9 per cent. In England and Wales, in 1970, 411 children under fifteen years of age were reported to have died from this disorder. A Department of Health and Social Security survey in the United Kingdom of three health areas for three years (1964–1967) revealed 679 post-natal deaths of infants aged one month to one year, 77 (11 per cent) of these were from gastroenteritis. The mortality rate for children admitted with acute gastroenteritis to the Queen Elizabeth Hospital in 1973, was 0·6 per cent (Gribbin, Walker-Smith and Wood, 1976). Thus, gastroenteritis continues to have a significant mortality in developed countries such as Australia and Britain (Fig. 6.10).

The Department of Health and Social Security survey indicated that some of the deaths were sudden and unexpected. Sometimes infants who were. apparently making good progress under treatment collapsed and died. In other infants the onset of the illness was sudden and its course so fulminant that, even though they were brought quickly to hospital, they were moribund on admission. In only 11 of 77 deaths was it clear that progressive deterioration over a period of days had occurred at home. In some of these earlier cases specialist aid may have reduced the mortality but, in general, the unpredictability of the severity of this disorder in Britain makes it hard to design measures to further reduce its mortality.

SUSCEPTIBILITY TO GASTROENTERITIS

Children under the age of two years are more susceptible to this infection than older children in whom infection is not common except in outbreaks within a family or institution. Malnourished children also have a greater susceptibility than normal children.

It has long been known that breast feeding reduces the chance of an infant developing gastroenteritis but it does not abolish such a risk entirely, as documented by Kingston (1973) in West Africa. It is true, however, that gastroenteritis is uncommon in infants who are exclusively breast fed. Various reasons for this have been put forward, several of which have already been mentioned in chapter 1 (see page 24).

There has been discussion concerning the relative importance of specific and non-specific antimicrobial factors transferred in breast milk to the infant's gut. It seems probable that both are important

(Soothill, 1976). Specifically the IgA and lactoferrin content of breast milk (Bullen and Willis, 1971) are of particular importance for protection against enteropathogenic strains of *E. coli*. Robinson, Harvey and Soothill (1978) have also shown that macrophages and neutrophils from human milk phagocytose and kill *E. coli in vitro* after opsonisation by the aqueous phase of milk. This is likely to be an important protective mechanism *in vivo*.

The protective role breast-milk affords the suckling infant against the hazards of enteropathogenic *E. coli* enteritis have been dramatically demonstrated by Stoliar *et al*. (1976). These workers took colostrum from Guatemalan mothers 2 to 4 days post-partum and breast milk from both Guatemalan and North American mothers and found that both their milks inhibited the fluid accumulation in rabbit ileal loops that was induced when the loops were incubated with both *E. coli* enterotoxin and cholera enterotoxin. Furthermore, it was shown that the antitoxin activity of the mothers' milk correlated with its IgA content but not its IgG or IgM content. This provides vivid and clear evidence of the protective role breast feeding may provide.

It has, however, already been made clear that the protection breast feeding gives against gastroenteritis is not complete. Protection is diminished when the infant is being weaned onto solid food or cow's milk, i.e. when the baby is not exclusively breast fed. The risk is obviously far greater when these weaning foods are heavily bacterially contaminated. The problem posed by this in the developing world has been highlighted by Rowland, Barnell and Whitehead (1978) who have pointed out that traditional weaning foods used for young infants in West Africa can be hazardous bacteriologically. Thus, providing a breast-fed infant with such supplements under the prevailing conditions in the developing world may be dangerous. Indeed, because of such weaning practices with bacteriologically contaminated food, infantile infective diarrhoea can continue to be very common in a community, despite breast feeding. Commercial baby milks and feeding bottles in such an environment can also carry similar risk. In such traditional societies, however, infants remain relatively free from gastrointestinal disorders so long as they are exclusively breast fed.

Hence, the infant in the developing world is most at risk during the transition from breast feeding to a full diet. In such communities, all foods babies ingest, except breast milk, must be regarded as being highly contaminated potentially, and so a cause of weanling's diarrhoea. Jelliffe and Jelliffe (1978) suggest that the situation can be helped if attempts are made to improve lactation in mothers by improving their nutrition, by persuading parents to delay introducing weaning foods to babies until the age of 4 to 6 months, by making the weaning foods more nutritious, and by using easy-to-clean plastic or metal feeding containers avoiding contamination.

PREVALENCE AND SEASONAL VARIATION

The peak prevalence of gastroenteritis in infancy is related to the age of weaning. In most countries in the developing world, this means that peak prevalence occurs in the second year of life, which corresponds to the peak prevalence in protein energy malnutrition. By contrast, in developed communities the peak prevalence occurs during the first year of life. This was the pattern observed during 1973, in the study by Gribbin *et al*. (1976) with the largest group of admissions under six months of age (*see* Fig. 6.15). More recently at the Queen Elizabeth Hospital, there has been a trend for children of more than 6 months to be admitted with acute gastroenteritis. This runs parallel with the trend for more breast feeding in the community.

Gastroenteritis continues to be a problem of world-wide importance as the following facts indicate. In 1974, WHO showed that in 22 North American and European nations, gastroenteritis/diarrhoea was the overall sixth cause of death in 1 to 4-year olds. Furthermore, approximately 500 million episodes of diarrhoea have been estimated to occur in children under five years in Asia, Africa and Latin America in 1975 (Rohde and Northrup, 1975). Thus, gastroenteritis continues to be a problem of enormous importance in developing communities; for example, Papua–New Guinea, where gastroenteritis was the commonest cause of hospital admission in children aged 1 to 4 years in 1967 (Biddulph and Pangkatana, 1971). Its prevalence is a major factor in the genesis of protein-calorie malnutrition in such communities. In South Africa, Hansen (1968) has observed in a careful one year follow up of 80 admitted to hospital with gastroenteritis in Capetown, that 12 subsequently developed kwashiorkor, 37 had loss of weight and failed to improve during the year of observation, and a total of 62 children had recurrent diarrhoea of varying severity. Walker (1971) has estimated that 20 per cent of Australian aboriginal children in the northern part of the Northern Territory are admitted to hospital with gastroenteritis before their second birthday. There is, thus, a close interaction between malnutrition, gastroenteritis and chronic diarrhoea in developing communities, and gastroenteritis continues to be a very important health hazard among children from such communities.

The total number of children admitted each year to the gastroenteritis unit at the Queen Elizabeth Hospital over the past 25 years has
tended to rise, although the number of children who have required
intravenous fluids has at the same time fallen, i.e. the indications for
admission to the unit have changed and many more children in recent
years have been admitted for social reasons. Figure 6.11 shows the
number of children admitted each week to the gastroenteritis ward
during 1970 at the Royal Alexandra Hospital, the annual total of
admissions for that year being 838.

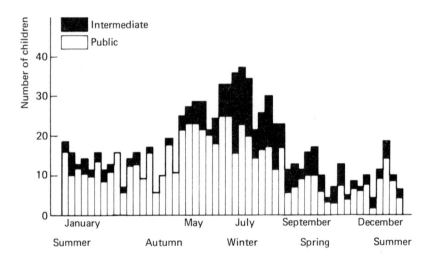

Fig. 6.11. Weekly admission number in the gastroenteritis unit at the Royal
Alexandra Hospital for 1970.
Black represents 'intermediate patients' and white 'public patients'.

From these observations it is clear that gastroenteritis in childhood
is still a common problem both in London and Sydney. It is true that
gastroenteritis continues to be an important problem in developed
countries, although its dimensions are not as great as in the developing
nations.

Gastroenteritis used to be considered an epidemic summer disease
in countries such as Britain, the United States and Australia. Figure
6.12 shows that in Sydney it is now a disease with a winter peak. Such
a trend to an increased prevalence in winter has also been reported by
Moffet, Shulenberger and Burkholder (1968) and others from the
United States. Ironside (1973) in Britain has also reported a similar

trend in Manchester, and it has also been observed at the Queen
Elizabeth Hospital in London (see Table 6.7). In contrast, Spencer
and Coster (1969) in South Africa have shown that gastroenteritis is
still a predominantly summer disease among the African population.

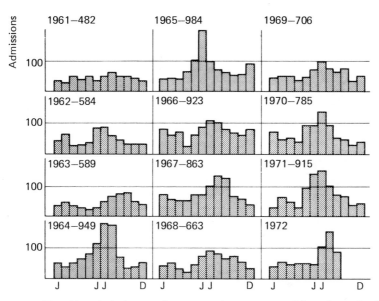

Fig. 6.12. Monthly admissions each year to the gastroenteritis unit at the Royal
Alexandra Hospital 1961–1972.

Dorman (1972) has studied the monthly number of admissions to
the gastroenteritis unit at the Royal Alexandra Hospital over a
ten-year period and has shown that the winter peak appeared for the
first time in 1964, and was associated with a large increase in the total
number of annual admissions. This pattern of admissions to the unit
has continued ever since (Fig. 6.12). During this winter peak, most
patients are infants and the percentage of bacterial isolations often falls
as low as 2–5 per cent. These observations suggest that a new,
probably viral, pathogen may have appeared in Sydney in 1964,
altering the pattern of gastroenteritis in the community. This is likely
to have been the rotavirus.

Gastroenteritis is often associated with poor housing, overcrowding
and low standards of hygiene, but the Sydney survey in 1970 showed
that many of the patients during the winter months were 'intermediate
patients' (*see* Fig. 6.11), i.e. children from the upper socio-economic

groups. A geographical survey of Sydney showed that children with gastroenteritis came from all sections of the community, rich and poor alike. Thus, it must be assumed that the mere improvement in living standards will not lead automatically to a disappearance of gastroenteritis. Such measures may simply result in a change in its aetiology.

However, it does seem clear now that gastroenteritis has a very low prevalence in rural areas in countries such as Britain. Crowding, a condition of urban life, may be a factor in the continuance of gastroenteritis in children of large, developed cities. Although rotavirus has not been found yet in throat washings, etc., Reiman *et al.* (1945) showed that inhalation of nebulised filtered throat washings from patients with acute gastroenteritis were capable of producing disease in volunteers. Urban spread of gastroenteritis therefore may be related to droplet infection rather than to the ano–oral route alone.

GASTROENTERITIS SYNDROMES ASSOCIATED WITH SPECIFIC PATHOGENS

Shigellosis

This is an acute enterocolitis due to infection with one of the organisms of the shigella group. The incubation period is 24–72 hours.

Chantemesse and Widal in France, in 1888, were the first to associate the shigellae with dysentery but a more complete description was given in Japan by Shiga in 1898.

There are four main sub-groups, namely, *Shigella sonnei*; *Shigella flexneri*; *Shigella boydii*; and *Shigella shiga* (the dysentery bacillus).

Shigellae unlike salmonellae are restricted to man as their host. In experimental studies fewer organisms are needed to transmit shigella infections than infections due to salmonellae or enteropathogenic E. coli. It has been established that an entero-toxin is produced, so far, only by *Shigella shiga*.

This shiga enterotoxin differs from cholera toxin in that it does not appear to activate mucosal adenylate cyclase *per se*. At present, therefore, the physiological significance of this toxin and the mechanism whereby the small intestine secretes fluid in shigellosis is not clear (Formal *et al.*, 1976). However, it seems probable that in this infection the primary process is diarrhoea resulting from abnormal jejunal transport superimposed on a colonic disturbance. Severity of shigellosis appears to depend upon the penetration of the epithelium by the organism and its multiplication thereafter (Formal *et al.*, 1976).

The main types of shigellae found at the Royal Alexandra Hospital and the Queen Elizabeth Hospital are shown in Table 6.5.

Table 6.5
Shigella isolations

	R.A.H.C. 1970	Q.E.H. 1973
Shigella sonnei	14	7
Shigella flexneri	8	—

At present, shigellosis is a relatively mild disease in Britain and in Australia, but in developing countries it is still a very serious disease with a high mortality and, usually, with a peak frequency in the summer. The dysentery bacillus itself is now infrequently isolated in Western countries. Infection is caused by person-to-person spread.

Septicaemia is even more uncommon in children with shigella infections than it is in salmonellosis, but rare cases where blood culture has yielded *Shigella sonnei* have occurred in children. There have even been reports of *Shigella sonnei* septicaemia occurring in the neonate (Moore, 1974).

Salmonellosis

There are more than 1,000 types of organism that make up the genus salmonella, and infection with these organisms may cause a variety of illnesses in animals and in man.

Many infections with salmonellae in children arise from animal sources via contamination of food, but food may also be contaminated by the infected stools or urine of a person who is excreting salmonellae. The risk of hospital cross-infection with salmonella infections is considerable because of this infectivity of stools and urine. Small numbers of organisms can cause illness in a compromised host and, equally, very large numbers may have no effect in a healthy naturally immune host (Curry, 1976).

Salmonella infections are common in farm animals, particularly poultry. The increasing use of frozen foods, especially poultry, in developed countries may be an important factor in the observed trend of an increase of salmonellosis in such countries (Fenner, 1971). It is interesting to note the higher percentage of children with gastroenteritis who were found to have salmonellae isolated from their stools in Sydney (Table 6.6), where the trend to increased poultry consumption is more advanced, than in the East End of London where fewer children had salmonellae isolated. Incorrect cooking methods, for example, inadequate cooking of incompletely thawed frozen poultry, are responsible for such infections. The incubation period is 12–36 hours.

Table 6.6
Gastroenteritis survey Royal Alexandra Hospital for Children 5 Jan. 1970–3 Jan. 1971, 838 admissions salmonellosis (53 cases)

Salmonella typhimurium	34
Salmonella derby	3
Salmonella adelaide	3
Salmonella chester	2
Salmonella bovis morbificans	2
Salmonella anatum	1
Salmonella singapore	1
Salmonella kottbus	1
Salmonella newport	1
Salmonella muenchen	1
Salmonella bredeney	1
Salmonella senftenberg	1
Not typed	2

Some types of salmonella infection occur both in animals and in man whereas others such as typhoid fever due to *Salmonella typhi* occur only in man. The small intestine is significantly involved in typhoid fever as, characteristically, the lymph follicles of Peyer's patches are inflamed and as a result ulceration may occur. Uncommonly in children, but more commonly in adults, perforation and haemorrhage may result. However, both typhoid fever and paratyphoid fever are primarily septicaemic diseases that manifest primarily as systemic disease, but on occasion a child admitted to a gastroenteritis unit may have this organism cultured from his stool.

The other species of salmonella cause predominantly a gastrointestinal disorder, but occasionally blood stream infection may occur and in neonates this is more common than in older infants. Neonates may even develop meningitis due to a salmonella organism.

This vulnerability of the neonate to blood stream infection with salmonellae may be related to low levels of IgM in the neonatal period. This is particularly likely as it is known that antibodies against the O antigen of Gram-negative organisms are chiefly found in IgM. This may also account for the susceptibility of young infants to infection with enteropathogenic strains of *E. coli*.

Most salmonellae have two main antigens, the H or flagellar antigen and the O or somatic antigen. Some have a third antigen known as the Vi antigen, e.g. *Salmonella typhi*.

These various antigenic components may be used to identify the particular species of salmonella. Their number, as mentioned earlier, is large but *Salmonella typhimurium* is the commonest encountered in most series. Table 6.6 indicates the type of salmonellae encountered in children with gastroenteritis at the Royal Alexandra Hospital in 1970.

Other situations where blood stream infection may occur include sickle cell disease and chronic granulomatous disease. In both conditions osteomyelitis may develop and indeed may be the clinical mode of presentation of the salmonella infection.

Enteropathogenic E. coli Enteritis

Adam, in Germany, in 1923, identified special types of lactose-splitting strains of *E. coli* as a cause of severe infantile gastroenteritis (Braun, 1974) but this observation was not widely accepted and up until 1945 shigellae and salmonellae were the only bacterial pathogens to have been established as causes of infantile gastroenteritis. In that year, Bray at the Hillingdon Hospital in London published observations he had made concerning the isolation of enteropathogenic strains of *E. coli* from infants with summer diarrhoea. It has subsequently been widely confirmed that certain strains of *E. coli* are enteropathogenic. The criteria for accepting such enteropathogenicity usually includes the consistent isolation of a particular strain in an epidemic as the predominant coliform in the stools of affected infants and its relative rarity in the general community. The antigenic structure of each strain is recorded and reference criteria are developed for future recognition.

Several types of antigen are assessed in identifying the strains of *E. coli*. These include the O, K and H antigens. It is the O antigen that is particularly important in identifying enteropathogenic strains of *E. coli*. This antigen is a heat stable lipopolysaccharide associated with the bacterial cell wall. A number of B subtypes are recognised. The enteropathogenic strains known at present are as follows:

O26	O44	O55	O86	O111
O112	O114	O119	O125	O126
O127	O128	O142		

These strains of *E. coli* may colonise the small intestine, and their capacity to do so is an important factor in determining their enteropathogenicity. This appears, in turn, to be related to the ability of these organisms to adhere to the surface mucosa (McNeish *et al.*, 1975). Another critical factor in determining their enteropathogenicity appears to be the elaboration by some strains of *E. coli* of a diarrhoea-producing enterotoxin. *E. coli* in fact, has been shown so far to produce two types of toxin. First, there is the heat-labile (LT) enterotoxin that is antigenically and functionally similar to cholera toxin. It stimulates adenyl cyclase, as does cholera enterotoxin, and also produces an excess loss of water into the intestinal lumen, i.e. a secretory state. The second toxin is the non-antigenic heat-stable (ST) toxin whose mode of action is not yet clear but which may act via stimulation of another intracellular mediator (cyclic GMP) (Field, 1978). Our understanding of these mechanisms of enteropathogenicity have been considerably expanded by animal work, notably that of Williams Smith (1976). It has now been shown from such studies that the ability of *E. coli* to colonise the gut, adhere to mucosal surface, and to produce enterotoxin can be transmitted from one organism to another by transmissable plasmids. These are extra-chromosomal genetic elements. Thus, plasmids could transfer the potential to produce one of these capacities, e.g. enterotoxin production, to organisms not ordinarily regarded as pathogens. At present, enterotoxin can be demonstrated only by its effect on animal models or on cultured cells. The development of a simple laboratory procedure that would allow rapid recognition of such an enterotoxin would be a great advantage and might demonstrate the enteropathogenicity of hitherto unsuspected organisms.

Another critical factor that may determine the enteropathogenicity of *E. coli* strains is the ability of the organisms to invade the epithelial cells of the small intestine. Du Pont and his colleagues (1971) suggested that two different types of clinical illness could occur depending on whether an individual was infected with an enterotoxin-producing strain or an invasive strain. In the former, severe watery diarrhoea similar to that seen in cases of cholera occurred, whereas in the latter an illness similar to shigellosis occurred.

The relative importance of enterotoxin-producing and invasive strains of *E. coli* in Britain remains uncertain. Although enterotoxin-producing strains of *E. coli* that cause a severe disease with profound fluid loss, sometimes referred to as cholera infantum, may occur, such disease appears to be commoner in the developing world than in developed communities. The best evidence that these mechanisms of toxin production and invasion are causes of human disease comes from studies of *E. coli* strains that cause traveller's diarrhoea in adults. In fact, most studies of classical enteropathogenic *E. coli* serotypes have failed to show that those strains, associated with sporadic or epidemic cases of infantile diarrhoea, possess either invasive or toxin-producing properties. Levine *et al.* (1978) have shown that three enteropathogenic strains (0127, 0128, 0142) given to adult volunteers all cause diarrhoea, but despite this there is no evidence of toxin production or invasiveness of these strains in extensive laboratory studies. This suggests that the classic *E. coli* enteropathogenic organism may produce their effects by as yet unrecognised mechanisms, possibly via another type of, as yet, unknown toxin.

Neonatal infection with an enteropathogenic strain of *E. coli* is particularly dangerous and can spread very rapidly through a nursery of newborn infants and be associated with a very severe form of diarrhoea and even death. The significance of the isolation of such a strain during an epidemic of infantile gastroenteritis is quite clear but its isolation from the stool of the occasional symptom-free infant is uncertain. However, the isolation of such a strain from the stools of a child with diarrhoea under the age of two years is usually regarded as a significant finding.

Thus, to say the least, from the viewpoint of the practising clinician the present position concerning diagnosis and recognition of infection due to strains of enteropathogenic *E. coli* is most unsatisfactory. It is possible that invasive and toxin-producing strains of *E. coli* do exist and are not detected by conventional serotyping. It is also possible that conventional serotyping in sporadic cases is of little use. Indeed, there are those who are very sceptical of the value of present routine serotyping of *E. coli*. Much more research is clearly needed concerning the role of *E. coli* in the genesis of infantile diarrhoea in the nineteen seventies.

Ironside (1973) has speculated that the disease may be due to the temporary clinical upset that occurs when new strains of *E. coli* reach the gut of the infant. A similar change is considered to be one of the causes of 'travellers' diarrhoea'. He suggests that a 'baby's trip to the local nursery is the bacteriological equivalent of the adult's trip to Egypt'. The incubation period for infections with these strains is believed to be 24 to 72 hours.

Table 6.1 (p. 172) indicates the isolation rate for these organisms in three hospitals in different countries. Within Britain itself there has been a change since 1953 when the MRC trial of prophylactic antibiotics found that 37 per cent of children with gastroenteritis were infected with one of the only two serotypes then known to be enteropathogenic. This figure is much higher than the present figure at the Queen Elizabeth Hospital and the figure reported by Ironside, Tuxford and Heyworth in Manchester in 1970, namely 4 per cent. These findings suggest a continuing change in the aetiology of gastroenteritis.

Yersinia enteritis and enterocolitis

Yersinia enterocolitica is a gram-negative rod previously known as *Pasteurella pseudotuberculosis*. It may cause a zoonosis in several animals. It is more common in Belgium and Scandinavia than Britain, where it is an uncommon infection.

In children, it presents most often as acute gastroenteritis with diarrhoea containing blood and pus and fever, whereas in adolescents and adults, as acute terminal ileitis or mesenteric adenitis (Vantrappen *et al.*, 1977). It is believed that the effects of this infection are produced by invasion of the intestinal mucosa. *In vitro*, it has been shown that *Yersinia enterocolitica* invades cultured human epithelial cells (Maki *et al.*, 1978).

The diagnosis is usually made by isolating organisms from the stools or by rising titres of Yersinia antibodies. It can also be isolated from ileocaecal lymph nodes and resected appendices.

Despite the similarity of this illness to Crohn's disease, there appears to be no evidence that Yersinia infections ever result in Crohn's disease. The ulceration of the ileum and colon heal within a few weeks.

Barium studies may show abnormalities of the terminal ileum which could be confused with Crohn's disease, but Vantrappen *et al.* state that the radiological differential diagnosis is not difficult. Radiological abnormalities are mainly changes in mucosal pattern, and the superficial ulceration skip lesions of Crohn's disease are never seen.

Autopsy studies show that the entire alimentary tract may be involved by an ulcerative process, primarily at the site of lymphoid tissue. Apthoid ulcers may be seen in colon similar to Crohn's disease but no sarcoid granulomata or giant cells are ever found.

Campylobacter enteritis

Campylobacter is a micro-aerophilic vibrio which, until recently, was an uncommonly recognised cause of acute gastroenteritis. The increasing recognition of the importance of this infection relates to the introduction of selective culture techniques. Skirrow (1977) found 7.1 per cent of unrelated patients with diarrhoea grew campylobacter. The highest incidence was in young children and it was most common under a year. A healthy carrier state may exist. It now appears to be an important cause of gastroenteritis at the Queen Elizabeth Hospital. Meadows (personal communication) found it to be present in stools of 12 (6·4 per cent) of 185 consecutive admissions during a four month period in 1977.

The mode of transmission involves ingestion of the organism, carriage in the intestine, and sometimes invasion of the blood. Wild birds and chickens may be an important source of infection.

The clinical features can vary, but diarrhoea lasting several days with or without fever is most frequent. The diarrhoea, on the one hand, may be trivial, but, on the other, may be severe and watery, containing blood. Aching of limbs may also occur. Vomiting and severe, cramping abdominal pain may be a feature and the child may be admitted in the first instance to a surgical ward as a suspected surgical emergency.

Food-poisoning Organisms

When acute diarrhoea and vomiting rapidly follow the ingestion of bacterially contaminated food, the diagnosis of food poisoning is made. It may result from ingestion of bacteria *per se* or preformed toxin, e.g. staphylococcal enterotoxin, as well as the toxin of *Clostridium botulinum*, (classical botulism) fortunately a rare occurrence today. Clostridium perfringens continues to be an important cause of food-borne diarrhoea and can cause a fatal enteritis known as 'pig-bel' in the highlands of New Guinea. Classically, infection with salmonella may produce this syndrome but other organisms have now been associated with food poisoning. These include *Vibrio parahaemolyticus* and *Bacillus cereus*.

Vibrio parahaemolyticus is a gram-negative rod associated with the consumption of uncooked sea foods. Its incubation period is 12 to 48 hours. Acute gastrointestinal symptoms last a few days but rarely are serious.

Bacillus cereus is a gram-positive rod that can produce a toxin. Infection is most often acquired by eating food that has been stored before eating, e.g. Chinese fried rice.

ROTAVIRUS GASTROENTERITIS

Virus Morphology

The virus particle found in the stools of children with acute gastroenteritis is morphologically identical to the virus particles found in the stools of infant calves with acute diarrhoea. The virus occurs in two forms. One is about 70 nm in diameter with a double-shelled capsid structure having a sharply defined circular outline with the appearance of a rim of a wheel, hence the Latin name, rota a wheel.

Then there are smaller rougher particles which appear to be viruses that have lost their outer shell and are about 60 nm in diameter and have been reported to be uninfective. Empty shells are frequently seen. Electron microscopy may reveal large numbers of virus particles packed together or there may be only scattered virus particles. Concentrations of greater than 10^6 particles/ml are necessary for the agent to be seen (Tan *et al.*, 1974).

Pathogenicity of Rotavirus

Flewett (1976) has pointed out that one can hardly hope to fulfil all Koch's postulates before accepting a virus particle found in the stool as a pathogen. He has listed some of the evidence that may reasonably be expected. Some of it is fulfilled for this particle and includes the following. (1) *Particles found in material from patients with the disease but not from patients with other unrelated diseases.* This, in general, appears to be true so far for rotavirus. (2) *Prevalence of a particle in the population coincides with the prevalence of the disease.* Again, this appears to be true outside the neonatal period. Davidson *et al.* (1975a) found no particles in controls. Rodriguez *et al.* (1977) found them in 8 per cent of 76 control children. (3) *Presence of the particle corresponds with the duration of the disease.* Studies to date in general support this. (4) *Purified particles induce the disease in adult volunteers or experimental animals.* Infection induced in an adult volunteer has been shown by Middleton *et al.* (1974) and it has been transmitted to an infant monkey (Lambeth and Mitchell, 1975). Rotavirus has been identified by electron microscopy in the duodenal mucosa, duodenal juice and stools of children with acute gastroenteritis, but only occasionally in controls. Thus, at present there appears to be enough evidence to suggest that rotavirus is a significant pathogen causing gastroenteritis. This whole subject has recently been excellently reviewed by Schreiber, Trier and Blacklow (1977).

Seasonal Prevalence and Geographical Distribution

Rotavirus has been found in sporadic cases and in epidemic outbreaks of acute gastroenteritis in childhood. Reports have come from the developed world including Australia, Europe and North America but also from developing communities in Africa and Asia. Its worldwide distribution suggests that it is a major pathogen of international importance. Characteristically, this agent has been identified in the stools of children during the winter peak of gastroenteritis. A winter peak in the prevalence of non-bacterial gastroenteritis has been known for some time in developed countries both in the northern and southern hemisphere. As long ago as 1929, Zahorsky described winter vomiting disease and, more recently, two winter epidemics of non-bacterial gastroenteritis have been described in north-west London (Sinha and Tyrrell, 1973). A study of monthly admissions to a gastroenteritis unit in Sydney from 1961–1972 showed the sudden appearance of a winter peak in hospital admissions in 1964, which persisted in subsequent years (*see* Fig. 6.12). An association between this winter peak and rotavirus in the stools has now been reported from Melbourne (Davidson *et al.*, 1975b), Toronto (Hamilton *et al.*, 1976), Washington (Kapikian *et al.*, 1976), Birmingham (Flewett *et al.*, 1973) and London (Table 6.7), i.e. in cold and temperate

Table 6.7
Monthly admissions to the Gastroenteritis Unit at the Queen Elizabeth Hospital for Children

	Total G.E.	M.	F.	Ent. Coli	Shi.	Salm.	Stools for E.M.*	Rota*	% Stools examined
Aug. 1976	33	19	14	3	–	2	7	0	0%
Sept.	26	13	13	4	–	5	12	1	8%
Oct.	28	18	10	1	–	4	10	4	40%
Nov.	50	19	31	2	1	1	25	9	36%
Dec.	58	31	27	2	3	1	36	11	30%
Jan. 1977	67	42	25	2	2	1	36	18	50%
Feb.	52	25	27	2	–	1	26	13	50%
Mar.	56	32	24	1	0	0	21	3	14%
April	44	25	19	4	1	0	10	2	20%
May	40	21	19	4	1	0	8	1	12%
June	50	27	23	0	0	1	24	3	12%
July	40	25	15	0	3	1	12	0	0%
Total	544	297	247	25	11	17	227	65	28%

* Stools examined for rota virus at London School of Hygiene and Tropical Medicine by Dr R. Bird.

climates. The peak prevalence may approach 80 per cent among infants and young children during the winter months in North America (Kapikian *et al.*, 1976; Hamilton *et al.*, 1976). In some reports, the virus is not found at all during the summer months but in others it falls to a 20 per cent level or thereabouts. Maiya *et al.* (1976) found rotavirus in 13 of 50 children in tropical southern India (26 per cent), the virus being found only during the cooler months of the year. In a recent study in semi-tropical Northern Australia, Walker and Marshall (1977) have shown that infections occurred predominantly in the rainy season; 50 per cent of children admited to Darwin hospital with gastroenteritis in the 'wet' season were found to have serological evidence of rotavirus infection in contrast to only 13 per cent of the children admitted in the 'dry' season months. Thus, it is clear that seasonal variation may have a profound effect on the prevalence of this infection. The importance of rotavirus in temperate climates is clear but its importance in developing countries remains to be established.

Pathology

Rotavirus particles have been identified by electron microscopy in the small intestinal mucosa of children with acute gastroenteritis in studies in Australia (Fig. 6.13) (Bishop *et al.*, 1973; Holmes, Ruck and Bishop, 1975), Canada (Middleton, Szymanski and Abbott, 1974) and Japan (Suzuki and Konno, 1975). They were found in the epithelium of the villus and the crypts (Hamilton *et al.*, 1976). With the exception of the Japanese report, the particles have not been found in the lamina propria. Rotavirus was found in the enterocytes of 6 out of 9 children with acute gastroenteritis biopsied by Bishop *et al.* (1973) 1 to 5 days after the onset of symptoms. All biopsies revealed histological abnormality ranging from mild to severe but the intraepithelial lymphocyte count was normal (Ferguson, McClure and Townley, 1976).

The virus particles in the enterocytes were found in distended cisternae of the endoplasmic reticulum and in the cisternae between the inner and outer nuclear membranes. The microvilli were often irregular and distended. Abnormal infected enterocytes were found scattered among enterocytes that were morphologically normal.

The histological abnormality had reverted to normal and the virus particles had disappeared in three children Bishop *et al.* studied after recovery some 4 to 8 weeks later.

The virus appears characteristically to invade the proximal small intestinal mucosa but autopsy studies have shown that the infection

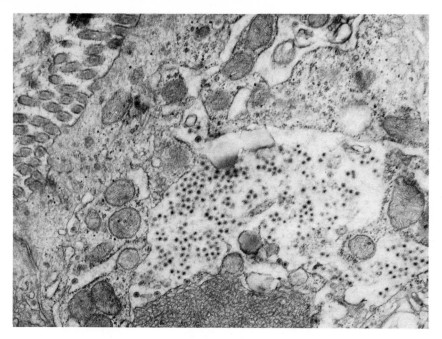

Fig. 6.13. Rotaviruses in the enterocyte of a biopsy from a child with acute gastroenteritis. (Reproduced by permission of R. Bishop and *The Lancet*.)

can spread along the entire length of the small intestine and even into the colon (Hamilton *et al*., 1976).

Pathophysiology

Mavromichalis *et al*. (1977) found rotavirus in intestinal aspirate of 6 out of 8 children with gastroenteritis who had rotavirus in their stools. All six had abnormal xylose absorption, whereas the two without rotavirus in the lumen had none, suggesting that small intestinal dysfunction related to mucosal damage occurred when the virus was found in the lumen.

To date, little is known in man of the mechanism of diarrhoea in rotavirus gastroenteritis but Hamilton *et al*. (1976) have studied an animal model using a virus in piglets. This is a corona virus, known as the transmissable gastroenteritis virus (TGE). It produces massive diarrhoea some 16 to 40 hours after infection, with high faecal electrolytes. At 40 hours they found decreased sodium and water flux, decreased mucosal activities of disaccharidases and sodium, potassium-APTase, but normal adenyl cyclase activity. Unlike enterotoxigenic diarrhoeas such as cholera, under these experimental conditions, sodium flux failed to respond to glucose. Ferguson and Snodgrass (1978) have gone on to study infection of one-day-old germ-free lambs with rotavirus. They found a state of accelerated epithelial cell turnover with functionally immature enterocytes clothing the villi. If a similar situation exists in rotavirus gastroenteritis in man, it is clear that the pathophysiology may be very different from the toxigenic bacterial diarrhoeas.

Gould (1977) has studied stool prostaglandin levels in 4 children with rotavirus gastroenteritis and 4 children with gastroenteritis but no rotavirus. Unlike ulcerative colitis, in which stool prostaglandin levels are elevated, he found that levels of prostaglandin the stools were well within the control range in both groups of children.

Age Range

Rotavirus has been found principally in the stools of children with gastroenteritis from the neonatal period up to five years but most are under 2 years of age. Most studies have reported a peak between 6 months and a year (Kapikian et al., 1976; Carr et al., 1976; Rodriguez et al., 1977), but Shepherd et al. (1975) found 43·3 per cent of their children under 6 months.

Although the disease is commonest in young children it may also occur in adults. Rotavirus has, indeed, been found in the stools of adults with acute gastroenteritis (von Bonsdorff et al., 1976). The virus may also occur in adults who are symptom free (Tallet et al., 1977).

Sex Ratio

As in earlier reports of non-bacterial gastroenteritis in which viral studies were not done (Gribbin, Walker-Smith and Wood, 1976; Tripp, Wilmers and Wharton, 1977), most studies of rotavirus gastroenteritis report that boys are more often affected than girls (Table 6.7). The reason for this male predominance is not yet clear, but it is most obvious in the younger children.

Incubation Period

The incubation period appears to be about 48 to 72 hours (Shepherd *et al.*, 1975).

Clinical Features

Most studies have described vomiting as the first symptom, often accompanied by diarrhoea but sometimes preceding it by several hours (Shepherd *et al.*, 1975). On occasion, there may even be no diarrhoea. The diarrhoea is typically acute in onset and often watery in character with usually less than ten stools each day. Pyrexia is a common but not a constant feature in all reports. A concurrent upper respiratory tract infection has been documented in 42 per cent in one report (Carr *et al.*, 1976) and 29 per cent in another (Rodriguez *et al.*, 1977). Most clinical reports of rotavirus gastroenteritis have described a relatively mild-self-limiting illness with dehydration, usually less than 5 per cent, present in about half or less of those children admitted to hospital. Rodriguez *et al.* (1977) described dehydration in 83 per cent of children with rotavirus gastroenteritis compared with 40 per cent in children who did not have rotavirus in their stools. But dehydration was mostly mild to moderate. It has, however, become clear that rotavirus gastroenteritis may on occasion be associated with a much more severe illness, and even death has been reported from Canada (Hamilton *et al.*, 1976) and Australia (Bishop *et al.*, 1973). Fatal rotavirus gastroenteritis does not appear to have been documented yet in Britain.

An initial study of 30 children with rotavirus gastroenteritis from the Queen Elizabeth Hospital for Children, London during the winter of 1974–1975, found a relatively mild illness (Shepherd *et al.*, 1975) but a second study of the winter of 1976–1977, analysing the features of 17 children, found a similar mild illness in 11, but in a further 6 a more severe illness (French *et al.*, 1979). Ryder *et al.* in Bangladesh (1976) have indeed found rotavirus in the stools of 12 out of 22 children, with severe dehydration due to diarrhoea, the degree of dehydration being comparable to that found in cholera, in their experience. In southern India, Maiya *et al.* (1976) found no difference in the clinical presentation of children with gastroenteritis in whom rotavirus was detected as compared with those in whom a bacterial pathogen was identified or no agent recognised. Thus, in developing communities rotavirus is associated with less characteristic clinical patterns.

So although rotavirus gastroenteritis seems most often to cause a relatively mild illness in developed communities, it may on occasion cause more severe disease and even death. However, it must be observed that all the reports to date have largely concerned in-patients and there is very little data available concerning the presumably clinically less severe and much commoner cases managed as out-patients.

Accompanying Pathogens

Any account of the severity of the clinical disease must try to take note of the possible role of accompanying pathogens, bacterial or viral. Several reports have described a more serious illness, when bacterial pathogens, especially enteropathogenic *E. coli*, are found in the stools at the same time (Shepherd *et al.*, 1975; Carr *et al.*, 1976). Madeley *et al.* (1977) have found rotavirus and other bacterial and viral pathogens occurring in different stool samples from the same infants and have found it difficult to determine whether one or all were significant pathogens.

Duration of Illness

The duration of illness ranges between 5 days to 3 weeks (Shepherd *et al.*, 1975) but usually lasts only 8 days (Tallett *et al.*, 1977). Most children present within five days of onset if they come to hospital.

Biochemistry and Haematology

An elevated blood urea on hospital admission has been described (Rodriguez *et al.*, 1977) and been related to the numbers of rotavirus in the stools (Carr *et al.*, 1977). Hypernatraemia may occur but is not characteristic. When there is dehydration it is likely to be isotonic. Lymphocytosis may be found.

Stool Microscopy

Characteristically, leucocytes are not present in the stools although they may be seen in some patients, 18 per cent in one series (Rodriguez *et al.*, 1977).

Infectivity

It appears to be a highly contagious disease, apparently spread by the faecal–oral route. Massive quantities of virus may be passed in the stools some 24 to 72 hours after infection. Outbreaks may occur in families and in institutions. In one study, 35 per cent of parents of children with rotavirus gastroenteritis had serological or stool evidence of rotavirus infection (Rodriguez *et al.*, 1977). It is also clear that adult staff members may play a role in transmitting rotavirus infections in children's wards.

Rotavirus in Neonates

A high incidence of rotavirus in the stools of asymptomatic neonates has been reported from Sydney (Murphy, Alberry and Crewe, 1977) and St Thomas's Hospital, London (Chrystie *et al.*, 1975). In one study, Murphy *et al.* found no less than 50 per cent of neonates by the age of three to four days were excreting virus. Only 24 per cent of these had diarrhoea. There was no seasonal variation. How the virus spreads in the neonatal nursery is not known but probably it is environmental within the nursery.

Despite the finding of rotavirus in asymptomatic neonates, Murphy *et al.* found that significantly more neonates with diarrhoea excreted the virus than in the symptom-free group. It does, in fact, seem likely that rotavirus can be a cause of gastroenteritis in the neonate, as suggested by Bishop *et al.* (1976), and a clue to why some with stool rotavirus do not get clinical disease is provided by Murphy *et al.*, who found that children who had in their stools viruses coated with an 'antibody-like' material did not get diarrhoea. It is known from the work of Matthews *et al.* (1976) that breast milk and cow's milk contain non-antibody virus inhibitor and this may play a role too.

Diagnostic Techniques

A number of techniques have been used. First has been electron microscopy of stools using negative staining, which has been used in many centres. This is a relatively simple technique provided an electron microscope is available. Second is the technique of counter-immunoelectrophoresis. This is a technique to detect viral antigen in the stool. (Spence *et al.*, 1975; Middleton, Petric and Hewitt, 1976). It appears to be about as sensitive as the electron microscope technique. Third is serum serology using a complement fixation technique. This was developed by Kapikian *et al.* (1975). With rotavirus stool antigen, these workers showed a rise in serum antibody titre with a complement fixation test using acute and convalescent sera. A related antigen, Nebraska calf diarrhoea virus, is more readily available. It is morphologically and antigenically identical to rotavirus. Fourth is an indirect immunofluorescent antibody technique (Davidson *et al.*, 1975b). This is a difficult technique but one that seems to be slightly more sensitive than the complement fixation test. Fifth is the ELISA technique mentioned on page 177.

Delayed Recovery

In the first detailed report of clinical features of rotavirus diarrhoea, Shepherd *et al.* (1975) described temporary sugar intolerance in 2 of 30 children with rotavirus gastroenteritis. Carr *et al.* (1976) found two such cases who had associated enteropathogenic *E. coli*. Four patients reported by Tallet *et al.* (1977) had recurrent diarrhoea but they found 'problems with absorption of sugar in a small proportion' only. Thus, so far, only a low frequency of sugar malabsorption has been reported. Yet in one period in the winter of 1976–1977, Lucas *et al.* (1978) found an unusually high frequency of temporary monosaccharide malabsorption coinciding with the winter peak of gastroenteritis; 6 out of 9 children with temporary monosaccharide intolerance who were examined had rotavirus in their stools. An association between sugar malabsorption and rotavirus would not be surprising in view of the damage to microvilli in infected enterocytes (Bishop *et al.*, 1973). In addition, it would appear theoretically possible that severe and extensive infection could temporarily damage a high proportion of lactase activity of the enterocytes and, perhaps, also cause a transient surface block to sugar absorption by temporarily damaging the brush border membrane which would cause a block in absorption to all sugars, as proposed by Walker-Smith, Kamath and Stobo (1972). The clinical severity would depend on the number of enterocytes damaged.

Finally, Holmes *et al.* (1976) have suggested that lactase is the receptor and uncoating enzyme for rotavirus. This would mean that infants with their high lactase levels may be more vulnerable, helping to explain the age of most affected individuals.

Immunity

Little is known yet about immunity to rotavirus infection. Repeat infection with rotavirus in childhood has been reported (Fonteyne,

Zusis and Lambert, 1978) but these authors recognise two types of rotavirus, namely type 1 and type 2. A different type was responsible for the second infection. There is indeed some evidence that there is more than one antigenic variety of rotavirus. Antibody levels tend to rise with age, reaching adult levels at two years (Kapikian *et al.*, 1976). Children with pre-existing antibody have become infected.

Infants aged 6 to 24 months appear more susceptible to infection regardless of the presence of antibody in their sera. Lower prevalence rates of rotavirus infection under 6 months may be attributable to immunity acquired from the mother. Bortulussi *et al.* (1974) found normal amounts of IgA in intestinal secretions during acute illness and in convalescence.

CLINICAL FEATURES AND DIFFERENTIAL DIAGNOSIS

As the definition of gastroenteritis makes clear, it is a disease characterised by the acute onset of vomiting and diarrhoea. Nelson and Haltalin from Dallas, Texas, in 1971 published a most useful summary of the clinical features of the different types of acute gastroenteritis that may occur in children. These are listed in Table 6.8 which is slightly modified from their original article.

When a child with acute vomiting and diarrhoea is first seen, the clinician's initial step in his assessment is to determine, on clinical grounds, whether the child has gastroenteritis or whether there is evidence that he has some other disease state that may manifest in a similar way. Listed in Table 6.9 are some of the disorders that may present with acute vomiting and diarrhoea, with features that may suggest the diagnosis of acute gastroenteritis.

Some of the disorders listed are relatively trivial, e.g. upper respiratory tract infection. The mechanism of diarrhoea and vomiting found in such infants is not clear and the illness resulting is usually mild. The author prefers to avoid the term parenteral diarrhoea because we need to look carefully at this group. It is now clear that a child with otitis media and acute diarrhoea may have a rotavirus gastroenteritis (Rodriguez *et al.*, 1977). It is also probable that adenovirus can cause both an upper respiratory tract infection and gastroenteritis.

Other conditions in this list are far more serious, and failure to make the correct diagnosis may have dire consequences for the child. An acute abdomen is the greatest risk, and those paediatricians who

Table 6.8
Clinical features of acute diarrhoeal disease useful in differential diagnosis

Clinical features	Shigella	Invasive enteropatho-genic E. coli	Salmonella (excluding typhoid fever)	Non-bacterial
Age	6 m–5 y (rare in neonate)	Less than 2 y	Any age	Any age
Diarrhoea in household	Common (>50%)	No	Variable	Variable
Onset	Abrupt	Gradual	Variable	Abrupt
Vomiting as a prominent symptom	Absent	Uncommon	Common	Common
Fever (over 102° F)	Common	Absent	Variable	Uncommon
Respiratory symptoms	Common (bronchitis)	Absent	Uncommon (except in septicaemic form)	Common (upper respiratory)
Convulsion	Common	Rare	Rare	Rare
Anal sphincter	Lax tone (rarely, rectal prolapse)	Normal	Normal	Normal
Time after onset when seen by doctor	Early	Several days	Several days	Early
Early course, untreated	Slight or no improvement	Persistent or relapsing	Persistent	Daily improvement

Permission of Nelson, from Nelson and Haltalin, 1971

care for a gastroenteritis unit are evermindful of the risk of failing to diagnose an infant with a surgical condition admitted to their unit. A detailed history carefully taken, coupled with a simple yet thorough clinical examination can usually exclude most of the conditions listed or at least indicate the appropriate investigations that need to be done immediately. These may include simple ward testing of urine, urine culture or a blood culture.

Danger signs on physical examination include abdominal distension, abdominal tenderness and a degree of 'toxicity' out of proportion to the child's state of hydration. Abdominal distension or tenderness suggest the possibility of an acute abdomen and a plain X-ray is always indicated. Sometimes gastroenteritis *per se* may cause such abdominal distension with a dilated gut. Nonetheless, such infants should be observed very carefully, even when there is no evidence of obstruction on X-ray of the abdomen.

Table 6.9
Differential diagnosis of acute gastroenteritis

Acute food intolerance
  e.g. cow's milk protein
    intolerance
Coeliac disease
	Metabolic disorders
	  diabetic pre-coma
	  haemolytic-uraemic syndrome

Systemic infections
  septicaemia
  pneumonia
  meningitis
  urinary tract infection
	Surgical disorders
	  acute appendicitis
	  intussusception
	  pyloric stenosis
	  various causes of incomplete intestinal
	    obstruction, including Hirschsprung's
	    disease

Upper respiratory tract
  infections
  otitis media
	inflammatory bowel disease
	  necrotising or non-specific enterocolitis
	  Crohn's disease
	  ulcerative colitis

Bloody diarrhoea, although it is a frequent accompaniment of bacterial gastroenteritis, should also alert the clinician to the possibility of intussusception and the haemolytic-uraemic syndrome in the small child, as well as ulcerative colitis and Crohn's disease more often in the older child.

The second step in clinical assessment of a child with gastroenteritis, once the diagnosis has been made, is to assess the child's state of hydration. The clinical signs and a rough clinical assessment of the extent of the dehydration are listed in Table 6.10.

When a child is assessed as 5 per cent or more dehydrated he will require intravenous fluids and so will need immediate admission to hospital, at least in developed countries. However, this is not the only

Table 6.10
Signs of dehydration

2–3% dehydration:	Thirst, mild oliguria
5% dehydration:	Discernible alteration in skin tone, slightly sunken eyes, some loss of intraocular tension, thirst, oliguria. Sunken fontanelle in infants
7–8% dehydration:	Very obvious loss of skin tone and tissue turgor, sunken eyes, loss of intraocular tension, marked thirst and oliguria. Often some restlessness or apathy
10% deyhdration: (and over)	All the foregoing, plus peripheral vasoconstriction, hypotension, cyanosis, and sometimes hyperpyrexia. Thirst may be lost at this stage

reason for hospital admission in a child with gastroenteritis and other possible reasons are listed below:

1. Children requiring I.V. therapy, i.e. 5 per cent or more dehydration.
2. Failure of outpatient management.
3. Uncertainty about the state of hydration, e.g. obese infants.
4. Uncertainty about diagnosis, especially if a surgical lesion is expected.
5. Children who have a severe history although not yet dehydrated.

Failure of outpatient management may often be for social reasons, which has been a common cause in both the Royal Alexandra Hospital and the Queen Elizabeth Hospital.

In 1973, Gribbin, Walker-Smith and Wood (1976) made a prospective study of the clinical features of all children admitted to the gastroenteritis unit at the Queen Elizabeth Hospital. There were 472 admissions, accounting for 6·8 per cent of the total admissions to the hospital in that year. Readmissions for recurrence of symptoms or for social problems were required for 45 of the 416 children admitted that year. Their ages ranged from two days to 8 years 10 months, but the majority were under the age of a year, the largest number being under 6 months. There was a clear male predominance in the youngest age group; 64 per cent of infants under 3 months were boys. The children admitted were divided into seven groups. Group A accounted for 240 admissions, for 233 children who had simple gastroenteritis as defined at the beginning of this chapter. Group B contained 126 admissions, for 120 children who, in addition to acute vomiting and diarrhoea, had evidence of infections outside the alimentary tract. These were mostly upper respiratory tract infections and otitis media. Group C consisted of a group of 41 children admitted with delayed recovery after gastroenteritis had been diagnosed elsewhere. Group D contained 27 children who had no gastrointestinal symptoms but who had bacterial pathogens in their stool, or had been in contact with such a pathogen. They were admitted for isolation reasons. Group E accounted for 8 children who proved to have surgical disorders despite their admission to a gastroenteritis unit (Table 6.11).

There was a small group, Group F, of 6 children admitted purely for social reasons, although in the other groups social factors clearly played a part in the reason for admission. Finally, Group G was a miscellany of 24 children in whom the primary diagnosis proved to be unrelated to gastroenteritis. It included 2 children who were found to have coeliac disease.

This study clearly illustrates the diversity of causes for the syndrome of acute gastroenteritis. At that time, unfortunately, stool electron microscopy was unavailable and so rotavirus was not identified. Table 6.1 indicates the aetiological agents diagnosed in that year, only 15 per cent having a bacterial pathogen from the total of 472 admissions. It would now seem that many children in Groups A and B with non-bacterial gastroenteritis in all probability had a rotavirus infection. Bacterial pathogens were found in all groups but most often in groups D and A. Thus, it was not possible to analyse clinical features in detail in relation to aetiology. Although fever was a common finding, many children in groups A and B did not have a fever. Dehydration was most common in Group A (36 per cent) less often in Group B (23 per cent). There was no consistent relationship between the degree of dehydration or fever and bacterial pathogens in the stool. Only 9 of 416 admissions were breast fed and of these only one infant fully breast fed. At that time the bottle-fed infants were being fed principally with high solute milks, and cereals were often introduced inappropriately early. In Group A, 14 per cent, and in Group B, 12·5 per cent of those children whose plasma sodium was estimated within 4 hours of admission, proved to have hypernatraemia.

Table 6.11
Surgical diagnoses in Gastroenteritis Unit, Queen Elizabeth Hospital for Children, 1973

Age	Sex	Diagnosis
12 days	M	Pyloric stenosis
1 month	M	Pyloric stenosis
2 months	M	Pyloric stenosis
1 month	M	Intussusception and peritonitis
9 months	F	Intussusception
12 months	M	Intussusception
2 months	F	Idiopathic perforation of caecum
14 months	F	Meckel's diverticulum

From this study it is clear that gastroenteritis is still a common problem at the Queen Elizabeth Hospital, but it is also clear that most children have a relatively mild form of the disease.

WATER AND ELECTROLYTE DISTURBANCES IN GASTROENTERITIS

The most important acute complication of gastroenteritis is dehydration which occurs when the child's overall output of fluid exceeds its input. As he becomes dehydrated, the volume and the electrolyte concentration of his intake usually become the primary determinants of the final state of the body's fluid tonicity, i.e. whether the dehydration is hypertonic, isotonic or hypotonic, but an increase of insensible water loss due to fever, hyperventilation, or a dry environment, may also play a role in influencing such tonicity. Insensible water loss is the volume of fluid that leaves the body as a result of the difference in vapour pressure between the skin and lung surfaces and the surrounding atmosphere. Plasma osmolality is normally 275–295 mosmol/kg.

The stool fluid losses in children with gastroenteritis are typically hypotonic, i.e. there is more than one litre of water per 150 mEq of Na^+ in the stools. Weil (1973) has emphasised that the actual tonicity of the extracellular fluid is determined most importantly, not by stool losses but by the volume and tonicity of the child's intake, although the ability of the kidney to excrete hypertonic urine is also an important determinant. In general, the tonicity of the child's intake is due to its content of salt.

Weil has described the sequence of events that occur in relation to fluid tonicity in infants with gastroenteritis who become dehydrated. Three of his examples will be briefly summarised since they help our understanding of the mechanisms that cause infants to develop dehydration of varying tonicity.

First, when no intake occurs the extracellular fluid tends to become hypertonic, but the kidneys can correct this by excreting hypertonic urine to restore isotonicity. There is also some movement of fluid from the intracellular fluid to the extracellular as a result of the osmotic gradient. However, as fluid loss continues the plasma volume falls and renal function begins to fail, and when this occurs the extracellular fluid becomes hypertonic.

Secondly, when there is a small intake of water and some sodium, the small intake acts as if the size of the insensible water loss is reduced but the Na^+ present adds to the work of the kidneys which makes hypertonic dehydration more likely.

Thirdly, when there is a large fluid intake that is essentially water or very dilute Na^+ containing, the end result is hypotonic dehydration because the net loss of Na^+ is in excess of the net loss of water.

Weil has concluded that the ideal time for initiating therapy for infants with gastroenteritis is when the intake of fluid is so balanced that an initial volume of fluid equivalent to the insensible water loss can be given in an essentially Na^+ free form. Any fluid over that volume will then contain a moderate amount of Na^+ and K^+ with a concentration approaching that in the diarrhoeal stool.

The importance of the volume and salt content of the infant's feeding in the genesis of the type of dehydration produced cannot be over-emphasised. It is clear that although a healthy infant's kidney can deal with a high solute load by producing more concentrated urine, high solute loads in the presence of gastroenteritis will lead to the kidney being unable to cope, resulting in hypertonic dehydration. Indeed, Colle, Aroub and Raile (1958) have shown that babies given feedings with high levels of sodium were, when they had gastroenteritis, more likely to develop hypertonic dehydration. Oates (1973) has shown in a study of 100 mothers of infants under six months of age in London, that 22 were making up the infant's milk formula in a more concentrated strength than that recommended. This was due to the use of heaped or packed scoops instead of level scoops of milk powder, or even by using extra scoops. This risk can be significantly reduced by maternal education concerning the risk of using over-concentrated feeds, the use of low solute milk formulae, and the promotion of breast feeding.

Hypernatraemic Dehydration

Hypernatraemia is defined as a concentration of sodium in the serum of 150 mEq/litre or greater.

This type of dehydration will be discussed in more detail as it has a higher mortality than the other types of dehydration. In addition, clinically significant damage to the central nervous system occurs more commonly and there are more hazards involved in its management.

Finberg in the USA in 1970, found that in his experience isonatraemic dehydration accounted for about 65 per cent of dehydrated infants with gastroenteritis, hypernatraemia for 20 to 25 per cent, and hyponatraemia for approximately 10 per cent. In 1973, he found, however, that the frequency of hypernatraemic dehydration had risen to 28–40 per cent of the annual number of admissions of infants with gastroenteritis seen in New York. In London, hypernatraemia was found in only 14 per cent of children with acute gastroenteritis at the Queen Elizabeth Hospital in 1973. In fact, following publication of the Department of Health and Social Security's Report *Present-day Practice in Infant Feeding* in 1974, and revised subsequently, there has been a remarkable fall in the prevalence of hypernatraemic dehydration. [This change relates to the replacement of high solute milks by low solute milks for most infants under six months in Britain.] Whaley and Walker-Smith (1977) observed a fall in the number of children admitted with hypernatraemic dehydration to the gastroenteritis unit at the Queen Elizabeth Hospital, and this trend has since accelerated. Davies, Ansari and Mandal (1977) also reported a similar change.

In this type of dehydration there are two physiological disturbances present, namely, a loss of body water and a maldistribution of water between the major compartments of body water. This variety of dehydration is sometimes incorrectly equated with hyperosmolar dehydration, but although hypernatraemia is the most frequent cause of hyperosmolality in infants, high blood glucose levels, for example, may also be the cause, and hyperosmolar dehydration may occur in diabetes mellitus without hypernatraemia.

Some of the factors predisposing to hypernatraemic dehydration are listed in Table 6.12.

Table 6.12
Factors predisposing to hypernatraemic dehydration

Prematurity	{ Small mass relative to surface area { Immaturity of renal function
Increased insensible water loss	{ Prolonged fever { Hyperventilation { Salicylate toxicity { Low humidity
High solute load in feeding Cessation of intake	

Finberg (1973) has reviewed hypernatraemic dehydration in detail and has observed that the relative preservation of the circulation and the early presence of neurological symptoms are hallmarks of the disorder.

The volume of the extracellular fluid tends to be maintained to a greater degree in hypertonic dehydration when compared with isotonic dehydration and so signs of circulatory collapse appear later. Their appearance is ominous because of the degree of water deficit by then apparent. In addition, the usual skin criteria for diagnosing dehydration are not accurate, the skin having a characteristic doughy consistency. The fontanelle is typically not sunken, and in many cases may even bulge. There is a clinical impression that this type of dehydration tends to occur more often in obese infants, and there is a risk in such infants that the signs of dehydration may be underestimated because of their obesity. The state of consciousness is usually depressed, and some infants with a severe degree of hypernatraemic dehydration may have convulsions, which may be related to brain shrinkage, a drop in CSF pressure causing haemorrhage in the central nervous system. Cerebral thromboses may also sometimes occur. Renal tubular necrosis and hyocalcaemic tetany are less common complications but hyperglycaemia may often accompany hypernatraemia and may lead to an incorrect diagnosis of diabetes mellitus being made. Such a phenomenon is transient and tends to occur when there is co-existent severe acidosis. Insulin should not be given because lowering of blood glucose levels may enhance the risks of developing cerebral oedema during treatment, as correction of the fluid and electrolyte balance may be too rapid.

Hyponatraemia and Hypokalaemia

These biochemical findings are more common in those infants who are already severely malnourished when they develop gastroenteritis. It is known that there is a predisposition for such infants to develop hypotonic dehydration. Abdominal distension and absent or markedly diminished bowel sounds strongly suggest K^+ depletion.

It is important to realise that the aetiology of gastroenteritis and the water and electrolyte disturbances that occur have a profound geographical variation. Observations made in one country or even in one region may not be appropriate to another country or to another region within the same country. While hypertonic dehydration is now common in the United States, as mentioned earlier, a high incidence of hyponatraemia and hypokalaemia has been reported from many places including the West Indies, Africa and among Australian aborigines. Kingston (1973) found that more than 80 per cent of infants in Liberia with gastroenteritis had hypotonic dehydration. He has emphasised the importance of recognition of hypokalaemia in these circumstances and its appropriate treatment. Kingston believes that continued intake of small amounts of breast milk at frequent intervals while diarrhoea continues is an important factor in the infants he described, as the sodium and potassium contents of breast milk are so low (Table 6.13). He considers that a different pattern of water and electrolyte disturbance is seen when gastroenteritis occurs in breast fed infants as distinct from formula fed children. Table 6.13

indicates the amounts of Na^+ and K^+ found in breast and cow's milk but the range for breast milk is very wide.

Table 6.13
Mean values for Na^+ and K^+ (mEq/l)

	Na^+	K^+
Breast milk	6	13
Cow's milk	23	37

The amount of Na^+ and K^+ in breast milk is far less than the average stool electrolyte losses (*see* Table 6.15) and so the net loss of Na^+ and K^+ is relatively in excess of the net loss of water in breast fed infants with gastroenteritis. This is a most unusual finding in Western countries where gastroenteritis is so uncommon in breast fed infants. These considerations have important implications in the management of gastroenteritis, which will be discussed later.

Acidosis

Various theories have been put forward to explain the aetiology of the metabolic acidosis that occurs in infants with severe gastroenteritis accompanying clinical dehydration. At present it seems that excessive intestinal losses of bicarbonate or non-absorbed organic acids are the most important causes in these children. In children with cholera, the intestinal loss of bicarbonate has been shown to be a major cause of their acidosis. Blood gas estimation together with the measurement of blood pH are useful investigations in a child who is severely dehydrated.

Acute Renal Failure

When this occurs as a complication of gastroenteritis, it may be due to oligaemia, producing reversible failure of renal function. This responds well to intravenous fluids. Much less commonly, it may be due to acute renal tubular necrosis. The prognosis of such a complication is often not good but it may respond to appropriate management.

MANAGEMENT

The successful therapy of gastroenteritis in children relies upon the maintenance or restoration of adequate hydration and electrolyte balance. In most children this may be achieved by manipulating the diet but when this fails and significant dehydration occurs intravenous fluids are required. Wheatley (1968) found that nine out of ten children could be managed successfully at home, and only one required hospital admission.

Diet Therapy

The principles of this management are to stop all solids and to replace the child's milk feeds with clear fluids or a dilute milk feed is given hourly or two-hourly for 24 hours. Usually, vomiting and diarrhoea stop under this regime. If it does not happen, the child is often admitted to hospital for observation because either the child has a severe form of gastroenteritis and will require intravenous fluids, or there is some other malady, or possibly his mother has not been giving him the oral regime as recommended.

There is no general agreement about the best oral feeding for the infant who is managed in this way, but it is clear that whatever is given the aim should be to provide a total fluid intake greater than about 20 per cent of the child's usual fluid requirements so that the input of fluid will keep pace with the fluid loss.

Table 6.14 indicates the theoretical fluid requirements in ml/kg at various ages throughout childhood.

Table 6.14
Fluid requirements in childhood

Age	Fluid requirements (ml/kg/day)
1st day of life	60
2nd day of life	90
3rd day of life	120
up to 9 months	120–150
12 months	90–100
2 years	80–90
4 years	70–80
8 years	60–70
12 years	50–60

A wide range of oral replacement fluids has been recommended for children with gastroenteritis. Table 6.15 shows a comparison of the sodium and potassium content of diarrhoeal fluid and some of these replacement solutions.

Weil has laid down certain guiding principles in relation to the oral feeding referred to earlier, but it is apparent from this table that very widely ranging solutions in relation to electrolyte content are used. Glucose has been recommeneded for many years, e.g. by Darrow and his colleagues in 1949, and evidence has now been produced to show that there are good reasons for using it. It has been established that there is coupled absorption and transport for glucose and sodium in the small intestinal mucosa and, as a consequence, the absorption of sodium and water is greatly stimulated by luminal glucose. Hirschhorn and his colleagues (1973) and others have found that glucose-electrolyte mixtures given by mouth or by intubation greatly diminish the intestinal loss of fluids and electrolytes in children with cholera.

They have extended this type of therapy to infants with acute diarrhoea due to other causes, with success. The solution they use in these circumstances is called Ge-Sol and its sodium and potassium composition is indicated in Table 6.15.

Table 6.15
Comparison of sodium and potassium content (mEq/l) of diarrhoeal fluid and oral replacement solutions

Fluid	Sodium	Potassium
Diarrhoeal fluid	50–100	20–40
Half-strength Darrow's	60	18
Electrosol tablets	46	17
Half-strength normal saline	74	—
Glucose-electrolyte mixture (MRC & QEH)	24	28
Sucrose-electrolyte mixture (OPEM & QEH)	24	28
Ge-Sol (Hirschhorn et al.)	81	18
WHO	90	20

The sodium content of this solution is within the range of the sodium content found in diarrhoeal fluid but it is higher in electrolyte content than the other solutions. Unless large volumes are taken there is a risk of hypernatraemia with this solution, except in communities where hyponatraemia is common, e.g. communities where there is a high incidence of protein-calorie malnutrition. Also, if diarrhoea ceases immediately, too much sodium can be given, especially in small infants. However, in view of the declining importance of hypernatraemic dehydration in developed countries, due to widespread use of low solute milks and better education, this risk may not now be so great.

Oral half-strength Darrow's solution is widely used in developing countries. Electrosol tablets when dissolved produce an adequate electrolyte solution for oral use, but as tablets, they do carry the risk of being given in excess dosage. Half-strength saline contains no potassium and significant potassium loss does occur in gastroenteritis, but in emergencies this solution flavoured with a little orange juice may be very useful until other solutions can be obtained.

The glucose-electrolyte mixture used at the Queen Elizabeth Hospital is based on one devised by the Medical Research Council in 1952 and modified for pharmaceutical reasons. Its composition is indicated in Table 6.16.

Table 6.16
Electrolyte composition of glucose-electrolyte mixture in mEq/l (QEH)

	Na^+	K^+	Ca^{++}	Mg^{++}	H^+	Cl'	Cit''	PO_4''
$CaCl_2$			4			4		
$MgCl_2$				4		4		
KCl		7				7		
NaCl	9					9		
K_3Cit		21					21	
Na_3Cit	10						10	
NaH_2PO_4	5				4			9
	24	28	4	4	4	24	31	9

This solution contains small amounts of Ca^{++} and Mg^{++} because of the occasional finding of reduced serum levels of these electrolytes in children with gastroenteritis. It contains 50 g glucose/litre.

One dissenting voice about the role of glucose is Ironside (1973), who cautions against the unrestricted use of glucose because of the risk of making up a hypertonic solution and so aggravating the clinical situation by producing more vomiting and diarrhoea due to osmolar effect. However, the glucose-electrolyte mixture has been used for many years with success at the Queen Elizabeth Hospital, for in-patients, and in view of this, and the theoretical advantage referred to earlier, the author used to feel that a glucose-electrolyte mixture was the ideal fluid to use for these children. However, glucose-electrolyte mixture (GEM) is a ready-made solution. Once opened for use it has a short 'shelf life' because of the risk of bacterial contamination. Hence, at the Queen Elizabeth Hospital, whereas in-patients have been given a glucose-electrolyte solution, out-patients have for many years been managed with a sucrose electrolyte solution, known as out-patient electrolyte mixture (OPEM). The electrolyte solution is supplied in a concentrated form and diluted five times with water; sucrose is then added at home.

In view of the theoretical advantages of glucose in cholera toxin induced diarrhoea and the experience of its use in diarrhoeal states not due to cholera, by Hirschhorn and colleagues (1973), as well as the theoretical drawback of using a sucrose solution because of the documented low sucrase levels found in the small intestinal mucosa in acute gastroenteritis (Barnes and Townley, 1973), on two occasions a clinical comparison of the use of glucose and sucrose additions to a basic electrolyte mixture in the outpatient management of acute gastroenteritis in children was undertaken (Rahilly *et al.*, 1976; Hutchins *et al.*, 1978). The osmolality of these two solutions are indicated in Table 6.17.

Table 6.17
Osmolality of 5% carbohydrate electrolyte solutions in milliosmoles per litre

Glucose electrolyte mixture (GEM)	351
Sucrose electrolyte mixture (OPEM)	261

These two studies at the Queen Elizabeth Hospital were carried out on out-patients attending casualty during the winter months, two years apart. Both showed that, in those given GEM (27 and 32 per cent respectively in the two studies) more children experienced failure with out-patient management and required admision compared with those given OPEM (10 and 18 per cent). As social reasons often contributed to failure in outpatient management, these studies can only be cited as evidence that a sucrose electrolyte solution appeared to be at least as good as glucose in the out-patient management of acute gastroenteritis in a developed community.

The second study (Hutchins *et al.*, 1978) did, however, make it clear that it was easier to make an error when the solution was made up with glucose and could lead to unacceptably high levels of osmolality in some instances. Such high levels could contribute to out-patient management failure. The author considers that a sucrose electrolyte solution with its lower osmolality, ready availability, and economic advantages commends its use both in developed and also in developing countries, from which encouraging results have been reported, from Indonesia (Moenginah *et al.*, 1975) and also from Calcutta (Chatterjee *et al.*, 1977).

Experimental animal work from Hamilton *et al.* (1976) provides a theoretical basis for the view that there is no specific benefit in using a glucose electrolyte solution when there is viral gastroenteritis. Using a transmissable gastroenteritis virus (TGE) to study gastroenteritis in pigs, they have been able to study glucose-stimulated sodium transport which, in fact, falls to its lowest level at the peak of the diarrhoea. Thus, it seems probable that in viral gastroenteritis, carbohydrate electrolyte solutions merely provide calories and are unlikely to have a specific effect on sodium absorption.

After 24 hours of such a mixture, milk may be gradually reintroduced into the child's diet by a system of regrading. There is often some looseness of stools after gastroenteritis and it is usually recommended to grade the infant back on to his usual feeding formula. The rapidity of the regrading will be adapted to the child's circumstances and may be done in quarter or fifth strength increments. At the Queen Elizabeth Hospital the glucose-electrolyte mixture is used to dilute the feeding throughout this regrading period. Table 6.18 indicates the regrading regime.

Table 6.18
Table of suggested regrading of feeds

		Regrading by quarters ml/kg corrected weight
Day 1	GEM*	150
Day 2	GEM	115
	Milk feeding	35
Day 3	GEM	75
	Milk feeding	75
Day 4	GEM	35
	Milk feeding	115
Day 5	GEM	—
	Milk feeding	150

* GEM—Glucose-electrolyte mixture.

Once the child is on to the full strength formula, solids may be reintroduced to his diet.

It is important for mothers to realise that some looseness of stools may persist for several days after gastroenteritis and that it may take some weeks for the normal rate of weight gain to be restored. When significant diarrhoea and failure to gain weight persist, further investigations are warranted. This will be discussed later under the complications of gastroenteritis.

In communities where malnutrition is common it is important that there should not be any prolonged reduction of caloric intake following gastroenteritis and it is vital that a starvation diet for a long interval should be avoided. Except during acute water and electrolyte disturbance the diet of malnourished children should not be unduly restricted even though increased feedings may accentuate diarrhoea. Provided this does not lead to dehydration and further electrolyte disturbances in these children, it is important to continue with an oral feed containing an adequate amount of calories. Such malnourished infants tolerate further caloric restriction very poorly and diarrhoea may even become worse with the untoward consequences. This is a quite different situation from that of the previously well-nourished child who develops gastroenteritis.

Intravenous Therapy

Intravenous therapy for dehydration in man was first used by a Scottish general practitioner, Dr Thomas Latta, in 1832, with some success, but it was long before this treatment became accepted. Gamble (1953) reviewed the subsequent history of this technique, and it was indeed notably Gamble, and also Darrow and colleagues, who in the 1940s and 1950s put safe intravenous therapy in childhood, on the therapeutic map. The subject has been well reviewed by Weil (1969) and Finberg (1970).

Fortunately, in the developed world, despite the continuing importance of acute gastroenteritis, the numbers of children with severe dehydration requiring intravenous fluids is falling. In 1973, at the Queen Elizabeth Hospital, only 60 from the 353 children admitted with acute gastroenteritis in Gribbin and her colleagues' categories A and B required intravenous fluids. Nevertheless, when needed, the condition is often urgent, and in the developing world severely dehydrated children requiring intravenous fluids continue to be a common problem.

There are three important phases in intravenous therapy; namely, resuscitation, rehydration and maintenance. These will be outlined first of all for children with isotonic dehydration.

Resuscitation

If a child is shocked (i.e. he is pulseless or has a low blood pressure and peripheral cyanosis) he needs a rapid infusion of fluids as a matter of urgency. He may require up to 15 to 20 ml fluid per kilogram of body weight to be administered over 10 to 15 minutes, to rapidly restore his state of acute oligaemia. More often a child who needs resuscitation is not so severely ill and may just have some peripheral cyanosis and a history of oliguria. He should then have an initial infusion of between 40 to 80 ml/kg actual body weight given over four hours. Such an infusion is considered adequate if at least 10 ml/kg actual body weight of urine is passed within the first four hours of the infusion. If inadequate urine is obtained the infusion should be continued and the clinical situation reviewed. If anuria persists, then the child should be managed as for renal failure. This will be discussed further under management of complications.

Table 6.19 is a guide to the amount of fluid that should be given during this resuscitation phase.

Table 6.19
Volume to be given over four hours

5% dehydration	40 ml/kg
5–7% dehydration	60 ml/kg
10% dehydration	80 ml/kg

The infusion fluids given vary considerably from unit to unit but 0·45 per cent sodium chloride in 5 per cent dextrose or half-strength Darrow's solution in 5 per cent glucose are most often used. Hartmann's solution, a stable plasma protein solution, or an albumin solution may all be used (Table 6.20).

Table 6.20
Composition of intravenous fluids (mEq/l)

	Sodium	Potassium	Chloride	Calcium	Lactate
Isotonic or physiological saline	154	—	154	—	—
Half isotonic (dextrose 5%, sodium chloride 0·45%)	77	—	77	—	—
Quarter isotonic (dextrose 3·75% sodium chloride 0·225%)	38	—	38	—	—
Fifth isotonic (dextrose 4% sodium chloride 0·18%	30	—	30	—	—
Hartmann's solution	131	5	112	4	28
Half-strength Darrow's solution	60	18	52	—	25

Once the child's circulation has been restored and he is passing urine, care should be taken not to give him too much fluid. Constant reassessment, clinically, is necessary.

Rehydration

When the infant is not oliguric and there is no peripheral circulatory failure, an initial infusion is not required. He should be rehydrated according to a calculation based on a clinical estimate of his percentage dehydration. When the infant who requires resuscitation has had an initial infusion and he is passing urine he should then be reassessed and future fluid requirements calculated according to his current estimated percentage dehydration. Caution should be used in rehydration, for too rapid rehydration may lead to central nervous system disturbances with convulsions. An infant who is estimated to be 5 per cent dry, is rehydrated over 24 hours. The calculated amount of fluid for rehydration is given as half isotonic saline with dextrose, either 2·5 or 5 per cent, and this is added to his normal daily maintenance fluid requirement.

The volume of fluid given for rehydration in the first 24 hours should not normally exceed that calculated for a 5 per cent deficit. When greater deficits are present the aim should be to rehydrate the child over 48 hours or more.

Example: Child weighing 7·8 kg estimated to be 5 per cent dehydrated

Amount of fluid to be given:

$$\frac{5}{100} \times 7\cdot8 \times 1{,}000 \text{ ml} \quad + \quad 7\cdot8 \times 150 \text{ ml}$$

as half isotonic saline and glucose

as quarter or fifth isotonic saline and glucose

Intraveneous Therapy in Relation to the Aetiology of Gastroenteritis

In general, children require intravenous fluids when they are significantly dehydrated regardless of aetiology. Relative specifically to rotavirus gastroenteritis Hamilton *et al.* (1976) think that speedier cessation of diarrhoea may occur when intravenous fluids are used regardless of state of hydration. Certainly, Torres-Pinedo, Lavastida and Rivera (1966) have shown a sudden fall in stool electrolytes when milk is withdrawn from the diet of infants with gastroenteritis. There is a firm clinical impression that when intravenous fluids are given to these children with nil by mouth for a short period, recovery is rapid and uneventful. Nevertheless, it would not in general be our practice at present to use intravenous fluids unless the infant was 5 per cent or more dehydrated.

Maintenance

The usual daily maintenance fluid requirement ranges from 150 ml/kg of body weight for an infant a few weeks old to 50–60 ml/kg for a child aged twelve years (*see* Table 6.14) and it should be given as 0·225 per cent or 0·18 per cent saline with glucose.

Daily sodium requirements are of the order of 2 to 3 mEq/kg of body weight. Maintenance potassium requirements aproximate 3 mEq/kg of body weight. Administration of potassium should begin as soon as urinary output is satisfactory, care being taken not to infuse a concentration of potassium greater than 40 mEq/l except in a severely malnourished child (*see* page 231). N.B.: Hartmann's and Darrow's solutions both contain potassium but in practice this usually does not appear to be a problem when these solutions are used for resuscitation. Their continued use in a child with anuria should, however, be carefully reviewed.

Investigations

Serum electrolytes, blood urea and total serum protein levels should be estimated as a matter of urgency in all children who are shocked, and within twenty-four hours in all children who are given intravenous fluids, for evidence of any electrolyte level disturbances, especially hypernatraemia, and as a confirmation of the state of dehydration. The levels of blood urea and total protein are sensitive indices of dehydration. Other useful investigations include haemoglobin and also blood gas estimation when signs of acidosis are present.

Management of Complications of Fluid, Electrolyte and Acid-base Balance

Hypernatraemic Dehydration

The management of hypernatraemic dehydration is more difficult than that of isotonic dehydration and there is still controversy as to the best method.

The principal hazard of managing infants with hypernatraemic dehydration is the risk of water intoxication, with cerebral oedema. This may occur when rehydration is too rapid and may manifest as convulsions due to cerebral oedema.

Finberg (1973) has reviewed the best therapy for this condition. Firstly, when circulatory failure is present in these infants, rapid correction of the failure is the aim, as with isotonic dehydration. He recommends the use of plasma or an albumin solution. Secondly, when there are no signs of circulatory failure but the child is anuric he recommends an initial infusion of a solution containing sodium, 75 to 80 mEq/l in 5 per cent glucose, but no added potassium until urine is passed. Thirdly, as the next phase in management in these children, or the initial phase in those infants without either circulatory failure or anuria, he recommends slow rehydration over 48 hours with a relatively dilute solution and a sodium concentration of 25 to 40 mEq/l to which potassium is added. There are risks from giving the higher sodium solution too rapidly or for too long, and also from giving potassium too soon. Provided there is no circulatory failure and no anuria the guiding principle should be to rehydrate the child slowly to allow physiological adjustment to occur. The aim is to lower serum sodium slowly as well as slowly to restore hydration; rapid reduction of serum sodium by rapid rehydration with a dilute solution may cause cerebral oedema with convulsions.

Hyponatraemic Dehydration with Hypokalaemia

Despite the low sodium level when hyponatraemia is present in malnourished children, Garrow, Smith and Ward (1968) have shown that total body sodium is usually raised, hence 0·18 per cent saline (1/5 isotonic saline) is recommended for rehydration as well as maintenance. In the previously well-nourished child, the regime described above for isotonic dehydration is appropriate, except when levels below 110 mEq/l occur, when extra sodium may be required. When there is severe hypokalaemia (serum K^+ less than $1\cdot5$ mEq/l) in a severely malnourished child, large amounts of K^+ may need to be given, 80 or 100 mEq/l. This is because Kunin, Surawicz and Sims (1962) have shown that infusion of moderate concentrations of K^+ together with glucose leads to a further fall of serum K^+ due to re-entry of K^+ into the depleted intracellular space.

These differences in the management of dehydration which depend upon the type of dehydration present and the presence of pre-existing malnutrition, emphasise the importance of adjusting the type of management to the pattern of disease in a particular community. There is no universal way of managing all children with dehydration.

Acidosis

Partial correction of the acidosis with intravenous bicarbonate may be of great value in desperately ill infants, the aim being to correct half the calculated base deficit. Care should be taken not to give the bicarbonate directly into the child's veins too rapidly as there is then a risk of cardiac arrest. Further, it should be added to the other intravenous fluids. In less severely ill infants correction of the dehydration alone will restore acid-base balance and bicarbonate therapy is unnecessary.

Acute Renal Failure

Once acute oliguria, i.e. a urine output of less than 10 ml/kg, has been present for more than four hours after the intravenous fluids have been started, Wharton (1968) has recommended considering the use of frusemide intravenously. Frusemide, when given intravenously, may present minimal renal shut-down. A dose of 1 mg/kg may be given provided the blood urea *is not* more than 300 mg/100 ml, as it is in about 1 per cent of children with gastroenteritis. If this fails renal dialysis would then have to be considered.

Drug Therapy

Anti-diarrhoeal drugs and anti-emetics are not recommended for most infants and children with gastroenteritis. Although in the older child, where vomiting is the dominant symptom, intramuscular anti-emetics, e.g. Stemetil, given in an appropriate dosage may be useful. Stemetil suppositories should never be given as their absorption is unpredictable and the therapy may be complicated by dystonic reactions. The incidence of such side effects is much higher in children than in adults. Lomotil, morphine derivatives and preparations containing kaolin and pectin, appear to have little value in the small child with gastroenteritis, although they may afford symptomatic relief in the older child or adolescent.

Yet, despite lack of convincing evidence for their effectiveness, anti-diarrhoeal drugs continue in practice to be prescribed for infants and young children. The best evidence for their lack of effectiveness is provided by the study of 80 children, aged 3 to 11 years, with acute diarrhoea in Guatemala (Portnoy *et al.*, 1976). They found that kaolin and pectin preparations and Lomotil were no different from placebo in their effect on stool frequency, stool water content or stool weight, although kaolin-pectin concentrate did produce fewer liquid stools. However, this effect is purely aesthetic and of no value to the child. The use of these drugs in younger children should be resisted.

Antibiotics have little place in the management of children with gastroenteritis. This is because, firstly, in most children, no bacterial pathogen is isolated from the stools; secondly, antibiotics may sometimes prolong the carrier state, for example in salmonella infections (Dixon, 1965); thirdly, there is little evidence that antibiotics influence the natural history of the disease even when bacterial pathogens are present; fourthly, there is conflicting evidence that antibiotics eliminate these pathogenic organisms from the gut; fifthly, as a consequence, it is uncertain whether they can prevent the spread of infection from one child to another.

Antibiotics are indicated when blood stream infection occurs in children with salmonella infections, but obviously antibiotics should also be given if there is an intercurrent indication, e.g. co-existent otitis media. Their place in the management of enteropathogenic *E. coli* infections and shigellosis is controversial. Neomycin has been claimed by some authors to be effective in eliminating these organisms from the stools; intramuscular ampicillin therapy has been claimed by others to be more effective in shigellosis. There are also reports of neomycin-resistant strains of enteropathogenic *E. coli*, Colistin then being recommended as a substitute. There is no general agreement on the role of antibiotics in these infections and some authors are of the opinion there is no convincing evidence that antibiotics do the least good in such children. Ironside (1973) has commented that their indiscriminate use may lead to the transfer of antibiotic resistance to other coliforms and that their use is a form of environmental pollution.

COMPLICATIONS OF GASTROENTERITIS

Apart from the acute disturbances of water, electrolyte and acid-base balance that may complicate gastroenteritis, there are a number of problems that may follow acute gastroenteritis. These include problems at the time of re-grading and also long-standing problems associated with chronic diarrhoea and failure to thrive. These complications are listed in Table 6.21.

Table 6.21
Complications of acute gastroenteritis

Immediate
Dehydration
Electrolyte imbalance
    hypernatraemia
    hyponatraemia
    hypokalaemia
Acid-base disturbance
    acidosis

Protein losing enteropathy
On initial regrading
    monosaccharide intolerance
    disaccharide intolerance

Chronic diarrhoea (postenteritis syndrome)
Food intolerance syndromes
    monosaccharide intolerance
    disaccharide intolerance
    cow's milk protein intolerance
Chronic diarrhoeal syndromes of unknown aetiology
        may be associated with—
    persistent small intestinal mucosal damage
    alteration of bacterial flora (quantitative and qualitative)

Protein-losing enteropathy is not a common complication, but when it occurs it is usually brief and self-limiting. It may temporarily cause diagnostic confusion with other causes of protein-losing enteropathy such as small intestinal lymphangiectasia (*see* page 333).

The syndromes of sugar intolerance may manifest as a brief self-limiting problem at the time of initial regrading, but sometimes may persist. At other times the syndrome may present later, sometimes as part of a more severe syndrome with chronic diarrhoea and failure to thrive.

Food intolerance has been known for some time to be a sequel to gastroenteritis. Sunshine and Kretchmer (1964) described fat and sugar malabsorption as sequelae of gastroenteritis. Burke, Kerry and Anderson, in 1965, emphasised the importance of lactose intolerance as a cause of refractory watery diarrhoea in infancy. They described a group of infants who had transient lactose malabsorption following clinical gastroenteritis in association with an abnormal small intestinal mucosa and low lactase levels. In relation to protein intolerance, transient gluten intolerance and temporary cow's milk protein intolerance have been described following gastroenteritis. These two syndromes are discussed in chapter 5.

Sugar and/or fat malabsorption may manifest immediately after gastroenteritis. As a result, the term post-gastroenteritis malabsorption has been used to describe this condition, yet clinically detectable malabsorption may not always be present despite the presence of chronic diarrhoea and failure to thrive following an attack of acute gastroenteritis. It is therefore suggested that the term post-enteritis syndrome is a more useful term when defined as follows:

The post-enteritis syndrome is the clinical syndrome when a child who has had an attack of acute gastroenteritis subsequently has intermittent or chronic diarrhoea with or without failure to gain weight following the return to a normal diet.

In clinical practice two main groups of problems cause delayed recovery after acute gastroenteritis in infancy. First, there is an acute intolerance to the increasing concentration of milk, and secondly, there is a more chronic problem with persistent diarrhoea and failure to thrive.

DELAYED RECOVERY AFTER GASTROENTERITIS

With acute intolerance to milk there is a return of diarrhoea, which is often watery and copious and sometimes accompanied by vomiting. This syndrome is most often due to malabsorption of lactose and sometimes also of sucrose, but there may also be intolerance to cow's milk protein (*see* chapter 5). Sometimes, in addition, there may be monosaccharide intolerance (*see* chapter 7). It is often brief in duration but it may also persist.

Fat malabsorption may occur; indeed, some degree of temporary steatorrhoea is a frequent accompaniment of gastroenteritis. This can be demonstrated indirectly by estimating plasma vitamin A (a fat soluble vitamin) at the time of acute episode of gastroenteritis and after recovery. This will show a low level, and rise to normal on recovery (Araya *et al.*, 1975), although factors other than Vitamin A malabsorption may also play a part in this change in Vitamin A blood levels, such as decreased mobilisation of stores. Sivakumar and Reddy (1972) have shown impaired absorption of labelled vitamin A acetate in gastroenteritis, and steatorrhoea may also be demonstrated by a conventional fat balance.

The more chronic problem of persistent diarrhoea and failure to gain weight following gastroenteritis is more difficult to settle and may be confused with coeliac disease when the child's diet includes gluten. Indeed, the differential diagnosis of any child under two years with chronic diarrhoea and failure to thrive is an important problem. In these circumstances the following diagnoses need to be considered, namely, post-enteritis syndrome, coeliac disease, cystic fibrosis, giardiasis and cow's milk protein intolerance as well as an anatomical abnormality of the small intestine. Chronic diarrhoea without failure to thrive following acute gastroenteritis needs to be distinguished from toddler's diarrhoea in which there is chronic diarrhoea but no failure to thrive (*see* chapter 12). Sometimes long-term follow up is the only way to establish the diagnosis definitely. In view of this, when symptoms have been present for three weeks or more after gastroenteritis, and there is doubt about the diagnosis, a small intestinal biopsy should be considered. This will demonstrate whether there is any structural abnormality of the small intestinal mucosa that may account for the child's continuing symptoms (Fig. 6.14). Such mucosal damage may be a sequel to acute gastroenteritis or relate to another disease entity such as coeliac disease.

Indeed the mucosa is flat, the diagnosis of coeliac disease must be considered provided the child is eating gluten, even though it is known that gastroenteritis *per se* may cause a flat mucosa. Only reinvestigation at a later date after a period on a gluten-free diet, as outlined in chapter 4, will enable the final diagnosis to be made.

Why such persistent mucosal damage occurs in some children after gastroenteritis yet not in others is at present the subject of investigation since most children who develop acute gastroenteritis have a short illness from which they recover quickly. Indeed why some children develop delayed recovery after gastroenteritis and others do not is far from clear. Gribbin, Walker-Smith and Wood (1976) endeavoured to analyse the clinical factors that may predispose to the development of delayed recovery in a prospective study of the problem at the Queen Elizabeth Hospital in 1973. They found delayed recovery occurred in 74 of the 348 children in Groups A and B (page 214) admitted to the gastroenteritis unit who survived acute gastroenteritis (21·2 per cent), and went on to analyse the clinical factors that appeared to predispose to delayed recovery.

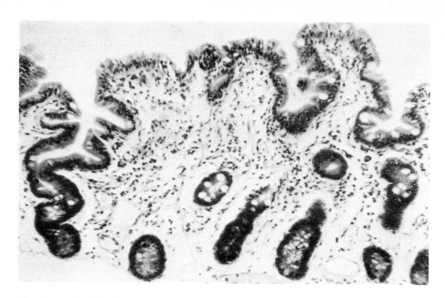

Fig. 6.14. Partial villous atrophy occurring as a sequel to gastroenteritis.

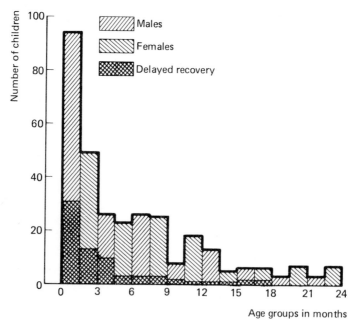

Fig. 6.15. Age and sex of children with delayed recovery after gastroenteritis under two years.

The prevalence of delayed recovery in 214 children under two years of age with simple acute gastroenteritis (Group A) (*see* page 214) admitted to the unit in 1973 is indicated in Fig. 6.15. This shows that delayed recovery was a problem confined to infants under eighteen months of age and particularly to those under six months. The largest group was under the age of 3 months at the time of the acute attack. In this youngest age group there was a clear male predominance. Analysis of more recent experience between 4th October 1976 and 20th January 1978 (Manuel, 1978) has shown a comparable prevalence of delayed recovery in the age group under 6 months, namely 30 per cent, compared to 27 per cent in 1973. There has, however, been a reduction in the total number of children admitted under 6 months, and a reduction particularly in those admitted under 3 months of age. The reason for this welcome change parallels the increase in breast feeding in the community and also the change in artificial feeding from high solute milks to low solute milks (*see* page 26) between 1973

Table 6.22
Admissions to Gastroenteritis Unit,
Queen Elizabeth Hospital

	1973	*1977*
Total	472	425
Under 6 months	212	121

and 1977 (Table 6.22). Nevertheless, delayed recovery is more likely to occur in infants who develop gastroenteritis under 6 months, and also, it is more likely to be a more serious problem within that age range.

Gribbin, Walker-Smith and Wood (1973) also found that there was a higher incidence of delayed recovery in infants whose weight on admission, corrected for dehydration, was below the 3rd percentile. This was related to the ethnic origin of the children concerned (Table 6.23).

Thus, the incidence of delayed recovery was more than doubled when the weight was under the 3rd percentile compared with those over the 50th percentile. Weight on admission reflects nutrition. So nutrition appeared to have an important influence. Nevertheless, there were 11 children who developed delayed recovery whose weight was above the 50th percentile on admission.

Table 6.23
Incidence of delayed recovery according to weight* on admissions

Ethnic origin	I Below 3rd percentile			II 3rd–50th percentile			III Above 50th percentile			Total		
	DR	NR	Total	DR	NR	Total	DR	NR	Total	DR	NR	Total
North European	5	15	20	15	72	87	6	43	49	26	130	156
Asian	7	5	12	11	15	26	1	7	8	19	27	46
Negro	1	2	3	3	24	27	4	7	11	8	33	41
Mediterranean	1	—	1	2	3	5	—	3	3	3	6	9
Total	14	22	36	31	114	145	11	60	71	56	196	252
Percent delayed recovery	39%			21%			15%			26%		
Chi-square (P)	I-II: 4.73 (0.1<P<0.05)			II-III: 1.05 (n.s.)			I-III: 7.3 (P<0.01)			I-II+III: 6.75 (P<0.01)		

Weight on admission corrected for dehydration; children with birthweights under 2,500 g or twins were excluded.
DR: delayed recovery. NR: normal recovery.

The relationship of delayed recovery to ethnic origin in their study as a whole is indicated in Table 6.24. Apart from a numerically small mediterranean group, the Asian infants, that is infants originating

Table 6.24
Relationship of delayed recovery to ethnic origin

Ethnic origin	Total number of children with acute gastro-enteritis	Delayed recovery following acute gastroenteritis	
		Number of children	% ethnic total
North European	208	48	23·0
Asian	72	24	33·3
Negro	58	10	17·2
Mediterranean	12	7	58·3
Mixed parentage	17	4	23·5
Total	367	93	25·3

Table 6.25
Possible factors influencing delayed recovery after gastroenteritis

1. Type of feeding—breast or bottle— influencing age of presentation and size of problem.

2. Age at time of acute gastroenteritis— influencing severity and size of problem severer problems under 6 months.

3. Nutrition— undernutrition may predispose.

4. Ethnic group may predispose— ?nutrition ?genetic.

5. Sex. Male sex more vulnerable in early infancy.

from the Indian sub-continent, had the highest incidence of delayed recovery. It is likely there may be both a genetic and nutritional reason for this. Asian children have a high incidence of lactase deficiency (see page 240), and undernutrition is more common in this group.

Table 6.25 summarises factors that may predispose to delayed recovery.

The categories of delayed recovery recognised in the study of Gribbin *et al.*, are listed in Table 6.26. Persistent diarrhoea was a consistent feature of all three categories but disaccharide intolerance was a simple and easily resolved problem (*see* chapter 7). The other two categories with persistent diarrhoea, some of whom also had evidence of sugar intolerance, and were a more difficult and intractable problem, were grouped together as the post-enteritis syndrome (*see* page 272).

Table 6.26
Categories of delayed recovery
(Gribbin *et al.* 1976)

1. Disaccharide intolerance	38
2. Prolonged diarrhoea	14
3. Failure to thrive	36

Disaccharide Intolerance

Of infants prospectively observed after acute gastroenteritis, 9·9 per cent developed disaccharide intolerance. Table 6.27 indicates the relationship to ethnic origin.

Table 6.27
Disaccharide intolerance related to ethnic origin

Ethnic origin	Total number of children	Children showing disaccharide intolerance (children receiving special feeds in brackets)	
		Number of children	% of ethnic total
North European	208	16 (11)	7·7 (5·3)
Asian	72	15 (9)	20·8 (12·5)
Negro	58	4 (3)	6·9 (5·2)
Mediterranean	12	1 (1)	8·3 (8·3)
Mixed parentage	17	2 (2)	11·8 (11·8)
Total	367	38 (26)	10·3 (7·0)

It is clear that Asian infants were most often affected. There was a wide variation in time interval before diarrhoea with excess reducing substances appeared after there was a return to a milk-containing diet. Most often the interval was a week or less, but sometimes it was as long as a month.

Post-enteritis Syndrome

The postenteritis syndrome as defined earlier (*see* page 234) developed in 50 children in Gribbin's study.

Why did this syndrome occur? In some patients (14 out of 25 biopsied) small intestinal biopsy indicated that there was a mucosal abnormality, i.e. a post-enteritis enteropathy (Fig. 6.16). In the remainder the small intestinal mucosa was normal, although it is possible that a biopsy in these circumstances could miss a patchy lesion. This, however, was less likely when the double port capsule was used (*see* page 46). The fact that there is an important difference between those with and without enteropathy was shown by Gribbin *et al.*, who found that those with an enteropathy were in-patients for 3 weeks to 7 months, only 2 for less than 6 weeks, whereas those without an enteropathy were in-patients for 2 days to 10 weeks (a mean of 3 weeks). Thus, the presence of an enteropathy was clearly associated with a more severe illness.

The cause of post-enteritis enteropathy is uncertain but one explanation is that there is an allergic or hypersensitivity reaction, i.e. there may be an immunological explanation. What evidence is there, that such a hypersensitivity reaction is present in the small intestine of those children? To find evidence for such a reaction Dr Anne Kilby at the Queen Elizabeth Hospital studied the number of plasma cells in the lamina propria of small intestinal biopsies taken from children with the post-enteritis syndrome, using an immunofluorescent technique (Kilby *et al.*, 1976). She found increased IgA cell numbers in the lamina propria, as found in coeliac disease, when the mucosa was abnormal in this syndrome but not when it was normal (Fig. 6.16).

She also found similar increases in IgM and IgE cell numbers (Figs 6.17, 6.18), but normal numbers of IgG cells and normal numbers of intraepithelial lymphocytes were found (*see* Fig. 6.19).

The possibility that the IgE-containing cells are not in fact plasma cells but mast cells coated with surface IgE has been raised by Mayrhofer (1977) from observations in the rat. He has concluded from these studies that mucosal mast cells actually contain IgE in addition to surface bound IgE.

This study therefore showed that there is some similarity between postenteritis enteropathy and the enteropathy of coeliac disease, namely, increased IgA and IgM cell numbers, and dissimilarity in that there is no increase in intraepithelial lymphocyte count (Fig. 6.19). In addition, post-enteritis enteropathy was, in general, less severe than

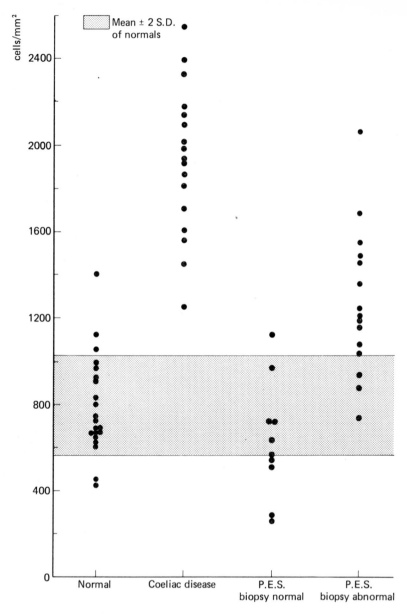

Fig. 6.16. IgA-containing plasma cells in the lamina propria of small intestinal mucosa of children with normal histology, coeliac disease, post-enteritis syndrome (PES) with normal mucosa and post-enteritis syndrome with abnormal mucosa. (Permission Kilby.)

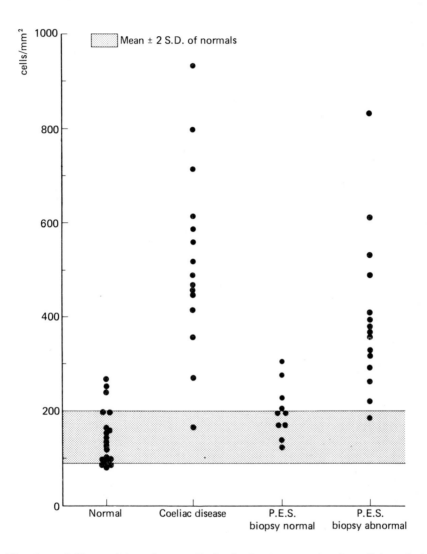

Fig. 6.17. IgM-containing plasma cells in the lamina propria of small intestinal mucosa of children with normal histology, coeliac disease, post-enteritis syndrome (PES) with normal mucosa and post-enteritis syndrome (PES) with abnormal mucosa. (Permission Kilby.)

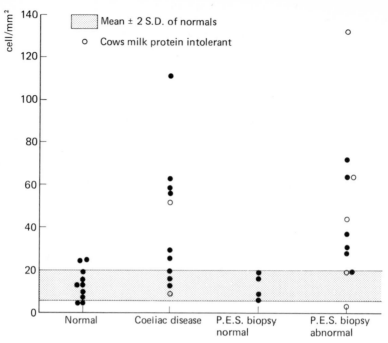

Fig. 6.18. IgE containing plasma cells in the lamina propria of small intestinal mucosa of children with normal histology, coeliac disease, post-enteritis syndrome (PES) with normal mucosa and post-enteritis syndrome (PES) with abnormal mucosa. (Permission Kilby.)

that found in coeliac disease. This demonstration of an increase in IgA, IgM and possibly IgE plasma cell numbers does not, of course, mean that they cause the lesion. Their increase may merely reflect the presence of local inflammation leading to increased traffic of plasma cell precursors to the small intestine, but the findings are at least consistent with an allergic reaction occurring in the small intestinal mucosa.

The main conclusion of such biopsy studies is that children with the post-enteritis syndrome may be divided into those with an enteropathy and those without. Zoppi, Garello and Gabarro (1977) made a similar conclusion and found 19 out of 48 children with post-enteritis diarrhoea had an abnormal small intestinal mucosa.

Two questions immediately arise—

1. What is the cause of this enteropathy?
2. What is the cause of the diarrhoea in those who do not have an enteropathy?

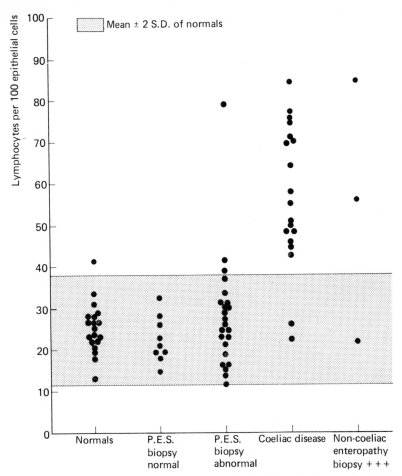

Fig. 6.19. Intraepithelial lymphocyte counts in children with normal histology, coeliac disease, post-enteritis syndrome (PES) with normal mucosa and post-enteritis syndrome (PES) with abnormal mucosa. (Permission Kilby.)

Post-enteritis Enteropathy

The persistence of an enteropathy following acute gastroenteritis, could be due to sensitisation to a variety of food protein, bacterial, and viral antigens. Considering the role of food allergy (i.e. a hypersensitivity state to a food protein that produces an allergic reaction in the small intestinal mucosa which manifests clinically as one of the syndromes of dietary protein intolerance, chapter 5) there is indeed clear evidence, that acute gastroenteritis can be followed by cow's milk protein intolerance (*see* pp. 145, 154). Why don't all infants who develop acute gastroenteritis develop this complication? One partial answer may be because there is an immunodeficiency state in those who do, allowing more antigen to enter, or there is a failure to deal with antigen that does enter the small intestinal mucosa (*see* Table 5.3). In 8/20 cases of cow's milk protein intolerance complicating acute gastroenteritis, described by Harrison *et al*. (1976), at diagnosis, the serum IgA levels were low, rising to normal levels with recovery. These data suggest that a temporary IgA deficiency may predispose to cow's milk protein intolerance. Poor nutrition may also be associated with deficient immunity and account for the predisposing role that undernutrition has. Not all children who develop this complication, however, have undernutrition.

So, in summary, food allergy or dietary protein intolerance may play a role in the genesis of postenteritis enteropathy and a transient immunodeficiency state, namely IgA deficiency or an as yet recognised immunoincompetence of the immature small intestine may play a role, with undernutrition also playing a part. The role of sensitisation to bacterial and viral antigens is at present largely unknown.

Post-enteritis Syndrome without an Enteropathy

Turning attention now to the mechanism of chronic diarrhoea in children with this syndrome who do not have an enteropathy, the role of disturbed immunological function must also be considered. Avigad *et al*. (1978) have investigated the flora of the small intestine in children with the post-enteritis syndrome. They cultured duodenal juice and the homogenised duodenal mucosa from children with the post-enteritis syndrome, children with other causes of chronic diarrhoea, and a control group of children without diarrhoea. They found no significant difference in bacterial flora as measured by total bacterial flora within these three groups. The role of bacterial colonisation of the small intestine and enteric disease was discussed briefly in chapter 1. Its role in this syndrome is not yet clear but Avigad *et al*. (1978) using an immunofluorescent technique were able to demonstrate mucosal antibodies against the bacteria grown from the luminal fluid or mucosa of the same children from children with the post-enteritis syndrome, and other causes of chronic diarrhoea. The finding of such antibodies was unrelated to the presence or absence of an enteropathy. Mucosal antibody to these non-pathogenic bacteria, obtained from the duodenal juice or homogenate culture, was present in 8 of 9 children with the post-enteritis syndrome regardless of whether an enteropathy was present. Antibody was also found in 3 children with other causes of chronic diarrhoea, but antibody was not present in the control group who did not have diarrhoea at the time of biopsy, except in one child who had previously had an enteropathy, and possibly one doubtful case who also had had a previous enteropathy. The role of such small intestinal mucosal antibodies against non-pathogenic organisms cultured from the small intestine of these children is not clear in relation to the pathogenesis of chronic diarrhoea in children, but clearly warrants further study.

Phillips *et al.* (1978) have used the scanning electron micriscope to study the surface of small intestinal lymphoid follicles obtained on proximal small intestinal biopsy (*see* Fig. 6.20). Normally, there appear to be no bacteria adhering to the surface of such follicles but, as shown in Fig. 6.20, there can be adhesion of rod-like bacteria to the surface, whereas bacteria were not adhering to the rest of the biopsy. This was a specimen taken from a child with post-enteritis syndrome shown to be producing antibody to rod-like bacteria. This preferential adhesion of bacteria to the surface of the lymphoid follicular region is interesting because there is now good evidence that antigen entry occurs through the epithelium overlying lymphoid follicles, and that immunoblast cells are primed at these sites prior to migration to the lamina propria of the gut mucosa where they secrete immunoglobulin (*see* chapter 1). Thus, adherence of bacteria to the overlying epithelium of the lymph follicle may be related to antibody production and may have significance in the pathogenesis of this child's continuing diarrhoea. It is clear that a great deal more research is required into the genesis of post-enteritis diarrhoea. This is an important subject both in the developed and developing communities, but in the latter it is a problem of enormous size.

MANAGEMENT

The management of such infants may be difficult. If there is evidence of mucosal damage and also disordered handling of fat as shown, for example, by an abnormal fat load test, the use of a feeding based on medium chain triglycerides such as Pregestimil is indicated. This feeding contains glucose as its carbohydrate. It contains as protein,

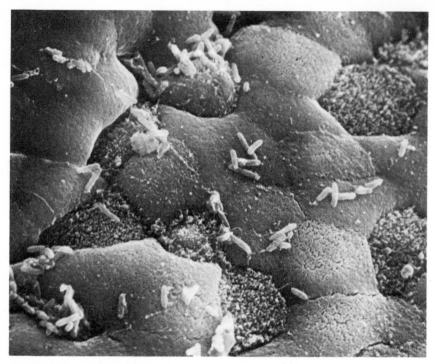

Fig. 6.20(a). Scanning electron microscope of lymphoid nodule in a small intestinal biopsy from a child with chronic diarrhoea demonstrating rods adherent to the surface of the mucosa, ×5,500. Reduced to ×3,300 by reproduction. (Permission of Phillips.)

casein that has been enzymically hydrolysed to reduce allergenicity. Thus, it is an effective feed for children who have disaccharide intolerance and many children with cow's milk protein intolerance.

If the child continues to fail to thrive, Caloreen may be added to the diet to supplement the calorie intake. Consideration may also be given to the need for a gluten-free diet because of possible transient gluten intolerance. If such a diet is introduced, long-term follow up and reinvestigation will be required as outlined in chapter 5.

Some children with acute food intolerance following gastroenteritis are intolerant to all the commercially available milk feedings and may be too ill for a small intestinal biopsy to be performed. In these circumstances, provided there is no evidence of lactose intolerance, expressed breast milk when available or a feeding based on chicken meat (*see* Appendix) may be of great value. Occasionally, any feeding by mouth is not tolerated and a period of intravenous alimentation is

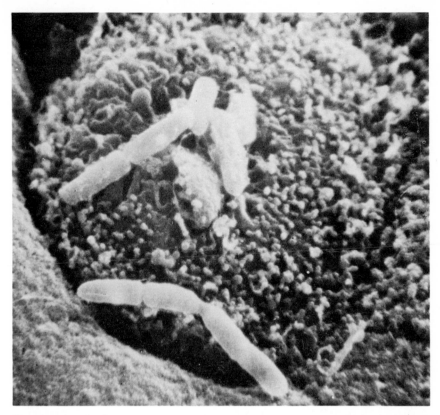

Fig. 6.20(b). Surface single cell ×19,350. Reduced to ×14,000 by reproduction. (Permission of Phillips.)

indicated (*see* chapter 11). A detailed account of the management of these more serious variants of the post-enteritis syndrome characterised by intractable diarrhoea is given inchapter 12, page 351.

7

Sugar Malabsorption

Defective digestion and absorption of ingested carbohydrate are common and important problems in infants and children. They may result from a primary inherited enzyme defect and thus be a permanent disorder, or they may be a secondary phenomenon of temporary duration and a sequel to small intestinal mucosal damage or to colonisation of the small intestine with bacteria.

DIGESTION AND ABSORPTION OF SUGARS

To understand the clinical syndrome associated with sugar malabsorption it is essential to have some knowledge of the principal dietary carbohydrates and their mode of digestion and absorption in man. These matters will be briefly reviewed here but the reader is referred to the bibliography, which he should consult for more detailed accounts.

Simple Chemistry of Carbohydrates

D-glucose is the most important carbohydrate in the diet and in the intermediate metabolism of carbohydrate in man. It is found in the blood of all animals and in the sap of all plants.

It is a hexose, i.e. a six carbon sugar molecule. It is usually represented according to the Haworth formula (Fig. 7.1).

Carbon atom one has an aldehyde group and so alpha and beta stereo-isomers are possible. It is important not to confuse stereo-isomerism with D and L rotation, which refers to the rotation of polarised light.

When one glucose molecule is joined to another to form a disaccharide or a polysaccharide the link may be between C_1 of the first molecule and C_4 of the second molecule (1–4 linkage) or between C_1 and C_6 (1–6 linkage). This linkage is via an oxygen bridge with either an alpha or a beta bond, depending on the stereo-isomer. These bonds are referred to as alpha or beta glycosidic bonds. When the bonds are 1–4, the arrangement of molecules is linear, and when 1–6, the arrangement is branched.

Hexoses such as glucose are called monosaccharides. Sugars with two monosaccharide units are called disaccharides and those with 2 to 10 units are known as oligosaccharides. Sugars with more than 10 units are polysaccharides.

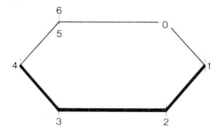

Fig. 7.1. Haworth formula

Carbohydrates in Diet

The principal carbohydrates in the diet of man are the storage polysaccharides (starch, glycogen and cellulose), the disaccharides, lactose and sucrose, and, to a lesser extent, the monosaccharides, glucose and fructose. Cellulose is not digested or absorbed in man, and in the adult, starch is the most important carbohydrate ingested.

The critical importance of the type of linkage between glucose molecules is illustrated by this difference in digestibility between starch and cellulose. Both are polysaccharides and have 1 to 4 linkages, but the linkages are of the alpha configuration for starch, and beta for cellulose.

In the milk-fed infant, lactose is usually the sole dietary carbohydrate until solids are introduced, although some artificial milks also contain sucrose; for example, 'Full Cream' Cow & Gate milk which contains 3·3 g sucrose/100 ml as well as 4·2 g lactose/100 ml. The infant has to ingest relatively large amounts of milk. A milk intake of 550 ml at the age of two weeks is equivalent to an adult intake of 4 to 8 litres of milk each day! The infant's small intestine, therefore, has to work very efficiently to deal with this relatively large load.

It is interesting to ponder the question: Why is lactose the sole carbohydrate of both human and cow's milk? Todd (1974), has reviewed the possible answers to this question.

Lactose is not superior to sucrose as a source of energy but its presence in the gut favours the growth of *Lactobacillus acidophilus* and promotes calcium and phosphate absorption. Carbohydrate in the diet also plays a role in synthesis and detoxification.

In relation to synthesis, Todd points out that cerebrosides, found especially in the brain, contain large numbers of glucose and galactose molecules. Synthesis takes place from UDP-glucose and UDP-galactose. In the newborn infant the brain grows rapidly and at this time nature provides galactose very generously in his diet. It is interesting to note that breast milk contains about twice as much galactose as cow's milk and that the brain grows twice as fast in the human infant compared with the calf, although body weight gain is far less.

In relation to detoxification, Todd observes that both glucose and galactose are involved in detoxification of toxic substances of metabolic, food or drug origin, but a galactose molecule entering the portal vein has a 10 to 20 times greater affinity for a liver cell than has a glucose molecule. In the newborn liver, galactose is an important source of UDP-glucose.

Starch, the plant storage form of carbohydrate, is made up of two main components, namely amylose and amylopectin. Amylopectin accounts for 80 per cent of ingested starch. Amylose is made up of a chain of glucose units with a screw-like form, linked via a 1–4 alpha glycosidic bond. Amylopectin is also made up of a chain of glucose units but in addition to the 1–4 alpha linkages, there are 1–6 alpha linkages at a number of branching points, approximately every 25 glucose units, along the chain. Glycogen, which is the animal storage form of carbohydrate, is also composed of a chain of glucose units with branching points at 1–6 linkages but it is of little dietetic importance in man.

The disaccharide lactose has a beta glycosidic bond linking a molecule of galactose to a molecule of glucose via a 1–4 linkage. The other disaccharides of clinical importance, namely sucrose, maltose and iso-maltose, are linked via an alpha glycosidic bond. Maltose consists of two glucose molecules linked by a 1–4 bond, whereas isomaltose, also consisting of two glucose molecules, is linked via a 1–6 bond. Sucrose (cane sugar) consists of a molecule of glucose linked to a molecule of fructose via an alpha linkage on the glucose side coupled to a beta linkage on the fructose side (alpha glucosido-beta fructose).

Carbohydrate Digestion and Absorption

Salivary and pancreatic alpha amylases act on starch to yield maltose, maltotriose (an oligosaccharide with three glucose units linked by a 1–4 bond) and alpha dextrins (branched oligosaccharides with 1–6 linkages at the branching points, but otherwise 1–4 linkages, containing an average of eight glucose molecules). Thus, the initial stage of starch digestion does not produce disaccharides alone and, in fact, oligosaccharides are the chief end product (Gray, 1970).

Classically, the next step in digestion was, until 1957, considered to be hydrolysis of these oligosaccharides by the 'succus entericus'. In 1957, Borgstrom and his colleagues noted that the hydrolytic activity of the small intestinal contents was too low during digestion to account for adequate digestion of disaccharides.

Miller and Crane went on, in 1961, to demonstrate that disaccharide hydrolysis was localised within the brush border or microvilli of the small intestinal epithelial cell, i.e. disaccharidase activity resided there.

Subsequently, the disaccharidases, or more correctly oligosaccharidases, have been shown in man to be the beta glycosidase, lactase and the alpha glycosidases, sucrase, maltase and isomaltase. Isomaltase is sometimes called oligo 1–6 alpha glycosidase or alpha dextrinase as it acts upon the alpha dextrins released from starch digestion by amylase by splitting the 1–6 linkage. Maltase splits maltotriose as well as maltose and is sometimes called glucoamylase.

These human intestinal disaccharidases have been identified by heat inactivation experiments (Dahlqvist *et al.*, 1963) and G gelfiltration on Sephadex and chromatography (Semenza, Auricchio and Rubino, 1965). More than one mucosal protein for most of these enzyme activities has been identified. Semenza and his colleagues have isolated five maltase activities and two lactases have also been recognised. Not all these enzyme activities appear to play a physiological role in hydrolysis; for example, the second lactase does not appear to have such a role and it is in fact an intracellular enzyme.

The present conception of the steps in the digestion of carbohydrate are indicated in Table 7.1, and the intestinal intraluminal and surface hydrolysis of dietary carbohydrate is represented diagrammatically in Fig. 7.2.

The active transport mechanism for glucose and galactose is dependent upon the sodium pump for its function, i.e. it is dependent on the mechanism that continually removes sodium ion from the cell.

Studies of disaccharidase activity along the small intestine have

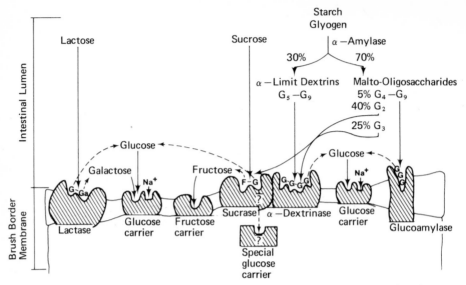

Fig. 7.2. Diagrammatic representation of intestinal intraluminal and surface hydrolysis of dietary carbohydrate
The oligosaccharides released from luminal action of amylase and the two dietary disaccharides are hydrolysed by specific enzymes imbedded in the brush-border membrane so that their active hydrolytic sites (shown as clefts in the molecule) are available at the brush-border surface. The released monosaccharides then bind to specific carrier sites in the initial stage of transport. G = glucose, with subscript indicating number of glucose units; Ga = galactose; F = fructose. (Permission of Gray from Gray, G. M. (1975) *New England Journal of Medicine*, **292**, 1220.)

Table 7.1
Steps in the digestion of carbohydrate

Alpha amylases in saliva pancreatic juice	Starch {	Maltose	Maltase $\longrightarrow$	Glucose + Glucose
		Maltotriose Alpha Dextrins	Maltase $\longrightarrow$	Glucose + Glucose
			Isomaltase $\longrightarrow$	Glucose + Glucose
		Sucrose	Sucrase $\longrightarrow$	Glucose + Fructose
		Lactose	Lactase $\longrightarrow$	Glucose + Galactose

revealed that it is well distributed along the length of the small intestine but lower levels are found in the proximal duodenum and the terminal ileum. Biopsies taken at, or just beyond, the duodeno-jejunal flexure are usually regarded as providing samples that will give representative values of intestinal disaccharidase activity.

All disaccharidases are present by the third month of gestation; the alpha disaccharidases reach a peak at the sixth or seventh month (Auricchio, Rubino and Murset, 1965), but lactase activity only reaches its peak level at about term. This accords with the observations of impaired lactose absorption in premature infants (Boellner, Beard and Panos, 1965).

After hydrolysis of oligosaccharides and disaccharides, the liberated monosaccharides are absorbed by active transport mechanisms. Glucose and galactose share one mechanism; fructose, on the other hand, has a different mechanism. It is believed that this site of active transport is in direct proximity to the site of disaccharidase activity in the brush border of the enterocyte. Only when these two intimately related sites of disaccharidase activity and active transport are negotiated are sugars truly in the cytoplasm of the enterocyte.

The products of brush-border hydrolysis, i.e. the monosaccharides, may not be adequately controlled by the active transport mechanisms of the same enterocyte because hydrolysis is so rapid (Gray, 1975). Hence, they may diffuse back into the intestinal lumen and so be absorbed subsequently at more distal sites. Thus, the small intestine manipulates the oligosaccharides presented to it by digestion, plus the dietary disaccharides, lactose and sucrose, by a two-step process (see Fig. 7.2). First, there is surface hydrolysis in the brush border to monosaccharides. Second, there is active transport of released monosaccharides either by the same cell on which hydrolysis has occurred or when diffusion of monosaccharide back into the lumen occurs by other enterocytes further along the small intestine.

Crane (1962) has also hypothesised that the active transport of glucose and galactose is carrier-mediated. He believes that glucose molecules and sodium ions bind to a carrier at separate sites and then are released from it after entry into the cell cytoplasm.

The carrier, a macromolecule is presumably a protein. It is considered that sodium ion binds to this carrier along with glucose but at a different binding site. As the concentration of sodium ion is low in the cell, the ion moves down the concentration gradient into the cell. As glucose accompanies sodium ion on the carrier, it is also taken in and released within the cell. Sodium ion is subsequently pumped out at the lateral membranes of the cell by an active process utilising energy derived from the hydrolysis of ATP and is dependent on sodium-potassium activated adenosine triphosphatase (Na^+-K^+)-ATPase. This enzyme catalyses ATP to ADP, releasing the energy for this sodium pump, and by this process glucose is taken into a cell where the glucose content may be already higher than in the lumen. It then passes out by simple diffusion into the portal capillaries. Thus, glucose movement can occur uphill because of its coupled absorption with sodium. The practical implications for this coupling of sodium and glucose transport in the management of cholera are outlined in chapter 6.

It has been considered in the past that fructose may have been absorbed passively, but observations in the experimental animal by Gracey, Burke and Oshin (1972) suggest that fructose too may be absorbed by an active transport system, albeit different from that used by glucose and galactose. This difference in the way these monosaccharides are absorbed has practical clinical importance.

SUGAR INTOLERANCE AND MALABSORPTION

Inherited and acquired defects of disaccharidase activity have been described in infants and children as well as a congenital defect of the active transport mechanism for glucose and galactose.

These disorders lead to malabsorption of various sugars, resulting in clinical intolerance to the offending carbohydrate when it is present in the child's diet and producing diarrhoea as the principal symptom. The diarrhoea is chiefly osmotic in origin, due to the effect of the presence of undigested disaccharides within the small bowel lumen (Laws and Neale, 1966; Launiala, 1968). This unsplit carbohydrate is fermented by bacteria in the large intestine forming lactic acid (Weijers et al., 1961) and short chain fatty acids.

Sugar malabsorption has also been described in infants with bacterial contamination of the small intestine via mechanisms (see chapter 10) at present unknown.

Although paediatricians in Vienna in the early part of this century described 'fermentative diarrhoea' treated by removal of carbohydrate from the diet, it is only in very recent times that sugar intolerance has been established as a real clinical entity in children. Interestingly, the clinical recognition of syndromes of sugar malabsorption occurred at the same time as significant advances in our understanding of sugar digestion and absorption were being made. Holzel, Schwarz and Sutcliffe in Britain (1959) and Weijers and his colleagues (1961) were among the first to describe these disorders in children.

Definition

There are terminological difficulties in describing disorders of sugar digestion and absorption but the clinical distinction between sugar intolerance, i.e. a treatable disorder, and sugar malabsorption which may not necessarily require treatment, is important.

Sugar intolerance is a clinical syndrome occurring in infants and children characterised by the development of diarrhoea and/or vomiting and failure to grow adequately when a particular sugar or sugars are ingested. Such a syndrome may be permanent, due for example to an inherited enzyme defect, or it may be secondary to temporary damage to the small intestinal mucosa.

Sugar malabsorption may be diagnosed when there is laboratory evidence of disordered sugar absorption, e.g. a 'flat' lactose tolerance test, but this diagnosis does not necessarily imply the presence of clinical sugar intolerance because there may be no symptoms when the offending sugar is ingested.

When sugar intolerance is diagnosed this should be looked upon as signifying the presence of clinically significant sugar malabsorption, which requires treatment.

Clinical Features

In infants and young children, watery diarrhoea is the cardinal symptom of sugar intolerance. This can be severe and produce significant dehydration. The stools are often so watery that they may be mistaken for urine. Such stools tend to soak into the infant's napkin and the severity of the diarrhoea may, as a result, be overlooked. If a stool is not available at the time of clinical assessment, in an infant in whom there is historical evidence of sugar intolerance, digital examination will usually lead to the production of a characteristic stool when sugar intolerance is present. Such a stool may be easily collected and tested for reducing substances. The diarrhoea may sometimes be accompanied by vomiting of variable severity. Sometimes the diarrhoea is less severe and so the diagnosis is delayed. This may lead to failure to thrive. In the older child and adolescent, the diarrhoea, although still usually watery, may be intermittent and sometimes lead to incontinence. Milk ingestion may produce not only diarrhoea but some colicky abdominal pain.

Diagnosis

The diagnosis of sugar intolerance should be suspected whenever loose watery stools are passed in young infants. A careful history including details of the child's dietary carbohydrate intake will usually suggest the diagnosis.

Table 7.2
Diagnosis of sugar intolerance

1. Stool reducing substances and pH
2. Stool chromatography for sugar
3. Oral sugar tolerance or loading test
4. Hydrogen breath test
5. Barium-lactose meal
6. Disaccharidase assay
7. Clinical response to sugar restriction

Table 7.2 lists the diagnostic test that may be of some value in the diagnosis of sugar intolerance.

Stool-reducing Substances and pH

The simplest clinical way to make the diagnosis of sugar intolerance is to demonstrate the presence of an excess of reducing substances (i.e. 0·5 per cent or more) in the infant's stools, using the Clinitest method of Kerry and Anderson (1964) as described in chapter 3. The importance of proper stool collection and examination of the fluid part of the stool cannot be over-stressed.

Although acid stools are often found in these children, stool pH is not a reliable screening test for sugar intolerance since stools that contain an excess of reducing substances are not always acid, and acid stools sometimes may not contain an excess of reducing substances (Soeparto *et al.*, 1972; Walker-Smith, 1973; Lindquist and Wranne, 1976). However, both tests provide different information as Ament and Perera (1973) point out. Stool pH may give an indication as to whether significant quantities of organic acids are produced, for example, from unabsorbed carbohydrate, whereas the finding of increased amounts of reducing substances indicates the presence of such unabsorbed sugar. Thus, both tests performed in conjunction may give useful information, but testing for reducing substances alone is the only satisfactory screening test for sugar intolerance.

Davidson and Mullinger (1973) cast doubt on the reliability of increased amounts of stool-reducing substances as markers of clinical lactose intolerance in the neonate, especially the breast-fed neonate, who normally passes partly liquid stools with an acid pH. Counahan and Walker-Smith (1976) have confirmed that 0·5 per cent or more reducing substances may be found in stools of normal neonates. They found 0·5 per cent or 0·75 per cent reducing substances in the stools of 16 out of 51 normal neonates aged between 5 and 16 days, both breast and bottle fed. None had more than 1 per cent reducing substances. Scheibe and Lentze (1973) have also found that total sugar excretion is high in normal neonates. It disappears rapidly in full-term neonates but is prolonged in premature ones. It was more common in breast-fed infants. Thus, there does appear to be a physiological malabsorption of lactose during the neonatal period which is not of nutritional significance. However, the presence of severe watery diarrhoea in a neonate with 1 per cent or more stool-reducing substances allows a clinical diagnosis of sugar intolerance to be made and indicates the need for treatment. The response to dietary management will then confirm or deny the diagnosis.

Neonates may, however, have abnormal amounts of oligosaccharides in their stools which give an abnormal result when testing stools with Clinitest tablets. Chromatography of such stools will establish the presence of these oligosaccharides. In stools of breast-fed infants they are presumably of bacterial origin and, when found, are of no diagnostic significance. In these circumstances the finding of increased amounts of stool-reducing substances is not an indication for treatment.

False negative results with Clinitest tablets may occur in children with sucrose malabsorption as sucrose is not a reducing sugar. Reducing substances will be present in the stools of such children only if colonic flora have first hydrolysed unabsorbed sucrose into glucose and fructose, or if the stools are preliminarily hydrolysed with dilute hydrochloric acid before testing, but this may not always produce reliable results. Stool chromatography is the only way to demonstrate, with certainty, the presence of sucrose in an infant's stool.

Table 7.3
Drugs causing false positive Clinitest results

Large quantities of ascorbic acid
Nalidixic acid
Cephalosporins
Probenecid

False positive results with Clinitest tablets may occur in neonates, as mentioned above and in children who are taking some drugs by mouth (Table 7.3).

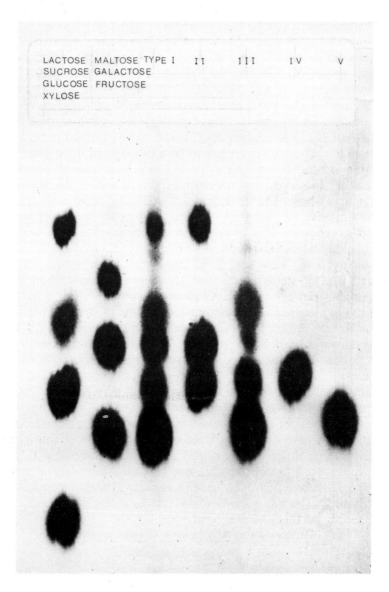

LACTOSE MALTOSE TYPE I   II   III   IV   V
SUCROSE GALACTOSE
GLUCOSE FRUCTOSE
XYLOSE

Fig. 7.3. Chromatogram of stools of children with the five patterns of sugar malabsorption compared with control sugars.

In addition, many drugs when given by mouth to infants may be administered in a sugar-containing vehicle or as tablets with a sugar base. Their continued administration to infants who are thought to be on a sugar-free diet may cause diagnostic confusion and sometimes therapeutic failure. Some artificial milks may contain variable amounts of lactulose which occur inadvertently during manufacture. This sugar cannot be absorbed and when present in large amounts could cause diarrhoea. Chromatography of stools would demonstrate its presence. The oral administration of this sugar to patients with hepatic coma produces an artificial fermentative diarrhoea and produces clinical improvement by at present, ill understood mechanisms.

Chromatography for Sugar

Paper chromatography for sugar of stools from children with increased amounts of reducing substances will determine the pattern of sugars present in an infant's stool. The technique is described in chapter 3. Figure 7.4 indicates the five principal patterns that may be seen. With knowledge of the child's dietary carbohydrate intake it is then possible to diagnose the type of sugar malabsorption present, as described by Soeparto and his colleagues in 1972.

Table 7.4
Approximate carbohydrate content in g/100 ml milk

	Total	Lactose	Other carbohydrate
Breast milk	7 (average)	7	Nil
Cow's milk	4·7	4·7	Nil
Cow and Gate V formula	7·0	7·0	Nil
Cow and Gate premium	7·0	7·0	Nil
Ostermilk complete	8·6	2·9	Malto-dextrins
Osterfeed	7·0	7·0	Nil
Nan	7·3	7·3	Nil
SMA	7·2	7·2	Nil
S_{26} (SMA Gold cap)	7·2	7·2	Nil
Similac	7·1	7·1	Nil
Enfamil	7·1	7·1	Nil

Table 7.4 indicates the carbohydrate content of commonly used milk feedings in Britain, Australia and USA.

Pattern I is characterised by the presence of lactose, sucrose, galactose, glucose and fructose in the stools of children having lactose and sucrose in their feeding, i.e. this is the pattern of lactose and sucrose malabsorption.

Pattern II is characterised by the presence of lactose, galactose, and glucose in the stools of infants having an ordinary cow's milk based feeding, i.e. this is the pattern of lactose malabsorption.

Pattern III is characterised by the presence of sucrose, glucose, and fructose sometimes with traces of other sugars. This is the pattern of sucrose malabsorption.

Pattern IV is characterised by the presence of glucose alone in the stools of an infant who is having a formula which only contains glucose, e.g. Galactomin 17.

Pattern V is characterised by the presence of fructose alone in the stools of an infant who is having a formula which only contains fructose, e.g. Galactomin 19, i.e. the pattern of fructose malabsorption.

It is of critical importance that stools should not be allowed to stand for any length of time before chromatography or before freezing for storage or, indeed, after thawing before chromatography (Lindquist and Wranne, 1976; Lifshitz, 1977). Lifshitz has even gone to the length of recommending a simple electronic device to signal the time of bowel movements to ensure that fresh stools are collected. The importance of this need for speedy testing has been clearly demonstrated by Lindquist and Wranne who showed that if disaccharides are added to sugar-free fresh stools the disaccharide and, indeed, all sugars have disappeared by 180 minutes later, the disaccharide disappearing after 30 minutes and being replaced by its component monosaccharides. This is due to the disaccharidase activity of the bacteria of fresh stools. Failure to take account of this time factor can lead to errors in the interpretation of stool chromatograms; for example, it is possible to have pattern IV in a child with lactose malabsorption if all the lactose has been split, for, in practice, the galactose also seems to disappear before the glucose.

Stool chromatography is of diagnostic usefulness in the neonate, particularly, as mentioned earlier, when false positive results with Clinitest tablets are due to the presence of oligosaccharides (short runners), and in any infant where there have been rapid changes in feeds with a different carbohydrate content and, as a result, uncertainty exists about the type of sugar malabsorption that is present when an increased amount of stool-reducing substances has been observed. A further value of stool chromatography is identification of lactulose, which is a non-reducing disaccharide composed of fructose and galactose that is found as an unwelcome byproduct of sterilisation procedures in some commercially made infant feeding formulae. It cannot be hydrolysed by human small intestinal mucosa because there is no appropriate enzyme there to split it. Ready-to-feed infant milks used in hospital practice in Britain and widely throughout the United States may, on occasion, have levels high enough to produce osmotic diarrhoea and a clinical picture identical to lactose intolerance, which can only be diagnosed by stool chromatography.

The total amount of reducing substances and the amount of individual sugars present in the stools may be quantitated but this information is usually unnecessary for adequate diagnosis. Detection of abnormal amounts of reducing substances in the urine of children with sugar intolerance has been advocated as a useful diagnostic test by Arthur and his colleagues (1966), but its role in diagnosis awaits further clarification. Prader, Shmerling and Hadorn (1966) suggested that such a disacchariduria was an expression of the severity of mucosal drainage, but attempts to devise a clinical test based on this hypothesis using the inert disaccharide lactulose (galactose-fructose) have proved unsuccessful (Muller et al., 1969).

Quantitative assay of stool lactic acid has also been used to diagnose sugar intolerance but this is not recommended for routine diagnosis. The finding of more than 50 mg lactic acid in a random sample of stool weighing 100 g has been taken as an indication of excess fermentation (Holzel, 1967).

In adults with sugar intolerance, nearly always lactose intolerance, testing of stools for pH and reducing substances has been shown to be unreliable by McMichael, Webb and Dawson (1965) as only very small amounts of sugar may be detected in their stools.

Oral Sugar Tolerance or Loading Tests

In older children, or in small children, after a period of sugar restriction oral sugar tolerance tests (sugar loading tests) may be useful diagnostically. An oral load of 2 g/kg is given to the fasting child and capillary blood specimens are taken at half-hourly intervals for two hours. Normally there should be a rise in the blood sugar level of 30 mg/100 ml within the two hours. More important is observation of the child for the onset of diarrhoea and the appearance of reducing substances in a loose stool after the oral sugar load. A 'flat lactose tolerance test' on its own without diarrhoea does not indicate a diagnosis of sugar intolerance, nor does treatment of the child with a special diet, but the appearance of diarrhoea with excess stool-reducing substances, and abdominal discomfort after a sugar load indicates the presence of sugar intolerance. In adults, Newcomer and McGill (1966) found an abnormal lactose tolerance test in 28 per cent of 18 healthy adults with normal lactose levels. Delayed gastric emptying may account for this finding. Harrison and Walker-Smith (1977) observed 30 children at the Queen Elizabeth Hospital aged from 2 to 38 months already on a milk-free, lactose-free diet who were being reinvestigated prior to a cow's milk challenge as outlined in chapter 5. No correlation at all was found in the group as a whole with, on the one hand, continuing lactose intolerance as diagnosed by the development of watery stools containing excess reducing substances after an oral load of lactose, and, on the other hand, maximal blood glucose rise during a lactose tolerance test, lactase levels and small intestinal morphology.

Barium–Lactose Meal

In older children a barium-lactose meal may be useful diagnostically. However, this is just a radiological way of demonstrating diarrhoea after an oral load of carbohydrate. It should not be used in infants and young children.

Disaccharidase Assay

Small intestinal disaccharidase activity rarely needs to be estimated in young children with sugar malabsorption because secondary lactase deficiency is the abnormality most often found, occurring secondarily to small intestinal mucosal damage. Lactase reduction occurs *pari passu* with reduction of sucrase, isomaltase and maltase activity, and the demonstration of a low lactase level is not synonymous with the presence of clinically significant lactose intolerance. However, lactase activity is more vulnerable to damage and takes longer to recover than the other disaccharidase enzymes.

The indications for disaccharidase assay are a clinical suspicion of the presence of congenital alactasia, or sucrase-isomaltase deficiency, i.e. when there is diagnostic uncertainty as to the cause of the sugar intolerance or before and after milk challenge as an aid to diagnosis of cow's milk sensitive enteropathy.

Lactose Hydrogen Breath Test

Hydrogen in the breath is the result of the breakdown within the intestines of substrates that have been eaten. Normally after eating, no hydrogen appears in the breath for one to three hours, i.e. until ingested substrate reaches the bacteria of the colon. A simple technique using the hydrogen breath test as a measure of lactose absorption in childhood has been described. An oral load of lactose is given and a small plastic tube in a nostril is used to sample the child's breath before and every half hour for three hours (Maffei *et al.*, 1977). A peak of hydrogen in the breath may occur in less than an hour when there is abnormal bacterial growth within the small intestinal lumen (Metz *et al.*, 1976). Higher levels of hydrogen than those normally found in the breath are found when carbohydrates, malabsorbed by the small intestine reach the colon, there to be fermented by colonic bacteria. Thus, in children who have carbohydrate malabsorption, the peak in breath hydrogen occurs one to three hours after an oral load of lactose. Douwes, Fernandez and Degenhart (1978), however, found a higher peak at an hour, and sometimes at less than an hour in children who were lactose intolerant, but they did not study small intestinal bacterial colonisation in these children. The role of such a test in routine practice has not yet been fully evaluated but children have been described who had abnormal hydrogen breath tests and responded well to a lactose-free diet yet did not have high levels of stool-reducing substances and other objective evidence of lactose intolerance. It may prove, in time, to be the most useful measure of lactose tolerance.

Clinical Response to Sugar Restriction

The *sin qua non* for the diagnosis of sugar intolerance is that the child makes a clinical response to removal of the offending sugar from his diet. The difficulties in making the clinical diagnosis of lactose intolerance has recently been demonstrated by the observations of Mitchell, Brand and Halbisch (1977) that weight gain was better in a group of Australian aboriginal infants who were given a pre-hydrolysed low lactose milk compared with those given a standard lactose containing milk powder, despite the fact that there was no consistent evidence of sugar intolerance as assessed conventionally in those doing well on a low lactose milk. The introduction of the expiratory hydrogen test may help to clarify this situation; Maffei *et al.* (1977) have found an abnormal expiratory hydrogen test to be a reliable guide to lactose intolerance requiring treatment. It is possible that stool analysis for reducing substances may be underestimating this diagnosis, nevertheless, the interpretation of Mitchell's data has been questioned.

To summarise, in infants and younger children sugar malabsorption can usually be adequately diagnosed by the demonstration of an abnormal amount of reducing substances in their stools while they are having feeds containing the offending sugar, but in older children, and sometimes in infants, other diagnostic methods may be used. The final clinical proof that the diagnosis of sugar intolerance is correct in these children will be provided by a clinical response to the removal of the offending sugar from the child's diet.

TYPES OF SUGAR MALABSORPTION

The varieties of sugar malabsorption that may occur in children are listed in Table 7.5.

Table 7.5
Varieties of sugar malabsorption

1. Disorders of disaccharide absorption
   (a) Primary: congenital alactasia
         sucrose-isomaltase deficiency
   (b) Secondary: e.g. post-enteritis, post-neonatal surgery, protein-calorie malnutrition
   (c) Later onset or 'racial' lactose intolerance

2. Disorders of monosaccharide absorption
   (a) Primary: congenital glucose-galactose malabsorption
   (b) Secondary: e.g. post-neonatal surgery, protein-calorie malnutrition

1. Disaccharide malabsorption

(a) (i) Sucrase-isomaltase Deficiency

Weijers and his colleagues in Holland in 1961 were the first to recognise that diarrhoea in infancy could be caused by a deficiency of the sugar-splitting enzymes, sucrase and isomaltase. These two enzymatic activities are attached to a protein that gives a peak with the same motility in a Sephadex column as a protein that has 85 per cent of maltase activity (Semenza et al., 1965). In this disorder there is complete absence of this peak. It is probable that all these enzyme activities represent one protein under a single gene control (Dawson, 1970). There is sufficient maltase activity in the other remaining proteins to ensure hydrolysis and normal absorption of maltose and maltotriose derived from dietary starch.

Definition: Sucrase-isomaltase deficiency is an inherited enzyme deficiency of the small intestinal mucosa, the mode of inheritance being as an autosomal recessive characteristic.

Incidence and Genetic Factors: The exact incidence of this condition in Western countries is unknown but a high incidence has been observed in the Eskimo population of Greenland where sucrase-isomaltase deficiency has been reported in 10 per cent of the population.

The autosomal mode of inheritance of this condition was suggested by Burgess and her colleagues at the Queen Elizabeth Hospital in 1964 and was established by Kerry and Townley in 1965, who performed small intestinal biopsies in four families of children with this disorder. They found that all parents had low intestinal sucrase and isomaltase levels.

Clinical Features: Symptoms will not appear until solids that contain sucrose are introduced into the child's diet. This usually occurs at about three months of age and the severity of symptoms will depend upon the amount of sucrose added to the infant's diet. Severe watery diarrhoea is characteristic in these infants, and is usually associated with poor weight gain, but in the older child and adults the symptoms may be much less severe. The condition may present with intermittent watery diarrhoea, and sometimes with incontinence with intermittent abdominal distension and crampy abdominal pain in the older child.

Diagnosis: Diagnosis is based firstly, on the demonstration of a 'flat' sucrose tolerance test coupled with the development of diarrhoea after the oral load of sucrose, and secondly, on enzyme assay which will demonstrate the characteristic sucrase-isomaltase deficiency in the small intestinal mucosa, which is morphologically normal.

Management: These children will respond clinically within twenty-four hours to a sucrose-free diet. There is no need to limit starch because of the small percentage of 1–6 linkages in the amylopectin of starch, as pointed out earlier. The need for dietary restriction appears to be permanent. Although it has been claimed that, with time, increasing tolerance to sucrose may occur, this apparent increasing tolerance is due to the patient's unconscious restriction of sucrose intake, even though he usually imagines he is still having a normal diet.

Reinvestigation studies of 9 children observed up to ten years after diagnosis at the Queen Elizabeth Hospital, have shown continuation of episodes of diarrhoea associated with sucrose ingestion (Kilby *et al.*, 1978). In those studied, there was also persistence of a 'flat' sucrose tolerance test. The marked improvement in sucrose tolerance with age, which some have reported (Auricchio *et al.*, 1963), probably occurs only rarely in the homozygous state, but it may be more common in heterozygous, sucrase and isomaltase deficiency where, although enzyme levels are depressed, they are not as low as the levels found in those who are homozygous for sucrase-isomaltase deficiency (Burgess *et al.*, 1964; Kerry and Townley, 1965).

(ii) Congenital Alactasia

This rare primary congenital syndrome was first reported by Holzel, Schwarz and Sutcliffe in 1959. It is characterised by diarrhoea from a few days after birth. In only a few children with this disorder has estimation of disaccharidase activity in a specimen of small intestinal mucosa been performed (Launiala, Kuitunen and Visakorpi, 1966; Levin *et al.*, 1970). In these, lactase activity is not always completely absent, i.e. there is hypolactasia rather than complete alactasia. Congenital alactasia appears to be recessively inherited.

The disorder may easily be confused with secondary lactase deficiency which is a far commoner condition, and some of the earlier reports of congenital alactasia may have confused this secondary type of lactase deficiency with primary alactasia. In primary alactasia the mucosa is morphologically normal and there is a specific depression of lactase activity, whereas in secondary lactase deficiency the mucosa is abnormal and the other disaccharidases also have reduced activity. True congenital alactasia unlike secondary alactasia is a permanent disorders.

(iii) Congenital Lactose Intolerance

This rare disorder, first described by Durand in 1958, is mentioned here as it may be confused with congenital alactasia. Holzel (1967) has pointed out that it is an entirely different clinical and pathological entity. The condition is often familial. It is characterised by vomiting, failure to thrive, and some diarrhoea associated with aminoaciduria and acidosis with lactosuria, and sometimes, over 1 g lactose in the urine each day; such lactosuria is not a feature of alactasia.

Untreated, this disorder may be fatal. However, after periods on a lactose-free diet the child may make a full recovery. The self-limiting nature of the disorder argues against its being an hereditary enzyme defect. It has been suggested that there is some temporary disturbance of small intestinal absorptive function with increased permeability of the small intestinal mucosa, but its true aetiology remains unknown.

(b) Secondary Disaccharide Intolerance

Disaccharide intolerance may occur as a transient phenomenon in a wide variety of diseases of the small intestine in childhood (Table 7.6).

The localisation of disaccharidase activity in the microvilli of the small intestinal epithelial cell renders them liable to be affected by any disorder that damages the small intestinal mucosa, and most of the disorders listed in Table 7.6 are associated with such damage.

Early studies of secondary lactase deficiency added cystic fibrosis to the list of causes but Antonowicz, Lebenthal and Shwachmann (1978) have shown that lactase deficiency in patients with cystic fibrosis is not related to the disease *per se* but may occur only when an enteropathy is present from some other cause. There was, indeed, a trend for patients with normal morphology to have elevated disaccharidase levels when cystic fibrosis was accompanied by pancreatic insufficiency.

Premature infants are predisposed to develop lactase deficiency because, as has already been mentioned, lactase is the last enzyme to attain mature levels during fetal development. Therefore, lactose intolerance complicates gastroenteritis more frequently in premature neonates who have gastroenteritis than in full-term neonates who develop this disorder.

The pathogenesis of this syndrome is believed to be based on a temporary deficiency, chiefly of lactase, but sometimes of sucrase, both deficiencies being secondary to mucosal damage. However, a lack of correlation between mucosal damage as assessed by light microscopy and disaccharidase levels has been described (Harrison and Walker-Smith, 1977). Indeed, a few children may have secondary disaccharidase deficiency despite a small intestinal mucosa that is histologically normal, but Phillips *et al.* (1978) have shown that disaccharidase activity (lactase) does correlate with microvillous surface area as assessed with the electron microscope. Hence, children with secondary lactase deficiency but with a histologically normal small intestinal mucosa, in fact have a reduced microvillous surface area. Thus, in some cases, morphological abnormality can be assessed only with the electron microscope, but in most cases as the mucosa recovers so also do the disaccharidase levels (Burke, Kerry and Anderson, 1965). However, in infants who have had surgery there may be no such depression of enzyme levels and the secondary sugar intolerance has then been attributed by some workers to bacterial colonisation of the small intestine. It has also been described, by Dubois and his colleagues (1970), in children with immunological defects.

Secondary disaccharide intolerance should be suspected whenever diarrhoea develops following a change or increase in the strength of the carbohydrate content of an infant's feeding, or in association with one of the disorders listed in Table 7.6, especially in the case of watery diarrhoea.

Secondary lactose malabsorption is the major problem but sometimes, especially after gastroenteritis, and also in children who have had surgery, sucrose malabsorption may occur. Children under the age of three months are most frequently affected by sugar malabsorption. In a survey of 110 children with secondary sugar intolerance at the Royal Alexandra Hospital over a two year period, 1970–1971, the greatest number were under the age of three months at the time of presentation (Fig. 7.4) (Bates, Walker-Smith and Stobo, 1972).

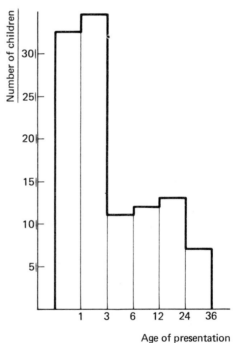

Fig. 7.4. Age at presentation, in months, of children with sugar malabsorption at the Royal Alexandra Hospital in 1970–1971.

Table 7.6
Causes of secondary lactose intolerance

Gastroenteritis
Coeliac disease
Giardiasis
Protein-calorie malnutrition
Following neonatal surgery
Cow's milk protein intolerance
Immuno-deficiency syndromes
Massive small intestinal resection

Sixty-five per cent of these children had secondary sugar intolerance as a sequel to gastroenteritis. Table 7.7 lists the numbers of children who had a bacterial pathogen, a parasite, a yeast, or fungus isolated from their stools.

Most children had no bacterial aetiological agent isolated from their stools.

Table 7.7
Stool isolations in children with gastroenteritis complicated by sugar intolerance

Specific bacterial pathogen	
Salmonella	4
Shigella	1
E. coli	6
Parasitic infestation	
Giardia	3
Yeasts and fungi	
Candida	2
No pathogen	57

Once a diagnosis of sugar intolerance is made, these children should be put on a lactose-free formula, i.e. a milk that contains only insignificant amounts of lactose. Some of these and their carbohydrate contents are listed in Table 7.8.

Care must be taken when using Galactomin feedings to add vitamins and trace minerals to the infant's diet, as these formulae are not complete foods.

The length of time an infant should remain on such a feeding is usually based on the clinical response. Once weight gain is satisfactory, normal feeds can be resumed or the sugar loading test performed and the effect on stools etc. observed.

It must be remembered, however, that infants with cow's milk protein intolerance may also respond in the same way to these lactose-free formulae as children with lactose intolerance, as the protein content of these milks has also been altered.

Harrison (1974) has found evidence of cow's milk protein intolerance occurring transiently as a sequel to gastroenteritis and associated with lactose malabsorption (*see* chapter 5). This cow's milk protein intolerance persisted after lactose tolerance had returned to normal.

Table 7.8
Lactose-free milk formulae

Special milk	Carbohydrate	Amount g/100 ml
Nutramigen (Australia)	Glucose	5·8
	starch	2·6
Nutramigen (UK and USA)	Sucrose	6·1
	Starch	2·7
Pro-Sobee	Sucrose	4·1
	Corn sugars	2·7
Velactin	Glucose	3·0
	Corn sugars	2·4
	Sucrose	0·3
	Soy starch	1·7
Galactomin 17	Glucose	1·25
	Maltose, dextrins and higher sugars	5·0
Galactomin 19	Fructose	7·3
Pregestimil	Glucose	6·3
	Starch	2·3
Isomil	Sucrose	3·1
	Corn sugars	3·7

The duration of sugar restriction in 110 children with sugar malabsorption from the Royal Alexandra Hospital is illustrated in Fig. 7.5. In most children the duration is only a few weeks or months but in a few it is far longer. In all, the need for dietary restriction is temporary.

The surgical disorders associated with sugar malabsorption are discussed elsewhere.

(*c*) *Later Onset of 'Racial' Lactose Intolerance*

An isolated deficiency of lactase is common in adults and a genetic aetiology has been suggested for this type of lactose malabsorption which may present in late childhood or adult life. It has been shown to

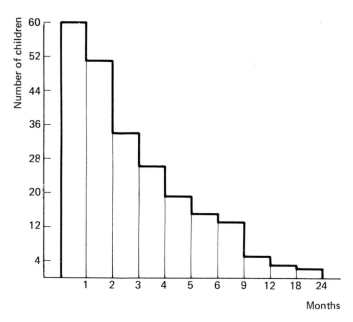

Fig. 7.5. Duration of special diet in children with sugar malabsorption at Royal Alexandra Hospital, 1970–1971.

be common in Africans, Greek Cypriots, Indians, Chinese, American Negroes, New Guinea natives and Australian Aborigines; indeed Caucasians are one of the few racial groups to maintain lactase levels in adult life. This observation has been explained either on the basis of a genetically determined fall of lactase activity (Cook, 1967) or as an acquired defect resulting from the lack of continued substrate challenge in the form of a low level of milk consumption (Bolin, Crane and Davis, 1968). Secondary damage to intestinal mucosa from gastroenteritis, protein-calorie malnutrition or parasitism could contribute to the severity of such a defect and thus hasten the onset of a genetic tendency for lactase levels to fall. As has already been emphasised, the demonstration of an abnormality of a lactose tolerance test does not prove that milk intolerance is present or indicate the need for dietary restriction, based on blood glucose levels during lactose tolerance tests. Habte, Sterk and Hjalmarsson (1973) found evidence of lactose malabsorption in 80 per cent of a group of Ethiopian children based on lactose tolerance tests, yet milk consumption in normal quantities (250 ml) was tolerated in all these school children including those who were shown to have 'flat' lactose tolerance tests. Some initially had transient symptoms with the ingestion of milk but all were able subsequently to tolerate the milk without any symptoms.

The practical importance of this 'racial' lactose intolerance may thus have been exaggerated in the past. Nonetheless, the older child of any race who has a history of watery diarrhoea with the passage of excess flatus and abdominal pain following milk ingestion should be investigated for possible lactose intolerance. If the diagnosis is established by a lactose tolerance test, which combines studies of blood glucose rise with observations of the stools for the onset of diarrhoea and the presence of excess reducing substances, or by a barium-lactose meal, treatment is then simple and highly effective.

2. Monosaccharide Malabsorption

(a) Congenital Glucose-galactose Malabsorption

A congenital disturbance of the active transport mechanism for the monosaccharides glucose and galactose has been described by Lindquist, Meeuwisse and Melin (1962) and later by others. It is a rare disorder inherited as an autosomal recessive characteristic. Renal tubular reabsorption of glucose may also be defective and so glycosuria may be found (Meeuwisse, 1970).

Infants with this disorder develop diarrhoea within a few days of birth and may rapidly become dehydrated. They can tolerate fructose, and diarrhoea immediately ceases when they are given a formula such as Galactomin 19 which is fructose-based. Both small intestinal histology and dissaccharidase activity are normal, but biopsies of the small intestine will show impaired uptake of glucose and galactose whereas fructose uptake will be normal.

Although the defect is permanent the child will be able to include some milk and sugar in his diet in later years but an unrestricted diet will lead to recurrence of symptoms and so the need for some dietary restriction is permanent.

(b) Secondary Monosaccharide Malabsorption

A temporary intolerance of monosaccharide as well as disaccharide was first described by Burke and Anderson in 1966 in a group of neonates following surgery to the gastrointestinal tract. They observed that neonates who had had surgery to the upper part of their alimentary tract, for example, and small intestinal resection for atresia, tended to become intolerant to all sugars. They postulated that an overgrowth of small bowel flora might account for the development of this sugar intolerance. As to management they suggested a period of total carbohydrate restriction followed by the gradual reintroduction of carbohydrate. Burke and Danks in the same year described infants in Melbourne who were temporarily unable to absorb any monosaccharide after a gastroenteritis-like illness and they postulated a similar pathogenesis to that described above.

Wharton, in 1968, described a temporary intolerance of monosaccharide in some children with kwashiorkor. This was usually an intolerance to glucose alone and the children tolerated a fructose-containing artificial milk, but some infants were intolerant to all monosaccharides including fructose.

Gracey, Burke and Anderson went on, in 1969, to describe the 'contaminated small bowel syndrome', where culture of duodenal aspirates leads to a growth of aerobic and /or anaerobic organisms. This syndrome occurs mainly in infants who have stasis of the passage of gut contents after surgery, but also in infants in whom there has been no surgical procedure (see chapter 10). Disaccharidase activity when studied in these children has been normal and there is no significant histological abnormality of the small intestinal mucosa. These infants with monosaccharide malabsorption slowly recover their ability to tolerate sugar as the colony counts of bacteria within the small intestinal lumen fall. They thus respond to a period of total carbohydrate restriction followed by cautious reintroduction of carbohydrate.

The pathogenesis of this disorder is not fully understood but Gracey and Burke (1973) consider that deconjugation of bile salts by organisms that ordinarily should not be present in the small bowel lumen may interfere with intestinal transport of monosaccharides.

At the Royal Alexandra Hospital over a two year period 1970–1971, 8 children were seen with monosaccharide malabsorption (Table 7.9). Most of these were children who had had surgery and in some the outcome was fatal. Some appeared to be intolerant to glucose but could tolerate fructose, similar to Wharton's (1968) experience with kwashiorkor.

Kilby et al. (1978) at Queen Elizabeth Hospital have studied the duodenal bacterial flora in 10 infants with transient monosaccharide intolerance. Five infants had a severe illness with protracted diarrhoea for some weeks following an episode of acute gastroenteritis, and five had delayed recovery just after an acute attack of gastroenteritis. Serial intubations were performed in 8 infants. Five infants surprisingly

Table 7.9
Infants with monosaccharide malabsorption

Child	Age at diag-nosis	Diagnosis	Presumed type of malab-sorption	Therapy	Initial diarrhoea response	Final out-come
S.T.	1 w	Pulmonary valvotomy with hypothermia	Glucose	Galacto-min 19	Good	Good
M.K.	2 w	TOF and duodenal atresia with duodeno-jejunostomy	Glucose	CF_1 and added fructose	Good	Good
H.A.	1 m	Aganglionosis of distal 2/3 small intestine jejunostomy	Glucose and fructose	CF_1	Good	Fatal
B.G.	5 w	Non-specific enterocolitis	Glucose	CF_1	Poor	Fatal
A.W.	6 w	Hirschsprung's disease with colostomy	Glucose	CF_1 and added fructose	Good	Good
R.B.	3 m	'Gastroenteritis syndrome' with recurrent acidosis and dehydration	Glucose and fructose	CF_1	Good	Fatal
A.W.	6 m	Veno-occlusive disease Hypogamma-globulinaemia	Glucose and fructose	CF_1	Good	Fatal
S.W.	2 y 9 m	Massive small intestinal resection. ? Subacute obstruction	Glucose and fructose	CF_1 and added fructose	Good	Good

proved to have duodenal bacterial counts within normal limits ($< 10^4$ organisms/ml). Again surprisingly, the bacterial count in 4 of these infants subsequently increased considerably at a time when monosaccharide tolerance had improved rather than the reverse. In the remaining 5 children there was evidence of bacterial colonisation. Thus, the role of bacterial colonisation in the genesis of secondary monosaccharide intolerance remains unclear.

Interestingly, in 3 of 5 children in this group who had their stools examined for virus particles, rotavirus was identified. Subsequently, at the Queen Elizabeth Hospital, Lucas *et al*. (1978) found during one period of the winter of 1976–1977 no less than 9 children with temporary monosaccharide intolerance complicating acute gastroenteritis of these, 6 had rotavirus in their stools, i.e. in the two series 9 out of 14 children with monosaccharide intolerance developed this as a sequel to rotavirus infection.

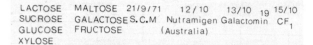

LACTOSE   MALTOSE 21/9/71   12/10   13/10 19 15/10
SUCROSE   GALACTOSE S.C.M Nutramigen Galactomin CF₁
GLUCOSE   FRUCTOSE   (Australia)
XYLOSE

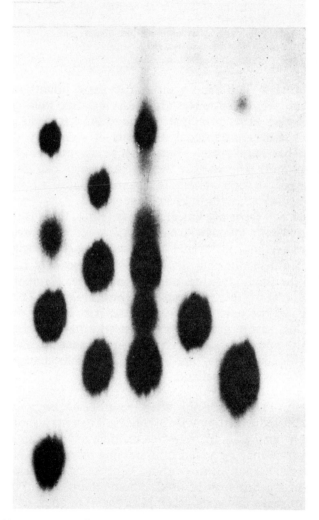

Fig. 7.6. Chromatogram of control sugars and then of stools from an infant, first showing lactose and sucrose malabsorption, then glucose and then fructose malabsorption and, finally, disappearance of sugars when given carbohydrate free feeding, CF_1.

Table 7.10 lists the conditions in which secondary monosaccharide malabsorption has been described.

Table 7.10
Secondary monosaccharide malabsorption

Following surgery in the neonate
Kwashiorkor
Following 'gastroenteritis-like illness' and
    rotavirus gastroenteritis
Hypogammaglobulinaemia

Clinical Features: The main symptom in these infants is diarrhoea, which either persists or recurs after a lactose-free milk containing a monosaccharide as its principal carbohydrate has been given to an infant on whom a provisional diagnosis of secondary disaccharide intolerance has been made. There may be an interval of some days before symptoms reappear, or the diarrhoea may continue unabated on the monosaccharide-containing formula. Figure 7.6 indicates the stool chromatographic findings in such a child.

There are two types of clinical severity. First, there is the group of patients in whom monosaccharide intolerance may present as the intractable diarrhoea syndrome and there may be associated malabsorption of other nutrients (*see* p. 348). There may be structural damage to the small intestinal mucosa on biopsy. Metabolic acidosis, often of a severe degree, is common in these children. They are often gravely ill and the outcome may be fatal (*see* Table 7.9). Secondly there is a less severe group of children who have a relatively brief episode of temporary monosaccharide intolerance following upon a gastroenteritis-like illness, and with appropriate management the prognosis for them is excellent.

Management: These children often require intravenous fluids to correct water and electrolyte disturbances. Then for a short time they need to be given a carbohydrate-free formula to which small amounts of carbohydrate may be added in increasing increments of 1 per cent up to a normal carbohydrate content. Glucose or the glucose polymer (caloreen) or fructose may be used. These infants should be observed carefully for signs of hypoglycaemia as they are often of low weight and have had periods of intravenous feeding. In the United States CHO-free is a suitable carbohydrate-free formula; in Australia CF_1 is available and in the UK comminuted chicken meat is often used (*see* Appendix).

Much more needs to be learned about this disorder.

8

Parasitic Infestation

Parasitic infestation in children is extremely common in many developing communities. It is very difficult to be certain of the possible pathogenic role of a given parasite in a particular illness. Two parasites that damage the small bowel mucosa in childhood have been clearly established. These are *Giardia lamblia* and *Strongyloides stercoralis*. Infestation with either parasite may be related to structural damage to the small bowel mucosa, but it has been suggested that intestinal bacteria may play a role (Leon-Barua and Lumbreras-Cruz, 1968).

A third parasite, namely *Ascaris lumbricoides*, may, rarely, cause intestinal obstruction, perforation or intussesception. Of the three, infestation with *Giardia lamblia* is the only one that is a significant cause of small intestinal disease in Britain and Australia.

GIARDIASIS

Giardia lamblia is a flagellate protozoon (Fig. 8.1) which was first discovered, by Antoni van Leeuwenhoek in 1681, in his own stool. It may infest the proximal small intestine in children and may be found in the glandular crypts of the duodeno-jejunal mucosa. Significant mucosal damage, usually partial villous atrophy but sometimes a flat mucosa, has been demonstrated in infestations with this parasite. However, the mucosa may sometimes be normal, morphologically, when the parasite is detected. In fact, Ament and Rubin (1972) have shown that the mucosal abnormality that occurs in giardiasis is a patchy lesion and that within the small intestine of one child serial biopsies along the small intestine may vary from a normal appearance to one that is severely abnormal.

Infestation is acquired through ingestion of cysts of *Giardia lamblia*,

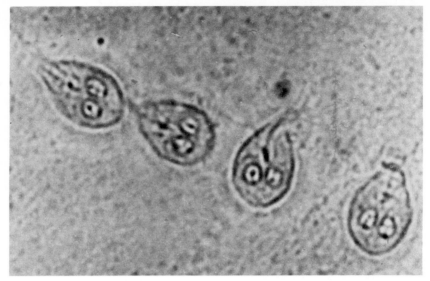

Fig. 8.1. Appearance of *Giardia lamblia* under the light microscope (trophozoite).

through personal contact with an infested individual, or via food or water that has been contaminated with infected faeces.

Pathogenesis

It has now been established that *Giardia lamblia* may cause diarrhoea, steatorrhoea and small intestinal mucosal damage in some children with giardiasis. Ochs, Ament and Davis (1972) have clearly documented this in a child with infantile X-linked agammag-lobulinaemia. This child had normal small intestinal mucosa and absorptive function six months before he developed malabsorption of fat, B_{12} and lactose, when he was found to have giardiasis. He then had a severely abnormal small intestinal mucosa which reverted to normal after eradication of giardia with metronidazole, *pari passu* with the disappearance of malabsorption.

   Why some children develop such a sequence of events when they are infested with giardia and others do not is unclear, but a number of factors are thought to predispose to the development of clinical symptoms and mucosal damage. They include bacterial interaction, alteration of bowel flora, malnutrition and a state of immunodeficiency. Barbieri and his colleagues (1970) have studied the electron microscope appearances of the small intestinal mucosa in children infested with *Giardia lamblia*. Electron micrographs revealed that a large number of parasites had their adhesive disc directed towards the epithelial cells. These discs were close to the cell surface, or directly applied to the mucoid coat of the microvilli. Similar appearances have been seen in a child studied at the Queen Elizabeth Hospital (Fig. 8.2).

These authors suggested that the malabsorption found in some children with giardiasis depended upon mechanical blockade of the epithelial cell surface, with thickening of the mucoid coat and alteration in the microvilli as well as inflammatory changes within the lamina propria.

Prevalence

The prevalence of giardiasis may be very high in children's institutions; for example 40 per cent in one series reported from Australia (Court and Stanton, 1959).

Carswell, Gibson, and McAllister (1973) have looked for *Giardia lamblia* in a large group of Glasgow children. They examined, first, a control group of in-patients who had no clinical evidence of either giardiasis or coeliac disease; secondly, a group of children with coeliac disease; and thirdly a group of children investigated for coeliac disease but in whom this diagnosis was excluded. There was no difference in the frequency of detection of giardia (16–17 per cent) in the stools of these three groups of children. Giardia was also sought in the duodenal juice and in small intestinal biopsy specimens from children in the second two groups and it was detected in a further 13 children. The protozoon was more common in males and in children from the lower socio-economic groups.

This high prevalence contrasts with the findings at the Queen Elizabeth Hospital in 1973 where on only one occasion out of 115 duodenal intubations was *Giardia lamblia* detected in the duodenal juice. At the Royal Alexandra Hospital, giardia was found on 6 occasions out of 120 duodenal intubations in 1971. The reasons for these differences in prevalence in different centres are not clear; identical methods of diagnosis were used in all three centres reported here.

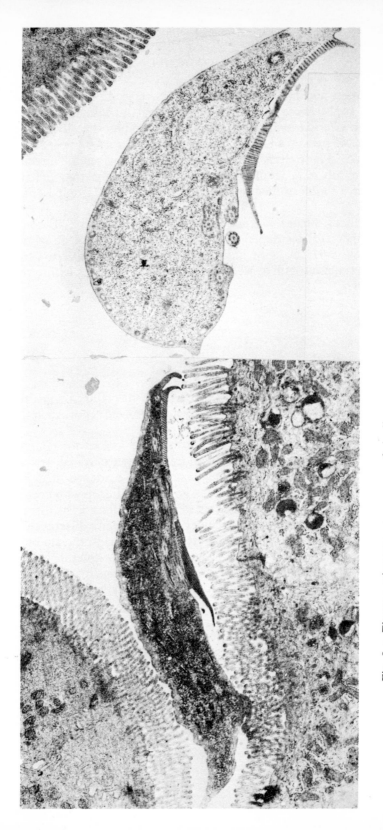

Fig. 8.2. Electron microscope appearance of giardia
Left: giardia with adhesive disc directed towards epithelial cell, with abnormal underlying microvilli.
Right: Parasagittal section with adhesive disc inferiorly and nucleus above it.

Clinical Features

Giardiasis may cause the syndrome of acute gastroenteritis, with acute onset of anorexia, nausea and watery diarrhoea, sometimes with crampy abdominal pain, an illness that usually has a self-limiting course.

Infestation with this parasite in children may produce chronic or intermittent diarrhoea and failure to thrive. Steatorrhoea may be absent and the whole clinical picture may closely resemble that of coeliac disease. Giardiasis may sometimes be complicated by secondary lactose intolerance.

There is a higher incidence of giardiasis in children with immunodeficiency syndromes such as acquired hypogammaglobulinaemia but some children who are infested with this parasite may be symptom-free.

Diagnosis

The diagnosis may be made by demonstration of *Giardia lamblia* in a child's stools but examination of the duodenal aspirate has a higher yield of positive results. Such specimens of juice need to be examined immediately, under the light microscope.

Barbezat and his colleagues (1967) found *Giardia lamblia* in the duodenal aspirate of 75 per cent of 52 children with protein-calorie malnutrition, while the parasite was identified in the stools of only 12 per cent of these children.

Small intestinal biopsy may also reveal the presence of the parasite on histological section, but serial sections may be necessary to demonstrate this.

Treatment

The standard treatment in the past has been Mepacrine but metronidazole (Flagyl) is now the most widely used drug therapy for this condition (Powell, 1968). The dosage is 250 to 750 mg/day depending on age. It is a highly effective form of therapy. Whenever *Giardia lamblia* is found in the duodenal juice of a child with an abnormal mucosa, a trial of metronidazole should be undertaken before other therapy is given.

STRONGYLOIDIASIS

Infestation with the nematode *Strongyloides stercoralis* is found not infrequently in aboriginal and part-aboriginal children in Australia, and tropical countries such as Brazil, but does not occur in Britain. During the life-cycle of this parasite, the larvae invade the mucosa of the proximal small intestine and develop into adult worms within the wall of the small bowel. However, unlike infestation with *Ascaris lumbricoides* the adult strongyloides worms are not usually found in the bowel lumen. The ova are laid in the gut wall and the hatched larvae subsequently migrate into the bowel lumen; with further maturation of the larvae autoinfection further down the small bowel may occur. In addition, the larvae may migrate into other organs such as the regional lymph nodes.

Adult and larval invasion of the intestinal mucosa may cause a catarrhal, oedematous or ulcerative enteritis (De Paola, Dias and da Silva, 1962). The usual clinical manifestations of such an enteritis are a severe watery diarrhoea producing a clinical syndrome similar to acute gastroenteritis. Ileal obstruction as a sequel to an oedematous enteritis has been demonstrated (Walker-Smith *et al.*, 1969). Strongyloidiasis may also produce malabsorption which is cured by eradication of the parasite (Booth, 1965).

Small bowel biopsy in children with strongyloidiasis may demonstrate parasitic invasion of the mucosa as well as partial villous atrophy. The diagnosis is generally made by demonstration of the larvae of *Strongyloides stercoralis* in stools or by duodenal aspiration. There is often an eosinophilia in the peripheral blood. Infestation with this parasite may be effectively treated with thiobendazole.

9

Crohn's Disease

This inflammatory bowel disease is found most often in young adults but it also occurs in older children and adolescents. While the small intestine is often involved, the colon, and indeed any part of the alimentary tract, may be affected. It is sometimes difficult to distinguish Crohn's disease from ulcerative colitis.

TERMINOLOGY

In 1932, Crohn, Ginzburg and Oppenheimer in the USA described a pathological and clinical entity in adults which they called regional ileitis, but when the disease process extends far beyond the ileum and the amount of diseased small and large intestine is extensive, the restricted term ileitis is obviously no longer appropriate. This is particularly obvious when it is realised that the colon may be affected without small intestinal involvement. Some authors have used the term regional enteritis and other granulomatous ileocolitis, but granulomata are not found in every case. The absence of a satisfactory clinico-pathological name which applies to the major manifestations of this syndrome has led many authors to prefer the term Crohn's disease, and at present this appears to be the one that is generally the most acceptable.

DEFINITION

As the aetiology of Crohn's disease is unknown, and the pathology variable, it is difficult to give a precise definition, but the following covers our present knowledge: a chronic inflammatory disorder that may affect any part of the alimentary tract, and that has a characteristic pattern of clinical and pathological features, many or all of which may be present but not one of which, individually, is essential for establishing the diagnosis (Lennard-Jones, 1970).

Some authorities have suggested that non-caseating or sarcoid granulomata are an essential prerequisite for this diagnosis, but if that view were adopted a number of patients would be left with chronic inflammatory bowel disease and no specific diagnosis. Until the aetiology of Crohn's disease is established, a precise definition will continue to pose problems as well as precise criteria for diagnosis.

INCIDENCE AND GENETIC FACTORS

Crohn's disease most often occurs in young adults aged between 20 and 40 years but it may begin in the first decade of life. The incidence of the disorder appears to vary from country to country and among different ethnic groups; for example, there is stated to be an increased incidence of Crohn's disease in Jews. Nonetheless, imprecise diagnostic criteria and confusion with ulcerative colitis make an accurate appraisal of the true situation difficult, but there is evidence that the disease is increasing both in Great Britain and Europe (Miller, Keighley and Langman, 1974; Bender, 1977). There is certainly a clinical impression among paediatricians that the disease is 'commoner' than it used to be, which has become obviously so at St Bartholomew's Hospital during the 1970s —see Table 9.1.

Table 9.1
New cases, age and sex distribution of Crohn's disease in childhood. Diagnosed at St Bartholomew's Hospital, 1973–1978

		Numbers		Age range at diagnosis in years
		Male	Female	
1973	1	1	–	10·4
1974	1	–	1	12·1
1975	2	–	2	13·5–12·0
1976	1	1	–	10·7
1977	8	7	1	6·2 –14·7
1978	8	4	4	9·75–14·0

Crohn's disease has been recognised most often in urbanised areas. It is found in American Negroes and West Indians in Britain, but has not so far been described in African Negroes. Discordance for Crohn's disease in twins has been described. If genetic factors are involved, these certainly are not straightforward and there are no known genetic markers to identify people at risk.

As with coeliac disease a familial occurrence of the condition has been recognised for some time, and different members of the same family may have Crohn's disease and ulcerative colitis. It is still uncertain whether or not the familial occurrence of Crohn's disease is related to genetic or to environmental factors, or possibly both.

AETIOLOGY

The cause of Crohn's disease is still unknown. Originally, Crohn's disease was confused with tuberculosis because of histological similarity between the two conditions, but there is no real evidence to incriminate *Mycobacterium tuberculosis* in the aetiology of Crohn's disease. Yersinia enterocolitica (Pasteurella pseudotuberculosis) can cause an acute terminal ileitis but this is distinct from Crohn's disease (*see* page 200).

Mitchell and Rees (1970) induced epithelioid and giant cell granulomata in the footpads of mice by inoculating tissue homogenates from Crohn's small intestine and lymph node tissue. These results have not always been confirmed, and in any event transmissability, does not prove infectivity. Slow clearance of, for example a virus, could account for this. Some viruses have indeed been found in some patients with Crohn's disease. Whorwell *et al.*, (1977) have isolated reovirus-like agents from patients with Crohn's disease, but Marshall and Walker-Smith (1978) who studied rotavirus complement-fixing antibody found low titres in 3 of 7 children studied.

The finding of circulating immune complexes in Crohn's disease is probably an epiphenomenon, the result of ulceration from exposure to antigen. It is possible that the granulomata are due to T-lymphocytes reacting to an unknown antigen or something not ordinarily acting as an antigen. There is an increase in plasma cell count in the lamina propria, particularly IgA and IgM cells (Green and Fox, 1973) paradoxically in uninvolved gut, whereas there is a gross diminution of IgA cells where the intestine is diseased.

There have been reports that delayed hypersensitivity reactions in Crohn's disease are reduced. These include loss of tuberculin reactivity, failure of cultured lymphocytes to respond normally to phytohaemagglutination and failure to sensitise patients to dinitrochlorobenzine (DNCB). Other authors have denied all these reports. In any event the failure of these responses appears to be a non-specific effect of chronic illness and not a significant factor in the aetiology of this disease.

Crohn and Yarnis, in 1958, noted that surgical diversion of the intestinal stream benefited patients with Crohn's disease. Thus, it has been postulated that some factor in the intestinal contents is one cause of Crohn's disease, but its nature is at present unknown, though it has been suggested that bacteria normally present in the alimentary tract may be a source of antigen participating in an immunological reaction. The eating of cornflakes as a breakfast food has even been implicated as a possible aetiological factor in adults with Crohn's disease (James, 1977), but this observation has not been substantiated.

Although sarcoid granulomata are found in the small intestine of patients with Crohn's disease, Scadding, in 1967, found no good evidence of small intestinal disease in a review of patients with sarcoidosis.

PATHOLOGY

Crohn's disease may affect any part of the alimentary tract, from the mouth to the anus. Duodenal and jejunal involvement is not common but seems more so in children than in adults. Indeed, extensive involvement of jejunum and ileum is more likely in children than adults. When disease is confined to the colon it may be difficult to distinguish it from ulcerative colitis. Table 9.2 indicates the major site of involvement in 15 children diagnosed at St Barth-

Table 9.2
Major site of involvement in 15 children with Crohn's disease (permission Campbell, 1978)

	Number
Colon only	5
Right colon and terminal ileum	4
Extensive small and large intestinal involvement	5
Perineal	1

olomew's Hospital. In this series no child had disease confined to the small intestine alone, and in the series reported by O'Donoghue and Dawson (1977) only 4 of 32 children had disease that was confined to the small intestine. Classically, the pathological lesions in Crohn's disease are stated to be discontinuous along the alimentary tract, i.e. so-called skip areas are a feature of the condition. Recently, a new concept has arisen, however, that Crohn's disease is really a diffuse lesion of the alimentary tract. Some of the evidence for this has been produced by Dunne, Cooke and Allan (1977), in adults. They showed that morphometric abnormalities and enzyme deficiences could be shown in apparently normal proximal jejunal biopsies from patients with Crohn's disease that is confined to the distal ileum or the large bowel.

Nevertheless, the pathological lesions in Crohn's disease are classically described as discontinuous along the alimentary tract, i.e. so-called skip areas are a feature of this condition.

Considering the gross pathology of the small intestine, the small intestinal wall, when involved, is thickened, which may lead to a narrowing of the lumen, i.e. stricture formation, and may sometimes produce complete obstruction. Often there is, in addition, longitudinal and transverse ulceration of the small intestinal mucosa. Microscopic sinuses, usually called fissures, may pass from the ulcerated mucosal surface deep into the small intestinal wall. The pathological lesion in Crohn's disease is typically transmural, although submucosal thickening is a characteristic. Hadfield (1939) attributed the thickening to obstructive lymphoedema and lymphoid hyperplasia. In many cases the lymph follicles contain sarcoid granulomata. In the submucosa, there may also be a diffuse inflammation, consisting of acute and chronic inflammatory cells, often but not always, with granulomata containing giant cells. A sarcoid reaction has also been described in the regional lymph nodes. Morson (1968) has suggested that the frequency with which the terminal ileum and anal region are involved in Crohn's disease is explained by the fact that both these regions are rich in lymphoid aggregations and that, probably, the primary lesion of Crohn's disease is in lymphoid tissue.

Mast cell degranulation has been found to be a prominent feature in a morphological study of the lesion of Crohn's disease by Dvorak et al., 1978, who investigated surgically resected specimens from 12 patients with Crohn's disease. They have suggested a role for the mediators released by mast cells in the pathogenesis of Crohn's disease. These are histamine, platelet activation factor, slow-reacting substance of anaphylaxis and eosinophil chemolactic factor.

CLINICAL FEATURES

The age of diagnosis is usually 10 years or over. In a large series, boys are affected as often as girls (Bender, 1977). Children less than 10 years of age may also be affected. Indeed, Crohn's disease has been reported in the neonatal period, but the relationship of this early disease and that found later in life is unclear. Although Crohn's disease in childhood and in adolescence may manifest in a similar way to the disease seen in adults, children with the disease may present without any gastrointestinal symptoms. Silverman drew attention to this in 1966 by describing 14 children aged 8 to 15 years at diagnosis, only 8 of whom had gastrointestinal symptoms at the time of diagnosis. These 14 children presented as cases of growth failure, pyrexia of unknown origin and pseudo-appendicitis. Chrispin and Tempany, in 1967, described 4 children aged 10 to 12 years at the time of diagnosis of Crohn's disease of the jejunum in whom there were few gastrointestinal symptoms. The dominant clinical features in these children were systemic.

O'Donoghue and Dawson (1977) have published the first detailed study from Britain of Crohn's disease in childhood. They reported the clinical features of 32 children at St Bartholomew's Hospital over a ten-year period whose disease started before their sixteenth birthday. Abdominal pain and diarrhoea were the common presenting symptoms but unexplained fever and failure to grow were also prominent, although in their series gastrointestinal symptoms were dominant. Indeed, the triad of pain, diarrhoea and weight loss, so characteristic of Crohn's disease in adult life, was commonly found. Fever occurred more often than in adult patients. In a further series of 15 children, Campbell (1978) (Table 9.3) again found that most children with Crohn's disease presented with gastrointestinal symptoms. Perineal ulceration is a well-known manifestation of adult Crohn's disease, but it is uncommon in childhood, although it may occur occasionally, diagnosis often being delayed (Wallis and Walker-Smith, 1976).

The gastrointestinal symptoms that occur in children with this disorder include abdominal pain, anorexia, nausea, vomiting and diarrhoea. The abdominal pain is characteristically peri-umbilical and colicky and it is often brought on by eating. Pain that is partially relieved by defaecation may also occur. The anorexia may be very severe and at times so gross as to suggest the diagnostic possibility of anorexia nervosa. Gryboski and her colleagues (1968) have drawn attention to the similarity of clinical features that may occur in the two disorders. Chronic constipation is also an important feature of some children with Crohn's disease.

Bender in a multicentre study involving paediatric gastroenterologists in Austria, West Germany and Switzerland analysed the clinical features of 155 children diagnosed as having Crohn's disease between 1972–1976. Abdominal pain was the commonest symptom (90 per cent) and anorexia next (84 per cent), followed by intermittent diarrhoea with mucus in 73 per cent of children.

Table 9.3
Clinical features of Crohn's disease in childhood, 15 children diagnosed at St Bartholomew's Hospital (permission Campbell, 1978)

Mode of presentation	Number of children	Delay in diagnosis (years)
Diarrhoeal illness	4	2·8
Unresponsive anaemia	3	1·9
Lethargy and weight loss	3	0·7
Recurrent abdominal pains	2	2·5
Perineal symptoms	2	2·5
Erythema nodosum	1	0·2
		(Mean delay 1·94 years)

Analysis of abdominal pain in childhood can be a difficult problem. Apley (1975) has pointed out just how common a symptom it is in children between the ages of 5 and 15 years and how, uncommonly, an organic cause is found. Clinicians must, however, be alert to the possibility that Crohn's disease is an important cause of this symptom.

The vomiting and diarrhoea found in some children with Crohn's disease may have an acute onset and suggest the diagnosis of acute gastroenteritis, but sometimes when there is bloody diarrhoea, due to colonic involvement, differentiation from ulcerative colitis may be very difficult. Occasionally, a child with Crohn's disease may present with a chronic malabsorption syndrome or with features of protein-losing enteropathy.

The syndrome of growth failure accompanied by unexplained fever, anaemia, and an elevated sedimentation rate in an older child, or a similar syndrome combined with delayed puberty in an adolescent, suggest that Crohn's disease should be considered as a diagnostic possibility. Other extra-intestinal features found in children with Crohn's disease include erythema nodosum, arthritis, uveitis and stomatitis.

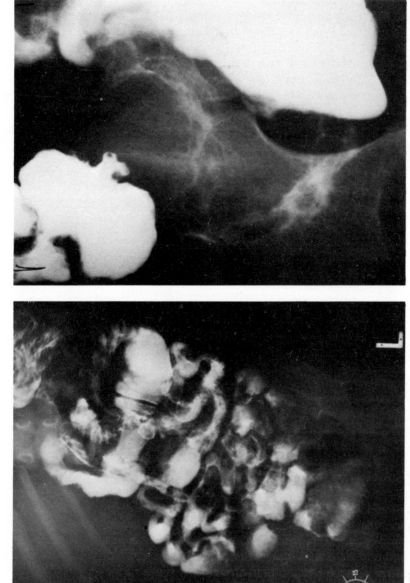

Fig. 9.1. Barium follow-through demonstrating: (left) abnormality of terminal ileum in a child with Crohn's disease, (right) generalised small intestinal involvement.

Physical examination of children with this condition may reveal retarded growth and development. Plotting earlier measurements of height and weight on a percentile chart may give information of diagnostic value. Evidence of malnutrition such as muscle wasting may be found. Sometimes an abdominal mass may be felt on palpation of the abdomen or there may be an area of tenderness or guarding. There may be one or more anal fissures with sentinel piles. Characteristically such fissures are relatively painless. A perianal abscess or a fistula-in-ano may also be found. Other features discovered on physical examination include erythema nodosum, finger clubbing and stomatitis. Occasionally, children with Crohn's disease may present with a severe attack and when first seen may have a striking pallor, tachycardia, and swinging fever with a general appreance often described as 'toxic'. Some children, however, on physical examination have no abnormalities whatever.

DIAGNOSIS

This depends chiefly upon strict criteria for evaluating intestinal morphology and radiology, and, to a lesser extent, on endoscopy and clinical features.

In the discussion concerning the terminology of Crohn's disease, at the beginning of this chapter, it was made clear that some authorities demand the demonstration of sarcoid-like non-caseating granulomata in the mucosa or submucosa but others are content with granulation tissue containing epithelial cells or giant cells but without definite granulomata.

A presumptive diagnosis may be made when radiological investigations demonstrate the typical abnormalities found in Crohn's disease in a child who has clinical features to suggest its presence (Fig. 9.1). A definitive diagnosis can be made when, in addition, the characteristic histology of the disease is observed in specimens of the small or large intestine obtained at laparotomy or in rectal mucosal biopsy specimens obtained at sigmoidoscopy or endoscopic biopsy. A rectal biopsy may show granulomata even in the absence of any apparent anal or colonic disease. Biopsy of anal lesions when present may also be valuable diagnostically (Fig. 9.2).

A provisional diagnosis of Crohn's disease in children is most often made by the former means, using a barium meal and follow-through, and a barium enema. However, routine barium studies may not be helpful in the early stages of the disease, and Silverman (1966) has emphasised that in such children very careful examination of the ileum at the time of barium studies is necessary to pick up minor abnormalities.

Crohn's disease needs to be distinguished radiologically from other disorders of the small intestine, particularly those that may affect the ileum. These include lymphoma, adenocarcinoma, tuberculosis, amoebiasis, strongyloidiasis, Henoch-Schönlein purpura with small intestinal obstruction, and Yersinia enterocolitica.

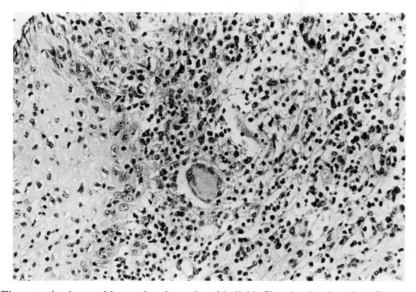

Fig. 9.2. Anal verge biopsy showing sub-epithelial infiltration by chronic inflammatory cells with multinucleate giant cells.

Colonoscopy is a useful diagnostic aid. In particular it enables histology to be taken from selected areas of bowel. The terminal ileum may also be examined with this technique and an ileal biopsy taken (Campbell, Williams and Walker-Smith, 1978). Endoscopic biopsies have been reviewed from 12 children at St Bartholomew's Hospital: 4 had characteristic granulomata, 3 had histology suggestive of Crohn's disease, 3 showed non-specific inflammation, and 2 had unhelpful histology.

The remarkable delay in diagnosis of children with Crohn's disease is shown in Table 9.3 which indicates that very often paediatricians are unaware of the clinical manifestations of this disease in childhood. Fortunately, with increasing awareness of this malady in childhood, coupled with better diagnostic techniques, the delay is now being reduced. It has fallen at St Bartholomew's Hospital from 2·9 years, in the cases of O'Donoghue and Dawson (1977) between 1965 and 1975, to 1·9 years in the cases of Campbell (1978) between 1975–1978.

INVESTIGATIONS

Anaemia may be found, sometimes related to folic acid deficiency, sometimes due to iron deficiency, but more often to a microcytic anaemia not due to iron deficiency and usually related to disease severity. Folic acid deficiency, when present, is in part dietary in origin, secondary to the anorexia which is a feature of this disease, but it may also be related to malabsorption when there is extensive mucosal abnormality. Although a Schilling test when performed in these children is often abnormal, megaloblastic anaemia due to Vitamin B_{12} deficiency is rare. The erythrocyte sedimentation rate is typically elevated, although not invariably.

There may be hypoalbuminaemia due to protein-losing enteropathy and there may also be evidence of malabsorption, e.g. steatorrhoea. However, Dyer and Dawson (1973) at St Bartholomew's Hospital have found in a group of patients with Crohn's disease, aged 14–71 years at diagnosis, who had severe nutritional abnormalities, that these abnormalities were accompanied only by relatively minor degres of malabsorption. This was insufficient to account for the severity of the nutritional disturbances observed and did not correlate with disease severity. Dyer and Dawson related the degree of nutritional disturbance to disease activity and they concluded that the two major factors accounting for this were, firstly, anorexia, and secondly, increased demands for essential nutrients secondary to the excess production and loss of inflammatory cells, which is a feature of Crohn's disease.

The commonest radiological signs in the small intestine are a thickened mucosa, areas of dilatation proximal to narrowed regions, rigidity of the walls and narrowing of the terminal ileum. The lesions seen are often discontinuous. In the colon there is eccentric involvement with incomplete haustral loss and normal patches within diseased areas. There may also be areas of apthous ulceration. In patients with extensive disease there may be an irregular outline of the bowel, referred to as a 'cobblestone appearance'. It is sometimes difficult to distinguish Crohn's disease from ulcerative colitis.

Study of bile salt metabolism in adolescents and adults with Crohn's disease has shown that the bile acid pool size is significantly reduced. This reduction was related to disease activity, suggesting that intestinal involvement from a functional viewpoint may be more extensive than is usually apparent from radiological studies (Vantrappen et al., 1977).

COMPLICATIONS

Intestinal obstruction, fistulae and abscess formation, as well as a stagnant loop syndrome secondary to incomplete obstruction, may occur.

Crohn's disease may clearly cause severe growth retardation, and delayed sexual maturation as an important complication. The cause of delayed growth is not clear. McCaffery et al. (1974) have shown an inadequate growth hormone response to a hypoglycaemic stimulus as in children with coeliac disease. Green et al. (1977) have studied one such patient and found a similar lack of response of growth hormone to hypoglycaemia and, also, an impaired plasma gonadotrophin response to luteinising hormone/follicle stimulating hormone-releasing hormone, which suggested hypopituitarism, but these abnormalities disappeared following a remission achieved by surgery. Clearly, the subject warrants further study.

Carcinoma as a complication of Crohn's disease in adult patients with long-standing small intestinal disease has been described. The risk involved has not yet been accurately determined.

TREATMENT

There is no curative therapy for Crohn's disease at present, the aim of therapy being to induce a remission which may not always be possible. The relief of symptoms is all that can then be achieved.

Approach to treatment will depend upon the initial severity of the illness. Severe illness or an acute attack usually warrants hospital admission with bed rest. A patient with less severe illness may be managed as an outpatient.

Treatment may involve the use of drugs, dietary manipulation or, in some cases, surgery (Table 9.4).

Drugs

There is no completely satisfactory drug treatment at present. Most often, drugs are used in an initial attempt to induce a clinical remission. Salazopyrin is usually the first drug of choice in children with Crohn's colitis. It is given in divided doses of 1–3 g/day, depending on age. It is not as effective as it is in ulcerative colitis. However, in some children it appears to induce a remission hence its being prescribed as first treatment in Crohn's colitis. So far, no carefully controlled trial has been carried out to establish the place of Salazopyrin in management in childhood. In fact, no drug has been adequately assessed in such a way in Crohn's disease in children which reflects the relatively small numbers of cases diagnosed until recently.

Table 9.4
Treatment of Crohn's disease in childhood

Drugs
Salazopyrin—Crohn's colitis
Steroids—induction of remission
Azathioprine—?maintains a remission
Metronidazole ?heals fistulae
Disodium cromoglycate—uncertain role

Nutritional
Elemental diet with constant rate external alimentation
Total parenteral nutrition

Surgery
Resection of localised lesions

Steroid therapy may be effective in the management of acute severe attacks to induce a remission, but it may not be as effective in inducing a remission in children with Crohn's disease as it is in ulcerative colitis. Steroid therapy does not alter the course of the disease. Three days of ACTH 1 u/kg/day) is recommended followed by rednisolone 2 mg/kg/day. The dose of steroids is slowly reduced when a remission has been achieved. After a time it may be helpful to administer prednisolone on alternative days. After several months an attempt should be made to stop steroid therapy completely.

Azathioprine in a dosage of 2 mg/kg/day may also be given to a child with a severe attack, the aim being to maintain the child in a remission once the steroid therapy has ceased.

Azathioprine was first recommended for this disease by Brooke, Hoffman and Swarbrick in 1969. A controlled trial of its use in adults at St Bartholomew's Hospital, by Willoughby *et al.* in 1971, has shown that the drug was more effective than a placebo in maintaining patients in a remission, once they were taken off steroid therapy. It may fail to be effective in some patients, and in others it is associated with toxic side effects. Long-term use of the drug in children does not appear to be associated with the same toxic effect on the reproductive system as has been described with cyclophosphamide. How long the child should be maintained on azathioprine is not at present clear.

Sometimes the drug is unsuccessful in maintaining a remission, and whenever steroids are stopped a relapse occurs. A situation of this kind is difficult to manage and other drugs such as salazopyrin and oral disodium cromoglycate (Nalcrom) have been used. The theoretical basis for the use of disodium cromoglycate in relation to degranulated mast cells has already been mentioned. Henderson and Hishon (1978) have described an adult patient who responded to this drug, but its role in childhood Crohn's disease if any, has not yet been established.

Metronidazole has been claimed to be of value, especially in healing fistulae (Hildebrand and Ursing, 1977). In adults, long-term use can cause peripheral neuropathy.

The decision to use such potentially dangerous drugs as steroids and azathioprine in these children, should be undertaken only after very careful appraisal of the clinical situation and a critical review of the indications for their use.

Cholestyramine resin may help relieve diarrhoea when ileal pathology is extensive, and malabsorption of bile acids results.

Codeine may symptomatically relieve the diarrhoea and abdominal pain, and sedation may play an important part in the management of this disease.

Dietary

Dietary management and symptomatic treatment should not be overlooked in the initial stages of therapy. Dietary management should not be neglected when anorexia is a major symptom. Vitamin therapy may be a valuable adjunct to management. When small intestinal mucosal involvement is extensive and there is significant steatorrhoea, a medium chain triglyceride feeding such as Pregestimil supplemented with medium chain triglyceride oil and Caloreen may lead to a significant improvement in nutrition.

Total parenteral nutrition may be used to close fistulae or for periods of gut rest during an acute exacerbation (Ricour et al., 1977). A new treatment using an elemental diet given constantly by nasogastric intubation, constant rate external alimentation (CREM) has been claimed to be of value for a period after total parenteral alimentation. It has also been used in severe malnutrition with anorexia and persistent digestive symptoms after usual medical therapy (Navarro *et al.*, 1977).

Surgery

Surgical treatment in children is usually reserved for complications of Crohn's disease, such as intestinal obstruction or for some of the ano-rectal manifestations. However, surgical resection of an involved area of gut does reduce the 'toxic mass' and appears to improve the patient's immediate outlook, although later, recurrence of the disease at the site of anastomosis is common, hence extensive resections of the small intestine should be avoided. Surgery may still have an important place in the management of Crohn's disease in childhood but assessment of the indications for its use depends upon the particular clinical situation and on the experience of the clinician concerned. Some authors commend its use in children.

O'Donoghue and Dawson (1977) recommend surgery, where resectable disease is present, at an early stage in those children whose growth is severely retarded or whose education is suffering because of time lost from school.

The management of Crohn's disease in childhood poses one of the biggest problems in paediatric gastroenterology. The children and their parents need much support and encouragement from their physician, who must be patient and understanding concerning their many problems. Quite often, psychosomatic symptoms may be overlaid upon organic symptoms and the distinction between organic and non-organic symptoms in these children may be very difficult to deal with. It can only be hoped that further research may provide better therapy than that at present available.

10

Surgically Correctable Lesions of the Small Intestine

Lesions of the small intestine that are surgically correctable may be divided into those that present during the neonatal period and those that present later, during infancy and childhood. A brief outline of some of the most important of these disorders is given here but for a more detailed account the bibliography and appropriate paediatric surgical texts should be consulted.

NEONATES

Surgically correctable lesions of the small intestine that present clinically during the neonatal period do so in four principal ways, namely, as neonatal small intestinal obstruction, small intestinal perforation, necrotising enterocolitis and gastro-intestinal bleeding.

Neonatal Small Intestinal Obstruction

Persistent vomiting, abdominal distension or failure to pass meconium, all may suggest the diagnosis of intestinal obstruction in the neonatal period. Vomiting from many causes is not uncommon in this age group, but bilious vomiting should always alert the clinician to the possibility of small intestinal obstruction (Middleton, 1969). Whenever such bilious vomiting is accompanied by abdominal distension, then the diagnosis of obstruction is highly probable. Although such obstruction is most often due to a congenital abnormality, it must be appreciated that some congenital lesions do not produce symptoms within the first twenty-four hours of life and may take several days and even many months to appear when the lesion causes only partial obstruction. The most important single diagnostic test for the investigation of a neonate with suspected intestinal obstruction is a plain X-ray of the abdomen taken in the supine, upright and erect lateral positions (Fig. 10.1). Sometimes a barium enema may also be necessary to differentiate between small and large intestinal obstruction. Table 10.1 indicates the principal causes of small intestinal obstruction in the neonate, and these will be discussed in more detail later.

Table 10.1
Neonatal small intestinal obstruction

Duodenal atresia or stenosis
Annular pancreas
Malrotation with or without volvulus
Jejuno-ileal atresia or stenosis
Meconium ileus
Duplications

Small Intestinal Perforation

Perforation of the small intestine may occur during the neonatal period although perforation of the stomach is more common. While peptic ulceration, trauma due to intubation, perforation proximal to a small intestinal obstruction, and perforation related to brain damage may occur, gastrointestinal perforation in neonates is most often spontaneous and of uncertain origin. Lloyd (1969) has undertaken a clinical and pathological study of 87 neonates with gastrointestinal perforation and 80 per cent of these infants had previously experienced a significant episode of asphyxia or shock. He therefore postulated local ischaemia as a cause of such perforation which was otherwise of unknown origin.

The symptoms of perforation include vomiting, abdominal distension and lethargy sometimes with cyanosis, laboured respiration, tachycardia and shock. Diagnosis is made by means of an upright plain X-ray of the abdomen. Once the diagnosis has been made, surgery is promptly indicated following restoration of hydration and correction of disturbances of electrolyte balance when these occur. The area of perforated small intestine should be resected, or if distal it may be exteriorised.

Necrotising Enterocolitis

Definition. Necrotising enterocolitis in the newborn is a condition in

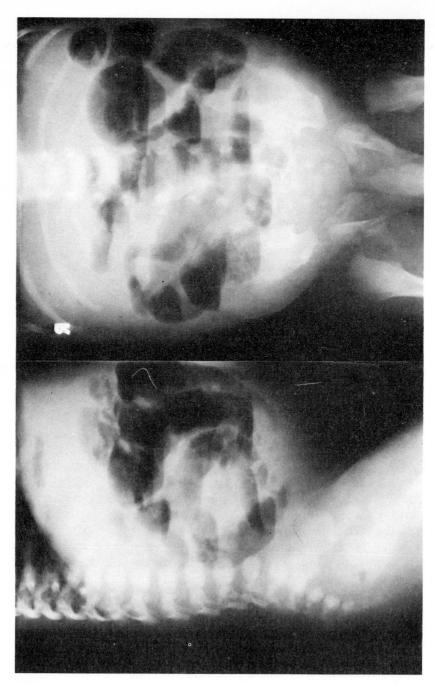

Fig. 10.1 Upright lateral and antero-posterior views of abdomen of infant with small intestinal obstruction (ileal volvulus in this case).

which there is a diffuse or patchy necrosis of the mucosa or submucosa of the small and/or large intestine. It is a syndrome which probably has a multifactorial aetiology.

Pathogenesis

Its pathogenesis is still a matter for debate. Many associated conditions have been recognised, namely, apnoea, hyaline membrane disease, a low apgar score, prior sepsis, premature rupture of the membranes, exchange transfusions, and the use of umbilical artery catheters. Most of those associations relate to prematurity and may be manifestations of either hypoxia or infection. Indeed, poor perfusion of intestinal tissue during the perinatal period, whether produced by asphyxia or not, has been considered an important factor in the pathogenesis of necrotising enterocolitis (Rowe, 1975). On the other hand, an infectious theory has also been put forward as outbreaks of necrotising enterocolitis are well recognised (Frantz *et al.*, 1975). In addition, enteric bacteria are necessary for the production of hydrogen gas which is the major constituant of the intramural gas characteristic of this disorder (Engel *et al.*, 1973).

Clostridium butyricum was found in an outbreak of necrotising enterocolitis in a hospital nursery, and normal full term as well as pre-term infants were affected (Howard *et al.*, 1977). This organism, in the ordinary way, is ubiquitous, but it may have acquired some enhancing factor to make it more pathogenic in this particular outbreak, and so become a major factor in the pathogenesis of necrotising enterocolitis. The type of infant feeding may also have a role in pathogenesis. Large volumes of hyperosmolor feedings have been incriminated. Necrotising enterocolitis has not been described in an infant fed only on the breast but it can rarely develop in an infant not yet fed. Breast feeding may have a major role in protecting against necrotising enterocolitis by virtue of its high secretory IgA content which provides passive protection, and its cell content (lymphocyte) immunity in the neonate. It is possible that in some instances cow's milk protein intolerance *per se*, may play a part in pathogenesis (dePeyer and Walker-Smith, 1977). Herbst (1975) has described evidence of milk intolerance, in particular excess faecal reducing substances, preceding the onset of necrotising enterocolitis, and this may be evidence of a cow's milk sensitive enteropathy preceding the disease. Thus, it seems probable that a number of aetiological factors are likely to be of pathogenetic significance in this syndrome.

Clinical Features

Necrotising enterocolitis presents usually on or about the second day of life with the sudden onset of abdominal distension, vomiting, and bloody diarrhoea. A plain X-ray of the abdomen reveals small intestinal distension, sometimes with a feathery appearance indicative of mucosal ulceration. There is, characteristically, also evidence of intramural gas, usually in the wall of the large intestine.

Surgical management is controversial but when there is perforation it is usually indicated. When it is not, some authors advocate a conservative approach with gastrointestinal suction, intravenous fluids and antibiotics; others advocate surgical resection of the abnormal bowel although this may necessitate a total colectomy in some patients. The survival rate varies from 10 to 50 per cent. The author favours a conservative approach, using a period of intravenous alimentation followed by expressed breast milk when available, unless lactose intolerance is present.

Gastrointestinal Haemorrhage

Most often, gastrointestinal bleeding in the newborn is due to a generalised tendency to bleed such as hypoprothrombinaemia, but it may sometimes be due to a localised lesion in the small intestine, such as a duodenal ulcer, haemangioma or a duplication. Laparotomy to seek a surgically correctable lesion should be considered only when a tendency to bleed has been excluded and bleeding continues despite a replacement blood transfusion.

SMALL INTESTINAL OBSTRUCTION IN INFANTS AND OLDER CHILDREN

Surgically correctable lesions of the small intestine in older children nearly always present as intestinal obstruction. Some of the important causes of this syndrome are listed in Table 10.2.

The syndrome needs to be distinguished from ileus which may occur in many situations including severe gastroenteritis, hypokalaemia and septicaemia. Classically, it presents, as in adult life, with colicky abdominal pain, nausea, vomiting, abdominal distension and constipation, but when obstruction is incomplete the signs may be less clear-cut and the child may present with features of the malabsorption syndrome related to stasis of gut contents with bacterial overgrowth (*see* stagnant loop syndrome, page 318).

Several of the more important surgically correctable lesions of the small intestine will now be discussed.

Table 10.2
Small intestinal obstruction in infants and older children

Intussusception
Inguinal hernia
Internal hernia
Malrotation with or without volvulus
Atresia and stenosis
Adhesions
Infection and abscess formation
Meconium ileus equivalent
Mesenteric cyst
Milk plug obstruction
Ascariasis
Strongyloidiasis
Lymphosarcoma
Aganglionosis of small intestine

Congenital Intrinsic Obstruction of the Small Intestine (Atresia and Stenosis)

Intrinsic obstruction of the small intestine of congenital origin presents most often in the neonatal period but when the obstruction is partial it may first present much later, in infancy and childhood.

Intrinsic small intestinal obstruction may produce either complete or partial obliteration of the bowel lumen. Complete obliteration may be due to a diaphragm occluding the lumen, or to a gap between the two ends of the small intestine which is complete, or there may be a connecting band between these ends. Such complete obstruction is known as atresia. When obstruction is incomplete it may be due to a narrowing of the lumen which is known as stenosis. An incomplete diaphragm may also occur, especially in the duodenum, partially occluding the bowel lumen and producing a clinical picture identical to that found in children who have stenosis. Small intestinal atresia is a more common finding than stenosis.

In an analysis of 42 consecutive admissions to the Royal Alexandra Hospital, atresia occurred most often and was found in 30 children. Stenosis occurred in the remaining 12.

The duodenum is most often involved, followed by the jejunum and then the ileum. These disorders are often associated with other abnormalities of the gastrointestinal tract as study of these 42 children revealed (Table 10.3).

It is clear that such abnormalities occur most often in association with duodenal lesions, those occurring in association with jejuno-ileal lesions being largely related to the pathogenesis of such lesions.

Table 10.3
Associated abnormalities of the gastrointestinal tract
Royal Alexandra Hospital

	Duodenum	Jejuno-ileum
No. of children	24	18
Malrotation of midgut loop	10	3
Meckel's diverticulum	1	3
Oesophageal atresia	4	—
Imperforate anus	2	—
Volvulus	—	4
Meconium peritonitis	1	2
Meconium ileus	—	2
Perforation	2	—
Annular pancreas	2	—
Atresia of bile ducts	3	—

Aetiology

Louw (1959) and Barnard (1956) have produced good experimental and clinical evidence to support the theory that a vascular accident occurring during intrauterine life is responsible for most atresias and stenoses of the small intestine. Tandler, in 1902, had suggested that a failure of recanalisation of the duodenum during the twelfth week of intrauterine life accounted for this disorder. However, the vascular insufficiency theory is more soundly based, although it does have to explain the fact that other abnormalities outside the gastrointestinal tract occur more often with duodenal lesions than with jejuno-ileal lesions (Table 10.4).

Louw believes that these associated malformations may be related to generalised fetal hypoxia and that local factors such as critical interference with blood supply to a segment of the bowel accounts for the local gut lesion. He points out that the second part of the duodenum is the most actively growing part of the gastrointestinal tract during the eighth and ninth weeks of pregnancy and so is the most vulnerable to the effects of hypoxia at that time.

Grob-Vontobel (1969) has reported evidence in a child that multiple atresias may be due to intrauterine volvulus associated with malrotation, thus supporting the vascular insufficiency theory.

A familial incidence with two or more members of one family affected has been described and, on the basis of this, inheritance as an autosomal recessive is proposed. An association with cystic fibrosis has also been reported.

Table 10.4
Associated abnormalities of the gastrointestinal tract
Royal Alexandra Hospital

	Duodenum	*Jejunum*	*Ileum*
No. of children	24	11	7
Genito-urinary	7	—	—
Musculo-skeletal	4	2	—
Down's syndrome	11	—	—
Cardiovascular	6	—	—

Santulli and Blanc, in 1961, described an uncommon variant of atresia known as the 'apple peel' small bowel. They reported atresia accompanied by severe prematurity and a total anomalous mesentery with 'apple peel' attachment of an unusually small distal bowel. It has been suggested that this is due to an obstruction to the superior mesenteric artery due to a secondary volvulus also associated with malrotation. Dickson (1970) reviewed 15 children with this uncommon syndrome and confirmed the pathological features. He also described a familial occurrence.

Clinical Features

Duodenal Obstruction: When duodenal obstruction is complete, vomiting usually occurs within a few hours of birth and is characteristically bilious, except when the obstruction is proximal to the ampulla of Vater. Vomiting does not occur when there is an accompanying oesophageal atresia, a well-recognised association of this disorder. Meconium at first may be passed normally and there may be no obvious epigastric distension. In view of the frequent association with other abnormalities such as mongolism mentioned earlier, these should be sought for carefully, once the diagnosis has been established.

When obstruction is incomplete the symptoms may be intermittent and the diagnosis delayed.

Jejuno-ileal Obstruction: Symptoms, typically vomiting and abdominal distension, usually occur within the first two days of life. When obstruction is complete, once the initial meconium has been passed, there is no further stool. In some infants no meconium is passed at all. When obstruction is incomplete the diagnosis may again be long-delayed and the child may present with intermitent vomiting, abdominal distension and even with features of malabsorption, and a clinical picture that may resemble coeliac disease.

Diagnosis

Plain X-ray of the abdomen is usually diagnostic in infants who present acutely. In duodenal atresia there is the characteristic 'double bubble' (*see* Fig. 3.1). When obstruction is incomplete there may be small amounts of air in the lower bowel. A barium enema may be useful to demonstrate associated malrotation which could suggest additional extrinsic pressure causing obstruction due to Ladd's bands, or it may suggest there is another atresia lower down, i.e. there may be multiple atresias.

When there is complete jejuno-ileal obstruction there are usually dilated loops of small intestine apparent on plain X-ray of the abdomen and there is no colonic gas. A barium enema may reveal a disused microcolon. When obstruction is incomplete a barium follow-through may be needed to establish the diagnosis. Rarely, laparotomy may be the final court of appeal.

Management

Delay in diagnosis leads to poor surgical results. Unfortunately, such delay sometimes occurs because of the lack of appreciation of the significance of bilious vomiting in the first 24 hours of life and, therefore, failure to ask for a surgical opinion.

Correction of fluid and electrolyte disturbances, if present, should precede surgery. At laparotomy, care should be taken to exclude any accompanying gastrointestinal abnormality. In duodenal obstruction, the operation of choice is duodeno-jejunostomy or duodeno-

duodenostomy. Some surgeons use a feeding enterostomy during the immediate post-operative period.

In jejuno-ileal lesions, resection is obviously indicated but as Gross (1953), Nixon (1955) and Louw (1959) have indicated, there should be adequate resection of the proximal dilated gut as, post-operatively, gut immediately proximal to an atresia may remain flabby and dilated with ineffective peristalsis. Louw recommends that 10 to 15 cm of the proximal blind end of jejuno-ileal atresias and 2 to 3 cm of the distal end should be resected. This reduces the great discrepancy in size between the two blind ends and so facilitates end-to-end anastomosis, although an oblique-to-end anastomosis is still often necessary (Dickson, 1970).

Despite these manoeuvres, post-operative diarrhoea may occur and this may be related to the stagnant loop syndrome producing sugar malabsorption acutely in the post-operative period or steatorrhoea months or even years later. This is discussed in more detail on page 318. Sometimes further surgery is necessary to correct this complication by resecting the area of proximally dilated bowel where there is stasis of gut contents above the previous anastomosis.

Duplications of Gastrointestinal Tract

These are congenital malformations that present most often in early infancy, may present later in childhood but far less often, and may even occasionally present in adult life.

Duplications are cystic or tubular structures whose lumen is lined by a mucous membrane, usually supported by smooth muscle. They occur most often within the dorsal mesentry of the gut. They are also sometimes described as enteric cysts, neurenteric cysts and reduplications, but the term duplications seems the most suitable, taking into account their probable embryological origin. Duplications may occur anywhere along the alimentary tract but they are found most often in relation to the small intestine, particularly the ileum. Only occasionally do they communicate directly with the gastrointestinal tract.

Their origin is believed to relate to an incomplete separation of the notochordal plate from the endoderm during embryological development leading to the drawing-up of the gut into a diverticulum. This may interfere with the growth of vertebrae and may thus account for the attachment of some duplications to the spinal cord and their occasional association with hemivertebrae which occurs most often with the tubular variety. Duplications may be found in association with intestinal atresias. Sometimes they may be lined by gastric mucosa and peptic ulceration and bleeding may occur.

Duplications may present in infancy as small intestinal obstructions, sometimes by the production of an intussusception. A palpable abdominal mass in infancy as well as rectal bleeding and volvulus may also be modes of presentation of this disorder. The clinical diagnosis is often difficult and the diagnosis may sometimes be made only on laparotomy. Occasionally, a techetium scan may be helpful diagnostically.

Meconium Ileus

This is a manifestation of cystic fibrosis, the disorder sometimes known as fibrocystic disease of the pancreas. Merconium ileus is the earliest mode of presentation of this disorder during the neonatal period. A similar syndrome in older children who have cystic fibrosis may occur. It is usually known as the meconium ileus equivalent.

The abnormally viscid consistency of the meconium is usually believed to account for this syndrome. It may result from several factors, including the lack of pancreatic enzymes during fetal life, which may, in turn, account for its high protein content, a characteristic of the meconium from these children. There is also evidence of reduced secretion of water and electrolytes in such infants which may further render the meconium more viscid. The meconium, because of its high viscosity, cannot be propelled along the bowel and so small intestinal obstruction results. This occurs most often in the distal ileum.

Clinical Features

The neonate with this disorder usually develops signs of intestinal obstruction within the first 24 to 48 hours of life, and with the classical signs of bilious vomiting, progressive abdominal distension and scant or absent meconium. Meconium ileus may be complicated by perforation of the gut, and when this occurs *in utero* small calcified areas in the peritoneum may be observed on plain X-ray of the abdomen, providing evidence of former meconium peritonitis. Such perforation may also occur in the neonatal period. Sudden acute abdominal distension, especially when accompanied by signs of tympany or ascites, strongly suggests this diagnosis. Plain X-ray of the abdomen may show a dilated bowel but unaccompanied by many fluid levels.

Sometimes there is a homogeneous shadow in the region of the lower ileum with a stippled appearance (Fig. 10.2). If a Gastrografin enema is done a microcolon, a consequence of disuse, may be demonstrated. The finding of such an X-ray appearance in the presence of a family history of cystic fibrosis makes the diagnosis of meconium ileus highly probable but the situation may be confused when there is an associated ileal atresia.

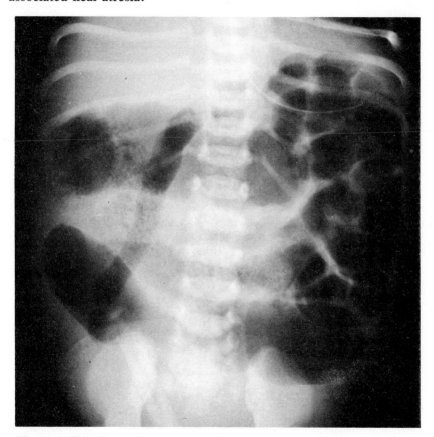

Fig. 10.2. Plain X-ray of abdomen of infant with meconium ileus.

Management

When meconium ileus is complicated by atresia or perforation, gangrene, peritonitis, or associated volvulus, surgical intervention is essential. In these circumstances resection of the affected segments with an end-to-end anastomosis is usually the treatment of choice, the distal end being brought to the surface as an ileostomy (Bishop-Koop). Various irrigations through the ileostomy have been advocated, including pancreatic enzymes, mucolytic agents such as acetyl cysteine, and the industrial detergent 'Tween 80'.

Non-operative treatment of uncomplicated meconium ileus, using enemata containing such agents, has been advocated for some time but only relatively recently has such non-operative management been widely employed with success. Noblett in Melbourne, in 1969, advocated the use of Gastrografin enemata to relieve intraluminal obstruction. Gastrografin is a radio-opaque hypertonic solution that contains a small amount of the wetting agent 'Tween 80' (0.1 per cent). This technique should not be used until: first, plain X-ray of the abdomen has failed to demonstrate any calcification, free gas or fluid in the peritoneal cavity; secondly, a contrast enema has excluded Hirschsprung's disease; and thirdly, the retrograde passage of contrast medium through the ileo-caecal valve has demonstrated an obstructing meconium mass with proximal dilated ileum, thus excluding ileal atresia.

Although there may be no signs clinically or radiologically of pulmonary complications at this stage, immediate cautious physiotherapy of the chest and inhalation therapy should be started and vigorous treatment of chest infections with antibiotics when they occur (as for older children with cystic fibrosis). A pancreatic enzyme preparation should also be started, at first in small dosage when milk feedings have begun.

The child's ultimate prognosis depends upon the prognosis of his cystic fibrosis. This diagnosis should be confirmed by sweat electrolyte estimations.

Annular Pancreas

This is a congenital disorder in which the pancreas grows around the second part of the duodenum. There is often accompanying intrinsic duodenal atresia, a duodenal diaphragm or sometimes malrotation with Ladd's bands. Some authors doubt whether this is a real disease entity.

The disorder presents in the same way as duodenal atresia and produces an identical plain X-ray appearance with the characteristic 'double bubble'.

The disorder should be managed in the same way as duodenal atresia by duodeno-jejunostomy and no attempt should be made to divide the annular pancreas at operation.

Small Intestinal Malrotation with or without Volvulus

Malrotation of the small intestine is due to disordered movement of the intestine around the superior mesenteric artery during the course of embryological development.

Two main abnormalities that produce clinical syndromes may occur. First, there is a gross narrowing of the fixation of the mesentery which may allow the midgut to twist around and cause a volvulus. This may occur acutely, causing complete obstruction, or it may occur intermittently, producing bouts of partial or complete obstruction which may at times release themselves spontaneously. Secondly, there may be partial duodenal obstruction from extrinsic compression of the small intestine by peritoneal bands (Ladd's bands) which extend from the caecum or hepatic flexure.

Malrotation may also be associated with annular pancreas and duodenal atresia or stenosis. It may also be found in association with diaphragmatic hernia, omphalocele and gastroschisis. However, malrotation may not produce symptoms and may sometimes be discovered only as an incidental finding on a barium study.

The majority of children who develop symptoms related to malrotation do so within the neonatal period, presenting with features of intestinal obstruction, complete or incomplete. When there is volvulus there may also be the passage of melaena stools and if the correct diagnosis is not made, perforation and peritonitis may result.

Those children with malrotation who present later in childhood may do so with features of intermittent obstruction such as episodes of vomiting and abdominal pain, but sometimes they may manifest with features of malabsorption and many clinical features suggestive of coeliac disease. This is due to intestinal stasis with bacterial overgrowth in the lumen of the small intestine. Such steatorrhoea may be accompanied at times by protein-losing enteropathy due to obstruction of the mesenteric lymphatics (Burke and Anderson, 1966), and sometimes chylous ascites may also be found.

Diagnosis

The diagnosis needs to be considered in the differential diagnosis of small intestinal obstruction in infancy.

Plain X-ray of the abdomen may be very useful, typically revealing some distension of the stomach and duodenum, but unlike duodenal atresia this is accompanied by some gas scattered through the lower part of the abdomen. However, volvulus of the mid gut may not be accompanied by any abnormality on plain X-ray of the abdomen and a barium meal and follow-through study may then be necessary to reveal the presence of a volvulus.

A barium enema may be useful to demonstrate the presence of malrotation of the colon by the position of the caecum and thus suggest accompanying malrotation of the small intestine, but a barium follow-through is often more useful, although in chronic cases repeated barium study may be necessary to make the diagnosis. Sometimes a diagnosis can only be made at laparotomy.

Management

Surgical intervention is indicated when symptoms occur and resection of the gut may be necessary when there is strangulation. Ladd's operation is usually the procedure of choice. This involves, in general, the placement of the caecum on the left and the small intestine on the right.

Milk Plug Syndrome

This is now a well-recognised syndrome which may be related in part to the ingestion of concentrated feeds. Dickson, Lewis and Swain (1974) have reviewed their experience of 17 children with the disorder at the Queen Elizabeth Hospital from 1964 to 1972. Over this period the milk plug syndrome accounted for 6 per cent of admissions for neonatal intestinal obstruction. It occurred more commonly in male infants and most were fed 'full cream' milk feeds. It should be suspected when an infant having such a feeding becomes obstructed on about the fifth day of life. Fifty per cent of these infants passed blood per rectum.

Diagnosis may be assisted by plain X-ray of the abdomen which shows small gut fluid levels, and replacement of the normal gas pattern in the right iliac fossa by an inspissated faecal mass which contains either bubbles of gas or has a ground-glass appearance. The management of such infants was at first regarded as operative but more recently Gastrografin, given orally or by enema, has been used with success. These infants may clinically be compared with those with Hirschsprung's disease, hence a Gastrografin enema may be useful both diagnostically and therapeutically. The wider use of low solute milks may lead to the disappearance of the milk plug syndrome.

Intussusception

This condition is more common in boys than girls and 50 per cent of cases occur within the first year of life. The most frequent type of intussusception is the ileo-caecal progressing to the ileo-colic variety. Other types are ileo-ileal and colo-colic. The apex of the intussusception is often the hepatic or splenic flexures.

Aetiology

In approximately 5 per cent of children with intussusception, precipitating lesions are present, but in the remainder there may be no such lesion. This contrasts with the situation in adults where intussusception is nearly always associated with a precipitating lesion.

In children, such lesions include polyps, foreign bodies, haemangiomata, Meckel's diverticula and ascaris worms. Intussusception may also occur in association with Henoch-Schönlein purpura when there is small intestinal involvement. It may also occur in children with cystic fibrosis, presumably related to the inspissated luminal contents which may be found in that disorder. Recurrent intussusception may occur in the Peutz-Jegher syndrome (Table 10.5).

Table 10.5
Features of Peutz-Jegher syndrome
Multiple polyps in the alimentary tract—chiefly small intestine

Inherited as a Mendelian dominant
Mucosal pigmentation—buccal mucosa and lips (Fig. 10.3)
Recurrent abdominal pain
Recurrent anaemia and gastrointestinal haemorrhage
Recurrent intussusception
Conservative management when possible

There has been speculation in the remaining children concerning its possible aetiology. The early introduction of cereals and hyperplasia of Peyer's patches secondary to adenovirus infections are among the suggestions that have been put forward, but there is no general agreement concerning the relative importance of such precipitating factors.

Clinical Features

The typical history is provided by a male infant aged three months to one year, who presents with screaming episodes associated with the

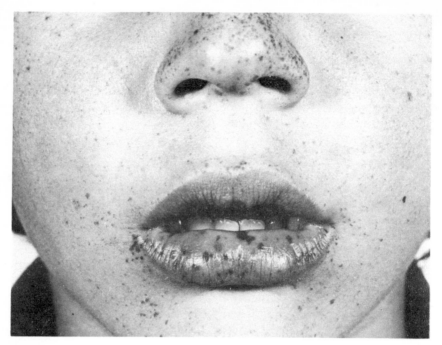

Fig. 10.3. Characteristic mucosal pigmentation of the lips in a boy with Peutz-Jegher syndrome.

drawing up of his legs due to abdominal pain, and often associated with vomiting and the passage of 'red currant jelly' stools. On examination he is characteristically feverish and has a tender distended abdomen, often with a palpable abdominal mass. Sometimes gastroenteritis may precede the onset of intussusception, and the passage of 'red currant jelly' stools may be confused with the bloody diarrhoea of bacterial enteritis.

Great care must be taken by those clinicians who are responsible for a gastroenteritis unit that the diagnosis of intussusception is not missed in children who are admitted to such a unit in error.

At the Queen Elizabeth Hospital in 1973, out of 472 consecutive admissions to the gastroenteritis unit there were three children admitted with intussusception.

Diagnosis

Early diagnosis is vital as necrosis of the bowel leading to perforation, peritonitis and death may occur when the diagnosis is missed. The first investigation that should be undertaken is plain X-ray of the abdomen which will usually reveal the presence of intestinal obstruction and may sometimes show the outline of an intussusception (*see* Fig. 3.2). Usually, the next investigation is a diagnostic barium enema, but immediate laparotomy may be proceeded with in some circumstances.

Therapy

Hydrostatic reduction at the time of the barium study may be undertaken if there is a history of less than twenty-four hours and there are no complications present. When there is shock or if there is evidence of perforation such reduction should not be attempted. In these circumstances laparotomy with the appropriate surgical correction should be undertaken. In addition, attempts at hydrostatic reduction should not continue if there is no progress for fifteen minutes or if the child's condition deteriorates. The barium solution used for hydrostatic reduction should drip by gravity and no extra abdominal pressure should be applied.

Inguinal Hernia

Once the neonatal period is passed incarcerated inguinal hernia is the most common cause of small intestinal obstruction. This diagnosis is suggested by the presence of a mass in the groin or scrotum which is painful and tender, in the presence of the clinical features of intestinal obstruction. As strangulation is uncommon many surgeons recommend reduction by taxis followed by herniotomy after two or three days.

Internal Herniae

These are rarer in children than in adults, but when they do occur they may present with recurrent abdominal pain and sometimes be confused with intussusception.

Primary Peritonitis

Although this is not strictly a surgically correctable lesion, it is sometimes diagnosed at laparotomy, and so is discussed here. The condition was once common in children, but is now quite rare. It is usually due to pneumococcal infection and occurs most often in children who have had a splenectomy or in children with severe nephrosis. The condition may sometimes be confused with appendicitis. The diagnosis is usually made by a diagnostic paracentesis, but sometimes only at laparotomy. With modern antibiotic therapy the prognosis is now good.

OTHER CAUSES OF SMALL INTESTINAL OBSTRUCTION

Localised infection within the peritoneal cavity, especially when an abscess has formed may produce complete or partial small intestinal obstruction. Such infection results most often from a perforated viscus such as a ruptured appendix occurring as a sequel to acute appendicitis. Multiple or single adhesions, the result of such infection or the consequence of abdominal surgery may also manifest as small intestinal obstruction.

A mesenteric cyst although usually asymptomatic may occasionally present with intestinal obstruction, or if it ruptures or bleeds.

Ascariasis and strongyloidiasis are rare causes of small intestinal obstruction outside tropical countries (*see* chapter 8).

Rarely, aganglionosis of the small intestine may occur in children with Hirschsprung's disease when the aganglionic area extends into the distal small intestine. If the involvement is extensive the prognosis is grave.

Another rare cause of small intestinal obstruction is lymphosarcoma which, when it involves the alimentary tract in children, most often affects the small intestine. It may present in other ways; for example, as a malabsorption syndrome with clinical features that may suggest the diagnosis of coeliac disease. In the past, such children were sometimes put on a gluten-free diet in error without having a small intestinal biopsy, the diagnosis of coeliac disease having been made on clinical grounds. The folly of such a course has been mentioned in chapter 4.

Stagnant Loop Syndrome

It has been known for some time that stasis of the small intestinal contents leads to bacterial proliferation and as a result features of malabsorption. This syndrome has been sometimes known as the blind loop syndrome but as a true anatomical 'blind loop' is often not present, the term stagnant loop seems more appropriate. Gracey and his colleagues in 1969 suggested the term 'contaminated small bowel syndrome' as they wished also to include in the one syndrome infants who appeared to have bacterial colonisation of the small intestine but no stasis of gut contents. Until the full significance of such a finding is determined, i.e. whether it is a primary or a secondary event, the term stagnant loop is preferred.

It is now well-known in adults that the normal small intestine has a sparse Gram-positive flora (Gorbach *et al.*, 1967) and others have reported a low concentration of coliforms (Hamilton *et al.*, 1970). Until recently there has been little comparable information in children but Challacombe and his colleagues in Birmingham (1974) found in 13 infants without diarrhoea that in 7 the duodenal juice was sterile and in the remainder organisms originating from higher up the gastrointestinal tract were present. No coliforms were found. However, in 14 infants with protracted diarrhoea, coliforms, especially *E. coli*, were often found in the duodenal juice. Whether their presence was primary or secondary still remains uncertain.

Classically, in adults the stagnant loop syndrome manifests with steatorrhoea and the malabsorption of vitamin B_{12} as its principal features. These manifestations may also occur in older children with this syndrome, as described for example by Bayes and Hamilton (1969); but in infancy, Burke and Anderson (1966) have described malabsorption of sugar as a sequel to intestinal stasis, occurring as a sequel to neonatal surgery for intestinal atresia or other abnormalities of the alimentary tract. They suggested that sugar malabsorption in these circumstances could be related to intestinal stasis with bacterial overgrowth, leading to a disturbance of sugar digestion and absorption (*see* chapter 7).

The frequency and importance of sugar malabsorption in these conditions has now been widely recognised in many paediatric surgical centres. There does seem, however, to be a remarkable variation in the frequency of this complication in different surgical units, which may be due in part to differing diagnostic criteria, but there is also a clinical impression that sugar malabsorption is a much less frequent complication of neonatal surgery in infants fed with expressed breast milk. As breast milk contains 7 g lactose/100 ml, this suggests that perhaps the sugar malabsorption in these circumstances may also be related to cow's milk protein intolerance, a subject that is being currently investigated (*see* chapter 7).

How bacterial colonisation of the small intestine can lead to sugar malabsorption is not clear. It does not appear to be related to small intestinal mucosal damage *per se* as the mucosa is usually morphologically normal. The presence of deconjugated bile salts has been

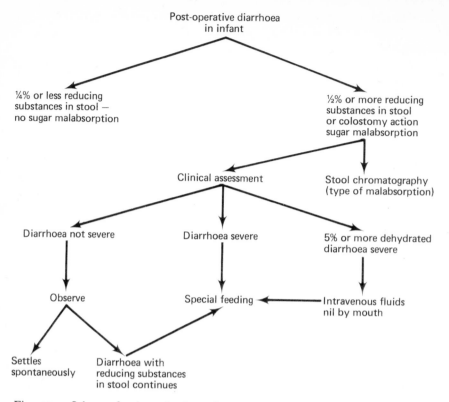

Fig. 10.4. Scheme for investigation of post-operative diarrhoea in a neonate, for sugar malabsorption.

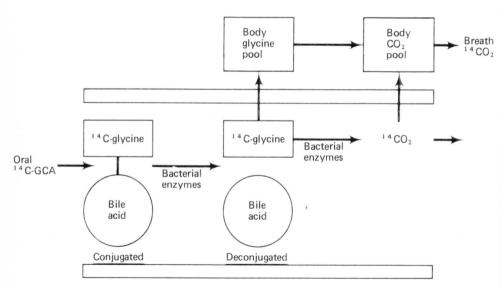

Fig. 10.5. Diagrammatic representation of ^{14}C glycocholate breath test.

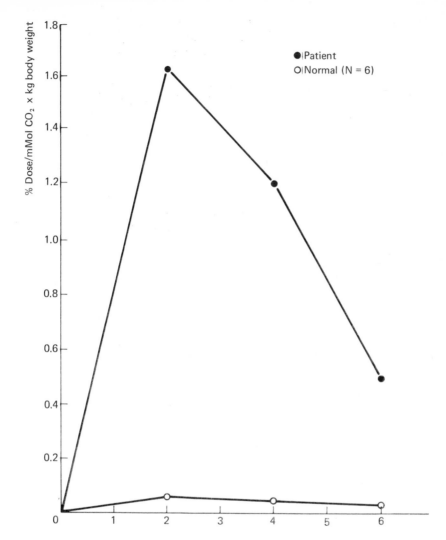

Fig. 10.6. Results of ^{14}C glycocholate breath test in a child with stagnant loop and a normal result.

suggested as a possible cause for the sugar malabsorption, deconjugation occurring as a result of bacterial colonisation of the small intestine (Gracey and Burke, 1973).

A simple scheme for the diagnosis and management of infants with diarrhoea following surgery in the neonatal period is illustrated in Fig. 10.4.

As mentioned earlier, in the older child, stasis of the small intestinal contents may cause steatorrhoea. This has been attributed to a fall in the level of conjugated bile salts related to an increase in the level of deconjugated bile salts in the lumen due to the action of bacteria that have colonised it. A useful way to diagnose an increase in the level of deconjugation of bile salts is to use the ^{14}C glycocholate breath test (Fromm and Hoffman, 1971), as illustrated in Fig. 10.5. This test can be used with co-operative children aged four or more. Figure 10.6 shows the results of such an investigation in a boy aged four years, with a stagnant loop proximal to an anastomosis for a resection of a jejunal atresia performed as a neonate (Kilby, Walker-Smith and Dickson, 1974). In these circumstances, when there is definite evidence of bile salt deconjugation or bacterial colonisation, coupled with steatorrhoea, surgical resection of the stagnant loop is indicated.

11

Massive Resection of the Small Intestine

Massive resection of the small intestine may be defined as a resection of more than 30 cm of the small intestine. As recently as 1955, Potts considered that a resection greater than 15 per cent of the length of the small intestine was incompatible with survival, yet Wilmore, in 1972, reported survival with only 15 cm of residual small intestine. Indeed, as the years pass, the number of infants and children who survive massive resection of the small intestine increases. Of course, it is not just survival that is important but the quality of survival. Nevertheless, recent advances in surgical technique, intravenous alimentation, and dietetics have enabled big improvements in this field to be made.

When a segment of the small intestine is resected it is more important to know how much small intestine remains *in situ*, rather than how much was removed. Measurements of the length of the small intestine at post mortem have revealed the wide range that occurs in children of varying ages. In a series of autopsies studied at the Royal Alexandra Hospital, neonatal small intestinal length varied from 68 to 386 cm with a mean of 243 cm (see Table 11.1 and Fig. 11.1).

Table 11.1
Length of the small intestine in childhood
A post mortem study of 100 children at the Royal Alexandra Hospital

Age	No.	Range in cm	Mean in cm
Neonates	42	68–386	243
One month to one year	40	104–591	344
One year to five years	11	232–485	396
Five to ten years	5	275–510	428
Over ten years	2	340–475	407

Resection in the paediatric age group usually occurs following surgical catastrophies in the neonatal period. These include volvulus neonatorum secondary to a developmental anomaly such as omphalocoele or malrotation; obstruction from multiple atretic areas requiring resection; necrotising enterocolitis and, on occasion, meconium ileus. Extensive Crohn's disease in the older child may sometimes require massive small intestinal resection.

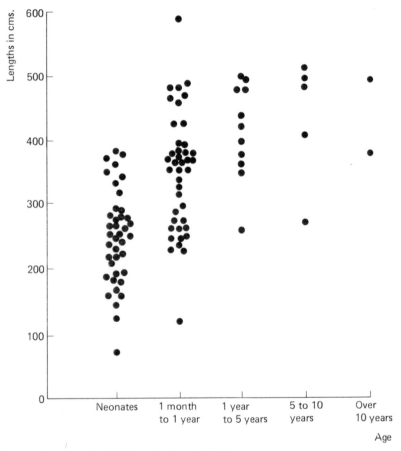

Fig. 11.1 Length of small intestine in 100 children at post-mortem.

The clinical syndrome that results from massive small intestinal resection is sometimes referred to as the 'short gut syndrome'. It is characterised by diarrhoea, and reduced absorption of all nutrients, minerals and vitamins. A congenital shortness of the small intestine producing a syndrome similar to that produced by surgery, has been described by Hamilton, Reilly and Morecki (1969). There is evidence that the untoward sequelae of massive small intestinal resection are not just the consequences of loss of the absorptive area *per se*, but are also the result of acid hypersecretion by the stomach, which begins within hours of resection (Sedgewick and Goodman, 1971).

The characteristic disabilities suffered by these children are, nevertheless, gross alterations in nutrient absorption. They have been reviewed by Parkinson and Walker-Smith (1973).

The problems encountered following massive small intestinal resection fall into two groups: first, the immediate post-operative problems, and secondly, the long-term problems. The immediate problems are chiefly severe diarrhoea with associated fluid and electrolyte losses, and the problems involved in retaining enough calories to maintain weight. The long-term problems relate more to the severity of the malabsorption state resulting from loss of absorptive capacity and the effect this has on nutrition and growth. On occasion, the tragic situation may arrive where enough small intestine may remain to sustain life but not enough to enable growth to occur.

ABSORPTION DEFECTS

The disturbances in function that result from massive small intestinal resection depend upon the site of the resection as well as the amount that has been resected. Defects in function are more severe following ileal resection. This relates to the interruption of enterohepatic circulation of bile salts produced by ileal resection as the ileum is the site of active absorption of bile salts (*see* Fig. 1.1). As a result, excess bile salts enter the colon and cause severe cathartic diarrhoea; in addition, there is a bile salt deficiency in small intestinal lumen which gives steatorrhoea. The severity of this bile salt deficiency depends upon the length of ileum resected and the liver's capacity to increase bile salt synthesis. The retention of the ileo-caecal valve has an important impact upon survival. If it is lost, mortality is significantly increased in infants (McMahon, 1966). Its loss may not only be associated with severe problems in fluid and electrolyte depletion but also with bacterial colonisation of the remaining small intestine.

Carbohydrate absorption is reduced because the surface area of the small intestine is smaller after resection, and there is less disaccharidase activity in what remains of the small intestine (Kern, Struthers and Attwood, 1963; Walker-Smith and Wyndham, 1967). Active absorption of monosaccharides is reduced because there are fewer cells, and the rate of glucose absorption induced by acid contents is slowed down (Goldenberg and Cummins, 1963). Acid hypersection itself produces irritative diarrhoea as well as malabsorption due to enzyme inhibition. Strauss, Gerson and Yalow (1974) have found high fasting plasma levels of 'big gastrin' in four adult patients following massive small intestinal resection. Dowling and Booth (1966) have also shown that, in adults, absorption of glucose is later increased. This increase in glucose absorption with time probably relates to compensatory hypertrophy, which appears to occur in the remaining small intestine.

Triglyceride digestion to fatty acids is grossly reduced and steatorrhoea results partly from this and partly from surface-area encroachment. Rapid gastrointestinal transit and bile salt deficiency when the terminal ileum is resected, further contribute to the steatorrhoea. Patients with severe steatorrhoea may also have troublesome watery diarrhoea due to hydroxy fatty acids produced by colonic bacteria acting on the colonic mucosa.

Protein malabsorption is proportional to the amount of bowel resected (Wilmore, 1969). Winawer, Broitman and Wolochow (1966) reported a 75 per cent loss of dietary protein intake in a patient with 18 cm of residual small intestine.

Water balance is usually a problem only during diarrhoeal periods at which time the electrolyte balance is also precarious. Calcium and magnesium balance is a problem because of steatorrhoea. Deficiencies of all vitamins have been reported, although prophylatic water soluble vitamin supplementation is usually effective. Parenteral administration of fat soluble vitamins A, D, E and K may be necessary. Vitamin B_{12} absorption may be sufficient if more than 5 cm of terminal ileum remains (Moe, 1964).

However, Valman (1974) has reported a long-term follow up of 10 children who had more than 45 cm ileum resected and, using a whole body counter technique, found that 7 had evidence of impaired absorption. One developed overt vitamin B_{12} deficiency at puberty.

Small bowel adaptation ensues between fifteen and eighteen months after resection. The residual intestine dilates, thickens and develops villous hypertrophy and epithelial hyperplasia (Wilmore et al., 1971; Porus, 1965). Epithelial hyperplasia, however, appears to occur only proximal to the enteroanastomosis in man, in contrast to rats, in which it is found throughout the residual small bowel. Increase in length may also occasionally be possible (McMahon, 1966). The pattern of intestinal peristalsis changes and as a result of these combined changes absorption increases, as may gastrointestinal transit time in due course.

Luminal nutrition and hormonal changes, which may be interrelated, appear to have a critical role to play in the adaptive changes that follow small intestinal resection.

Surgical intervention has been reported to help. Hypersecretion may be reduced by vagotomy and pyloroplasty, and colonic interposition and/or small intestinal segment reversal may slow transit time (Wilmore *et al.*, 1971), although results are unpredictable.

Dietary requirements change with time after resection (Wilmore *et al.*, 1971; Sedgewick and Goodman, 1971). Initially, massive diarrhoea may result from taking small volumes of water orally. After one or two months the condition improves and glucose in water, and then amino acid/sugar solutions, can be tolerated and absorbed (Dudrick, 1972; Sedgewick and Goodham, 1971). This 'elemental diet' can quite rapidly be changed to a low fat 'transitional' feeding. Codeine effectively controls diarrhoea; anticholinergics control the acid hypersecretion. The role of antacids is uncertain (Dudrick, 1972; Sedgewick and Goodman, 1971).

The value of amino acids *vis à vis* small peptides and protein hydrolysates in such an elemental diet has recently come under some scrutiny. It is known now that the products of the intraluminal digestion of protein, namely free amino acids and small peptides, are absorbed by two separate transport systems (Asatoor *et al.*, 1970). Silk and his colleagues at St Bartholomew's Hospital (1973) have produced evidence from intestinal perfusion studies in adults that dipeptides are more efficiently absorbed than their component amino acids. It thus seems probable that amino acids may not be ideal for such 'elemental diets' and protein hydrolysates may be preferable (*see* chapter 1).

The wide range of tolerances of glucose and fructose in these patients requires a feeding carefully tailored to the individual. Carefully graded increases in the diet content of these sugars must be made to reach the maximum tolerable content. The final 'transitional' feeding should be high in protein and low in fat as well as containing as much carbohydrate as can be tolerated. Disaccharides may be poorly tolerated and should be avoided. The diet should be supplemented with vitamins, calcium, magnesium and all electrolytes. The amount of supplementation should be monitored clinically or by serum levels. Large amounts of calcium, magnesium and fat soluble vitamins will be required because of steatorrhoea.

Medium chain triglycerides (MCT) are hydrolysed and absorbed as monoglyceride or free fatty acids via the portal vein. Substitution of MCT for normal dietary fat will help increase fat absorption and decrease steatorrhoea. The improvement may take 7 to 10 days.

However, such substitution may be poorly tolerated in 'short gut' patients as MCT is rapidly hydrolysed even in acid conditions. The resultant free fatty acids can produce diarrhoea both by direct irritation and an osmotic effect (Greenberger and Skillman, 1969).

Gastrointestinal tract adaptation is usually sufficiently well advanced by two months after resection to enable the transitional diet to be introduced. This adaptation seems to occur even when oral nutrients are withheld (Dudrick, 1972) and has usually stopped 15 to 18 months after resection. Sufficient adaption has usually taken place in 6 to 12 months (Lawler and Bernard, 1962; Moe, 1964; McMahon, 1966) to allow the change over to a low fat but otherwise more normal diet. At this stage codeine and anticholinergic drugs can be reduced or stopped (Dudrick, 1972).

One feature seen after intestinal resection is a reduction in body and organ mass to that which can be maintained by the residual bowel. The rapid weight loss and stabilisation at a more optimal level have been well recorded (Winawer, Broitman and Wolochow, 1966; Linder, Jackson and Linder, 1953; McMahon, 1966). Thereafter there may be weight gain.

Our goal when treating patients with intestinal resection should be long-term survival of an intact individual. In the adult, growth is complete and only maintenance is required. The neonate, however, requires sufficient nutrition from his residual small intestine to ensure growth, not just maintenance.

Neonatally starved infants function intellectually less well than socio-economically similar, well nourished controls (Klein, Habicht and Yarbrough, 1971). At present there is no evidence to associate this with brain underdevelopment although it is known that there are critical periods of neurone replication.

Valman (1976) in a follow-up study of 12 children with extensive resections of the ileum found that none had diarrhoea lasting more than a year after resection. They were able to tolerate a normal diet in all cases, although 4 of the 5 tested had steatorrhoea. The children tended to be shorter than their siblings but only two were below the third centile compared with the height expected from their parent's height. Young, Swain and Pringle (1969) also found the long-term prognosis in those who survived to be satisfactory. Wilmore (1972), too, found subsequent growth and development in 18 of 50 infants were mostly within normal limits for weight, once they had negotiated the first year.

After the first year of survival, persistent malabsorption and growth retardation may be due to a surgically correctable lesion, such as a stagnant loop, and should be investigated (*see* chapter 10).

Hyperoxaluria with its risk of renal calculi is a complication of massive small intestinal resection. Valman, Oberholzer and Palmer (1976) found hyperoxaluria in 4 of 10 children who had had ileal resections. McCollum *et al*. (1975) found that hyperoraluxia could occur in other small intestinal diseases such as coeliac disease, where it was reversed by a gluten-free diet.

The exact mechanism for hyperoraluxia is not clear but seems to relate to increased colonic absorption due to altered colonic permeability. From a practical view point these children should have their urinary oxalate levels monitored and be placed on an oxalate-free diet, if high levels are found, to avoid renal calculi. Such a diet is unpalatable and should be introduced only if there is a real need for it.

MANAGEMENT

Each case of massive small intestinal resection should be managed on its own merits. From the literature it seems that intravenous alimentation should be undertaken for at least two to three months in all infants left with 15 cm or more of residual small bowel and an intact ileocaecal valve after massive small intestinal resection. These infants have a reasonable chance of intact survival. Below this length of small bowel, chances of survival are at present extremely small. Intravenous alimentation may perhaps not be worthwhile in infants with less than 10–15 cm of small intestine, as at present only Dudrick (1972) has reported survival in such a case. Below 10 cm of residual small intestine, such artificial prolongation of life is hard to justify.

An 'elemental diet' should be gradually introduced after 1–2 months' alimentary rest. Codeine and an anticholinergic drug should be used to control diarrhoea and gastric acid hypersecretion. Antacids may also help control the effects of hypersecretion. When the 'elemental' sugar/protein hydrolysate solution is tolerated, a 'transitional' complete oral feeding should be started. CHO-free (Syntex), CF_1 (Nestlé) or comminuted chicken meat (Cow & Gate) (see Appendix) provide an excellent basis for this. Fructose and glucose can be added gradually to this. At the same time, the volume of oral feeding should be gradually increased. The final formula should be low in fat, high in protein and contain as much carbohydrate as can be tolerated without exceeding the patient's absorptive capabilities.

As oral intake increases, intravenous nutrition may be reduced but growth should continue unhindered. Intravenous nutrient augmentation should not be stopped until oral intake is sufficnet to at least maintain body mass. It may be necessary to resume intravenous augmentation during later intercurrent illnesses, especially enteritis. All changes in diet must be gradual as intestinal hurry will continue for several days after the initiating insult has been removed.

Sodium, potassium, chloride, calcium, magnesium, phosphate, water and fat soluble vitamin supplementation will be necessary in quantities sufficient to maintain normal body levels. Parenteral vitamin B_{12} as well as parenteral fat soluble vitamins may be required.

Antimonilial therapy is indicated whenever this pathogen is detected.

A more normal diet may be anticipated after 6 to 12 months of the individualised transitional diet. At this stage, codeine and anticholinergies may no longer be necessary and their dosages may be safely reduced.

The first report of growth and development in an infant fed continuously via intravenous alimentation came from Wilmore and Dudrick in 1968. Since then, this technique has been widely used in children. While it does sometimes have serious side effects, such as infection, it has proved to be an extremely valuable and at times life-saving measure, particularly in children who have had massive small intestinal resection. A detailed discussion of this technique is outside the scope of this book but one excellent account of the technique of intravenous alimentation is given by Harries (1971).

The long-term outlook of children who survive following massive small intestinal resection is being evaluated at present. However, it seems that once the first two years of life are safely negotiated the future looks favourable. The long-term consequences of the disruption of the mother-child relationship, due to prolonged separation during infancy, awaits full evaluation.

Miscellaneous Disorders of the Small Intestine

In this chapter a number of disorders will be briefly referred to. Some of them appear primarily to involve the small intestine but in others the small intestine is only secondarily abnormal, e.g. brief mention will be made of small intestinal abnormalities found in common systemic disorders such as protein-energy deficiency.

ACRODERMATITIS ENTEROPATHICA

Acrodermatitis enteropathica is a rare autosomal recessively inherited disorder. It is a disease of infancy, and is believed to be caused by a defect in zinc absorption.

It presents with chronic diarrhoea, characteristically beginning at the time of weaning. It only rarely appears during breast feeding. Sometimes the diarrhoea leads to dehydration and it may become intractable. There is a characteristic skin rash which affects the mucocutaneous areas around the mouth and the anus. The perianal rash is often confused with a napkin dermatitis. There may also be dermatitis of the fingers and toes, with dystrophic nails and paronychiae; alopecia is often present. Typically there are signs of malnutrition and growth failure.

There have been conflicting reports concerning the state of the small intestinal mucosa in this disorder as autopsy studies have described focal areas of degeneration and some biopsy studies have reported the mucosa as normal. Ultrastructural studies of small intestinal biopsies have demonstrated an abnormality of Paneth cells (Lombeck et al., 1974). The Paneth cell inclusions disappear with zinc therapy.

Kelly *et al.* (1976) have described a reversible small intestinal enteropathy in 3 children with this disorder. The mucosal abnormality was grade + or + + but the most characteristic finding was a change in the enterocytes. These were cuboidal with large nuclei and altered shape, the nuclear changes being attributed to abnormal synthesis of nucleoprotein, which is dependent on zinc-containing enzymes.

Untreated this disease is usually fatal. It usually presents at the time of first contact with cow's milk and return to breast milk will induce a remission. In the past, a remission was also induced by the halogenated quinoline, di-iodohydroxy quinoline (Diodoquin) but now treatment with oral zinc results in a dramatic and sustained improvement.

The aetiology of the disorder had been under investigation for some time before Barnes and Moynahan (1973), after careful analysis of the diet of a child with the syndrome, found a gross deficiency in the intake of zinc and also a low plasma zinc level. Moynahan (1974) went on to make the very exciting observation that zinc deficiency was fundamental to the pathogenesis of acrodermatitis enteropathica and, what was more, he found that clinically this disorder responded dramatically to zinc therapy. Evans and Johnson (1976) have gone on to postulate that these children cannot absorb zinc because they cannot synthesise prostaglandins which facilitate zinc absorption from the intestine. A low molecular weight zinc binding ligand is indeed essential for the maintenance of normal zinc absorption. From evidence in the experimental animal it is possible that this is a prostaglandin. Thus, Evans and Johnson (1977) assert that prostaglandin is essential for the maintenance of normal zinc absorption. Interestingly, human breast milk, unlike cow's milk, contains a zinc-binding ligand which they have identified as prostaglandin E_2. Hence, children with acrodermatitis enteropathica respond clinically both to breast milk and oral zinc supplementation.

Aggett *et al.* (1978) with *in vitro* studies have demonstrated that there is a defect in zinc uptake by the small intestinal mucosa in this disorder. Furthermore, using balance studies they have shown that the intestine is in a net secretory state with respect to zinc.

Other Causes of Zinc Deficiency

Zinc is absorbed throughout the small intestine and the colon but most rapidly in the proximal small intestine. An intraluminal ligand or binding factor originating from the pancreatic juice and breast milk, as well as mucosal ligand, facilitates its absorption. Zinc appears to share in the small intestine a common active transport mechanism with copper.

Zinc deficiency may thus occur in association with diseases of the small intestine such as coeliac disease and protein-losing enteropathy. It may also be found in infants who are having parenteral nutrition and insufficient zinc is being administered. Indeed, zinc and copper deficiency may both occur with parenteral nutrition for infants, especially those with necrotising enterocolitis who come to surgery when premature. This may lead to a severe napkin rash and neurological signs which are relieved by zinc therapy. Zinc deficiency may also occur in infants on synthetic diets when the addition of minerals has been inadequate. Soy preparations are low in zinc content and may occasionally precipitate clinical deficiency in states of relative zinc deficiency. It has also been described in association with pancreatic insufficiency and in haemolytic states.

All these secondary states of zinc deficiency may produce clinical manifestations similar to acrodermatitis enteropathica, with stomatitis and a perianal rash. They can also produce depressed cellular immunity.

PROTEIN-LOSING ENTEROPATHIES

These are a heterogeneous group of disorders in which an abnormal amount of protein is lost into the gastrointestinal tract. Tift (1977) has divided these disorders into (a) disease states that have altered gut permeability, and (b), those in which there is stasis of lymph flow. This is a helpful division, but in some disorders, e.g. Crohn's disease, both mechanisms may be operative.

Abnormal protein loss from the small intestine may occur in a number of disease states. Some of these are primary disorders of the small intestine *per se*, for example coeliac disease, while others are systemic disorders such as kwashiorkor in which the protein loss from the small intestine is one aspect of the generalised disturbances found in that disorder.

Table 12.1 lists the causes of abnormal protein loss from the small intestine in childhood.

The relative clinical importance of the protein loss in some of these disorders is variable, e.g. coeliac disease, but on occasion it may be a major problem in that malady. Some protein-losing states are brief in duration, e.g. those associated with acute gastroenteritis. Some respond rapidly to treatment, e.g. some cases of allergic gastroenteropathy which respond quickly to a milk-free diet (Waldmann *et al.*, 1967).

Table 12.1
Causes of abnormal protein loss from the small intestine in children

Primary lymphatic abnormality—lymphangiectasia
Secondary lymphatic abnormality, e.g. constrictive pericarditis
Acute gastroenteritis
Coeliac disease
Allergic gastroenteropathy
Crohn's disease
Hypogammaglobulinaemia
Nephrotic syndrome
Lymphosarcoma
Blind loop syndrome
Radiation enteritis
Chronic volvulus of malrotation

The diagnosis of protein-losing enteropathy should be considered whenever a child with chronic diarrhoea has unexplained hypoproteinaemia. The diagnosis may be definitively established by means of a radioisotope study. Intravenous Cr^{51} Cl_3, which binds to plasma protein *in vivo*, is a simple radioisotope test that may be used to diagnose abnormal enteric protein loss (Walker-Smith, Mistilis and Skyring, 1967). In practice, however, it is often unnecessary to resort to such a study because the protein-losing state is frequently temporary or responds rapidly to appropriate treatment once the primary diagnosis has been made, e.g. coeliac disease. However, it may be useful to perform this investigation when the diagnosis of lymphangiectasia is considered.

SMALL INTESTINAL LYMPHANGIECTASIA

The syndrome of idiopathic hypoproteinaemia without proteinuria and with normal hepatic function has been shown to result from excessive loss of plasma protein into the alimentary tract (Schwartz and Jarnum, 1959; Waldmann *et al.*, 1961; Jarnum and Petersen, 1961). Dilatation of the small intestinal lymphatics, usually known as lymphangiectasia has been a frequent finding in many patients with this syndrome, although histologically the appearance may on occasion be best described as a lymphangioma (Walker-Smith *et al.*, 1969).

Small intestinal lymphangiectasia has been described as a primary or congenital abnormality or as a secondary manifestation of some other disease process such as constrictive pericarditis (Petersen and Hastrup, 1963). The primary abnormality may be accompanied by generalised lymphatic abnormalities outside the alimentary tract, including lymphoedema, chylous ascites and hypoplasia, or aplasia of the peripheral lymphatic system (Jarnum, 1963; Mistilis and Skyring, 1966) but the lymphatic abnormality may be confined to the small bowel and its mesentery. It is usually, but not invariably, accompanied by hypoproteinaemia oedema (McKendry, Lindsay and Gerstein, 1957). Radioisotope studies in these children have demonstrated that the hypoproteinaemia is due to abnormal protein loss into the gut (Jarnum, 1963). The pathogenesis of the hypoproteinaemia in such children has been attributed to the rupture of dilated lymphatic channels or to protein exudation from intestinal capillaries via an intact epithelium, where there is obstruction of lymphatic flow (Waldmann, 1966).

Clinical Features

Children with this disorder may present throughout childhood, but most often in the first two years of life with diarrhoea and failure to thrive and, later, generalised oedema with hypoproteinaemia. The clinical picture may closely resemble coeliac disease.

Characteristically, these children are found on investigation to have lymphopenia in the presence of a normal bone marrow and extreme reduction of serum albumin and serum immunoglobulins, in particular serum IgG, and carrier proteins such as protein-bound iodine. Owing to the lymphopenia and immunoglobulin deficiency there is increased susceptibility to infection. The severe protein loss may be accompanied by enteric calcium loss leading to hypocalcaemia (Mistilis and Skyring, 1966). Steatorrhoea is also often found in this disorder.

It is a rare condition. Only three children with the syndrome were diagnosed out of 742 consecutive small intestinal biopsies performed at the Royal Alexandra Hospital from 1966 to 1972.

Diagnosis

The diagnosis is established definitively by demonstrating the characteristic lymphatic abnormality on small intestinal biopsy (Fig. 12.1). However, the lesion is patchy and one negative biopsy does not exclude the diagnosis.

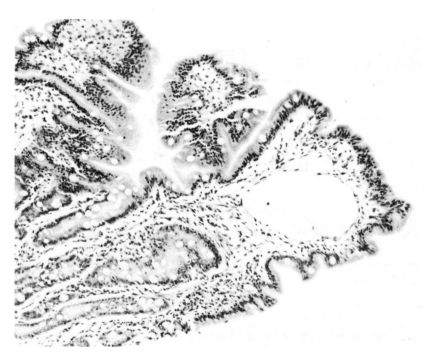

Fig. 12.1. Jejunal mucosa with a dilated lacteal.

The radioisotope demonstration of abnormal enteric protein loss using a technique such as intravenous $^{51}CrCl_3$ is helpful in diagnosis but is not, of course, specific (*see* Table 12.1).

Lymphangiography may establish the diagnosis when dye is injected into the lymphatics of one leg and subsequently shown to appear within the small intestinal lumen (Mistilis, Skyring and Stephen, 1965), but lymphangiography may be hazardous in children.

Barium studies in most cases show coarse mucosal folds without dilatation of the small intestine.

Pathology

Post mortem studies reveal a considerable variation in the distribution of the lymphatic abnormality along the length of the small intestine. Indeed dilated lacteals may occur irregularly along the entire length of the small bowel and there may be large globular structures which are made up of grossly dilated lymphatics projecting into the lumen (Fig. 12.2).

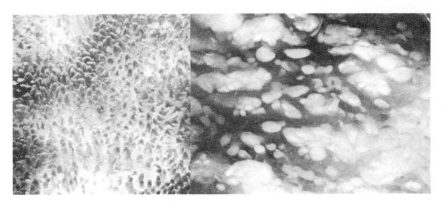

Fig. 12.2. Appearance of mucosa under dissecting microscope at postmortem in intestinal lymphangiectasia (right), and normal ileum (left).

Lymphatic proliferation and dilatation may also occur within the mesentery, as well as the serous, muscular and submucosal layers of the small intestinal wall (Fig. 12.3). This overgrowth of lymph vessels may also extend into the lymph nodes and occupy part of the nodal tissue (Fig. 12.4).

Treatment

This is usually dietetic, since the lymphangiectasia is rarely localised enough to allow surgical excision of the involved gut in order to effect a permanent cure. The basis of dietetic management is to limit the amount of long chain fat in the diet which is normally absorbed via the intestinal lymphatics. This leads to a reduction in the volume of intestinal lymph and to the pressure within the dilated lymphatics. It is best done by placing the child on a low fat diet (5 to 10 g/day) and adding medium chain triglycerides, instead of the usual long chain dietary fats, in unrestricted amounts. A milk containing medium

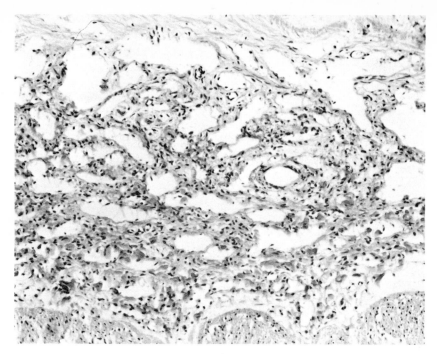

Fig. 12.3. Tortuous submucosal lymphatics.

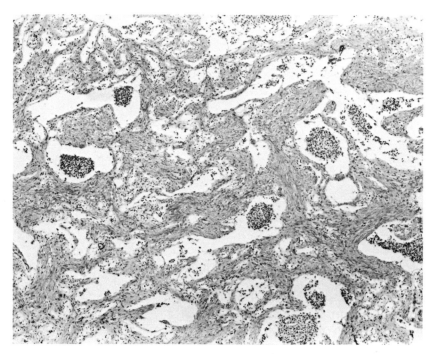

Fig. 12.4. Section of mesenteric lymph node with dilated lymphatics.

chain triglyceride such as Pregestemil may be used with medium chain triglyceride oil for cooking. A diet based on medium chain triglycerides usually leads to a clinical remission, but some children may be resistant to this dietetic therapy when the abnormality is very extensive and, on occasion, death may result despite therapy (Walker-Smith et al., 1969). Albumin infusions are of little value in management as their benefit is so transitory. Steroids have been advocated for severe cases but there is little evidence to justify their use in these circumstances.

A follow-up study of six children by Tift and Lloyd (1975) showed that although there was a continuing chyle leak, as evidenced by persistent lymphopenia and hypoalbuminaemia, the children had a rapid and sustained improvement in dependent oedema following the use of the diet recommended above, although asymmetrical oedema from peripheral lymphatic abnormalities was unaffected. Their growth rate improved on the diet. Clinical relapse occurred quickly when the diet was relaxed. Continued adherence to a strict diet, at least through puberty is, therefore, recommended. Indeed it seems probable that this is a life-long disorder and that dietetic management may usually need to be permanent.

Surgical resection can offer some hope when the lesions are localised to one part of the small intestine, but this may be difficult to determine even at laparotomy, and localisation seems to be an unusual event in this disorder.

ABETALIPOPROTEINAEMIA

Salt and his co-workers in 1960 described a syndrome in a child characterised by an absence of betalipoprotein, acanthocytes in the peripheral blood and steatorrhoea. Small intestinal biopsy revealed that the columnar epithelial cells were distended with lipid. This rare disorder, known as abetalipoproteinaemia, is inherited as an autosomal recessive characteristic. The small intestinal epithelial accumulation of fat is attributed to a failure of chylomicron formation with consequent retention of fat in the enterocyte. Betalipoprotein is an essential component for chylomicron formation and without it chylomicrons cannot be formed. As explained in chapter 1, absorbed long chain triglycerides are transported as chylomicrons along the thoracic duct. Failure of the mechanism leads to fat retention in the epithelial cell.

This disease usually presents in early infancy as failure to thrive, often accompanied by features of malabsorption with a clinical appearance similar to that of coeliac disease. Later in childhood ataxia and retinitis pigmentosa may develop.

The diagnosis may be suggested by small intestinal biopsy. The overall morphology of the small intestinal mucosa is normal but the enterocytes are engorged with fat droplets which may be identified, by appropriate stains, as triglycerides. This appearance is not specific as it can be seen in patients who do not have abetalipoproteinaemia. Further evidence in favour of the diagnosis is provided by a low serum cholesterol, a very low plasma triglyceride level, and by the presence of acanthocytes on examination of the peripheral blood, but again this is not specific. The diagnosis is established definitively only by a demonstration of the absence of betalipoprotein in the plasma.

The steatorrhoea found in this disease may be effectively treated by substituting in the diet medium for long chain triglycerides. Medium chain triglycerides are absorbed via the portal vein rather than the thoracic duct. Other manifestations of this disease are not affected by this therapy.

The disorder needs to be distinguished from familial hypobetalipoproteinaemia (Fosbrooke, Choksey and Wharton, 1973) which is inherited as an autosomal dominant. It seems unlikely that this disorder is merely the heterozygote of abetalipoproteinaemia but a distinct one.

SELECTIVE DEFECTS OF SMALL INTESTINAL ABSORPTION

Several rare disorders of absorption of specific nutrients from the small intestine may present during childhood and some that have not been discussed elsewhere will be briefly reviewed here.

Hartnup Disease

This is an uncommon disease that is inherited as an autosomal recessive characteristic. Clinically, its typical features are cerebellar ataxia, a pellagra-like skin rash and photosensitivity. There is a defect of absorption of neutral amino-acids from the small intestinal mucosa (Milne et al., 1960), and there is also a renal tubular defect for reabsorption of the neutral amino-acids (Baron et al., 1956). The diagnosis is therefore usually based on the demonstration of a gross and specific type of aminoaciduria. The clinical manifestations are due to malabsorption of the amino-acid tryptophan, producing nicotinamide deficiency which is responsible for the clinical features.

It has been shown in Hartnup disease that when tryptophan and phenylalanine are given orally as a dipeptide, the absorption is far greater than when each amino-acid is given individually. Thus, it is a specific disorder for amino-acid rather than dipeptide absorption (Navab and Asatoor, 1970).

Cystinuria

Children with cystinuria have a selective malabsorption of the amino-acid cystine and the basic amino-acids lysine, ornithine and arginine. There is also a renal tubular defect for these amino-acids characterised by aminoaciduria. As cystine is insoluble in normal urine, renal calculi develop.

Rosenberg and his colleagues (1966) have described three biochemically distinct types of cystinuria of varying severity.

Primary Hypomagnesaemia

Friedman, Hatcher and Watson in 1967 reported generalised convulsions in a neonate due to hypomagnesaemia, with associated hypocalcaemia that were unresponsive to calcium. A specified defect in the absorption of magnesium was suggested.

Stromme and his colleagues, in 1969, reported two brothers with this syndrome and produced evidence of malabsorption of magnesium. They proposed the name 'familial hypomagnesaemia'.

The nature of the defect awaits elucidation.

Menkes's Steely-hair (Kinky-hair) Syndrome

Recent evidence shows that a specific defect in the absorption of copper occurs in Menkes's steely-hair syndrome which is a rare, recessively inherited disorder characterised by retardation of growth, peculiar hair and focal cerebellar degeneration that presents in early infancy (Danks et al., 1972; Menkes et al., 1962). Despite low plasma total copper and caeruloplasmin levels and evidence of copper malabsorption from radioisotope studies, Danks and his colleagues (1973) have shown that the small intestinal mucosa in children with this syndrome contains increased levels of copper. They have suggested a fault in the egress of copper from the small intestinal mucosal cell to the blood stream. Intramuscular copper EDTA has been shown to raise plasma copper levels to normal in these children (Walker-Smith *et al.*, 1973) but no clinical improvement resulted. Indeed, there is now evidence in Menkes's steely-hair syndrome of a more generalised defect of copper transport throughout the body as well as a defect in copper absorption, unlike acrodermatitis enteropathica in which there is a specific defect of metal absorption. This accounts for the failure of parenteral copper therapy to lead to clinical improvement, as has been reported by most observers. There is, however, one report by Grover and Scrutton (1975) of some clinical improvement with very early diagnosis followed by immediate treatment with parenteral copper.

The description by Hunt (1974) of a very similar disorder in mice (the mottled mouse syndrome) has led to investigations of copper metabolism in this disorder as a model for the human syndrome. Both have an X-linked inheritance. Danks, Camakaris and Stevens (1977) have shown that, mutant fibroblast cells cultured from the skin of children with Menkes's steely-hair syndrome, and lung cells as well as renal epithelial cells from mice with the mottled mouse syndrome, all accumulate copper in excess. This suggests that in both disorders there is a common problem in transporting copper by these cells, which may be an irreversible binding to an altered intracellular ligand.

Much more work is needed to clarify the nature of the defect of copper metabolism in Menkes's steely-hair syndrome, but study of 'the mottled mouse' may help throw light on the problem.

Selective Malabsorption of Vitamin B_{12}

This disorder was first described in 1960 by Imerslund and by Grasbeck and his colleagues independently. It is characterised in children by familial megaloblastic anaemia due to an isolated defect of B_{12} absorption and is often accompanied by proteinuria. Such children are not achlorhydric. General malabsorption is not a usual feature, but Bell and his colleagues (1973) described steatorrhoea reversed by B_{12} therapy in a child with this disorder. An ileal mucosal defect of absorption for vitamin B_{12} seems most likely, but Mackenzie and his colleagues have shown that B_{12} complexed with intrinsic factor was taken up normally by a homogenised biopsy taken from the ileum of a patient with this disorder. Again, it seems there may be a defect of egress of an absorbed nutrient, this time vitamin B_{12}, from the enterocyte, but at present this is still speculative.

Congenital Malabsorption of Folic Acid

An extremely rare disorder of folic acid absorption has been described, characterised by megaloblastic anaemia, convulsions, ataxia and mental retardation, apparently due to a specific defect of folic acid absorption.

SMALL INTESTINAL ABNORMALITIES IN HENOCH-SCHÖNLEIN PURPURA

Henoch-Schönlein purpura may be accompanied by serous or haemorrhagic effusions into the wall of the small intestine, leading to abdominal pain and the passage of melaena stools. The clinical picture may be confused with intussusception and acute appendicitis. A barium study may reveal localised narrowing of the small intestinal lumen and distortion of the mucosal folds. The radiological appearance may be confused with Crohn's disease.

Steroid therapy has been advocated for this syndrome when the abdominal manifestations are severe but there is no convincing proof of their benefit in management and there is the real risk of administration masking the signs of intestinal obstruction and perforation. Conservative expectant management is all that can be advocated at present and, fortunately, the outcome is usually satisfactory.

SMALL INTESTINAL DISEASE IN CHILDREN WITH IMMUNE DEFICIENCY SYNDROMES

It has already been made clear that defects of immunological function may occur in a number of diseases of the small intestine in childhood and that, furthermore, immunological abnormalities may be major factors in the pathogenesis of many of them. Gastrointestinal symptoms are, however, common in children with primary immunodeficiency syndromes and in a number of them there is evidence of disease of the small intestine.

Soothill (1977) commenting on the high incidence of immunopathological disease in patients with immunodeficiency has proposed that the mechanism whereby damage results may itself be normal, but is overstimulated by excess antigen contact. This is because another mechanism has failed to eliminate or exclude the antigen, rather than that the disease results from overactivity of the damaging mechanism. Normally, antigen is eliminated by antibody, complement and phagocytes. Defective function of one of these, either as a primary abnormality, possibly involving a genetic factor, or as a secondary one could lead to defective elimination. These mechanisms may be interrelated, e.g. IgA may activate the alternative pathway of complement and when there is transient IgA deficiency, as may occur in early infancy, it may parallel an transient deficiency of suppressor T cells.

In clinical practice, it may be difficult at the initial presentation to know whether an infant with chronic diarrhoea has a primary or a secondary immunological disorder. Indeed, on occasion, it may be only after a number of investigations and the passage of time that it becomes clear that an infant with intractable diarrhoea has a primary or a secondary immunodeficiency state (*see* page 348).

Primary Immunodeficiency Syndromes

These are a heterogeneous group of diseases that are characterised by impairment of the B-cell system, the T-cell system, or both. Impairment of the B-cell system's normal development and function will produce deficiency in immunoglobulin synthesis. Impairment of the T-cell system will lead to defective cell-mediated immunity.

The World Health Organisation has produced a classification of these primary immunodeficiency syndromes, and their gastrointestinal complications have been reviewed by Ochs and Ament (1976) and by Katz and Rosen (1977). Table 12.2 summarises these syndromes and describes the small intestinal involvement in each.

The incidence of small intestinal disease in these syndromes is variable. It is rare in the congenital antibody deficiency syndromes such as X-linked agammaglobulinaemia but is very common in children with severe combined immunodeficiency.

Small Intestinal Morphology in Immunodeficiency Syndromes

The lesions of the small intestinal mucosa obtained on biopsy are often patchy and could be missed if only one biopsy were taken. Three principal morphological abnormalities may be noted.

1. Decrease or Absence of Plasma Cells in Lamina Propria. Plasma cells are absent from the lamina propria of children with agammaglobulinaemia and there is usually a reduced number of plasma cells in

Table 12.2
Primary immunodeficiency syndromes and small intestinal disease

Type of immunodeficiency	Small intestinal disease
I B-Cell Defects	
1. Infantile X-linked agammaglobulinaemia	Absence of plasma cells in lamina propria but gastrointestinal complications are unusual
2. X-linked immunodeficiency with increased IgM	Lymphoma of small intestine (Katz and Rosen)
3. Selective IgA deficiency	Coeliac disease, giardiasis
4. Transient hypogammaglobulinaemia of infancy	Diarrhoea and malabsorption
5. Variable immunodeficiency (acquired hypogammaglobulinaemia)	Reduced plasma cells in lamina propria, nodular lymphoid hyperplasia Giardiasis
II T-cell Defect Di George's syndrome (Thymic hypoplasia)	Diarrhoea and intestinal candidiasis
III B & T Cell Defects	
1. Severe combined immunodeficiency (a) autosomal resessive (b) X-linked (c) sporadic	reduced plasma cells in lamina propria Severe diarrhoea, sometimes intractable
2. Immunodeficiency with thrombocytopenia and eczema (Wiskott-Aldrich)	Malabsorption

small intestinal biopsies taken from children with hypogammaglobulinaemia. The overall morphology of the small intestinal mucosa is usually normal in children with congenital immunoglobulin deficiency but it may be abnormal with partial villous atrophy and even a flat mucosa in children with acquired hypogammaglobulinaemia.

2. Lymphoid Nodular Hyperplasia, i.e. large lymphoid follicles within the lamina propria that cause protrusion of the overlying mucosa. This was first described by Heremans, Huizenga and Hoffman (1966). This is most often found in adult patients with late onset and antibody deficient syndromes, and has only rarely been found in childhood (Ochs and Ament) although Roy and Dubois (1971) studied five such children. *Giardia lamblia* has been identified in most patients and symptoms have been relieved by eradication of the parasite.

3. Mucosal Abnormality. A flat mucosa or varying degrees of partial villous atrophy may be found in some children with these syndromes. Coeliac disease may occur in children with selective IgA deficiency (*see* chapter 5) (Savilahti, Pelkonen and Visakorpi, 1971). The only difference between these children and other children with coeliac disease but no IgA deficiency is that IgA deficiency persists in the children on a gluten-free diet, despite the return of the mucosa to normal, whereas in the others on a gluten-free diet all immunological abnormalities return to normal. More often the small intestinal mucosa is found to be normal in children with isolated IgA deficiency.

A flat mucosa and reduced lamina propria plasma cells in patients with acquired hypogammaglobulinaemia in adults, has been described, which only rarely responds to a gluten-free diet.

Mucosal abnormality may also occur in severe combined immunodeficiency but more often the mucosa is normal in these children and in children with thymic hypoplasia.

Functional Disorders of the Small Intestine in Immune Deficiency Syndromes

Damage to the small intestine, if severe and extensive, will lead to malabsorption. Malabsorption, particularly steatorrhoea, has been well documented in children with congenital and acquired hypogammaglobulinaemia. Clinically, it is uncommon in the congenital group and is more severe in the acquired type (Dubois *et al.*, 1970). Steatorrhoea may be associated with coexistent Giardia infestation. Appropriate therapy with metronidazole may lead to a dramatic improvement with disappearance of steatorrhoea and rapid weight gain.

Dubois and his colleagues (1970) have demonstrated disaccharidase deficiency in some children, in a variety of primary immunodeficiency states occurring either as an isolated lactase deficiency or a generalised disaccharidase deficiency. Monosaccharide malabsorption may sometimes also occur in such children. The cause of the disturbances of sugar digestion and absorption is still to be clarified. It does seem probable that in most cases it occurs secondarily to small intestinal mucosal damage. Its relevance to clinical management in most children is also unclear.

Clinically, it seems that the severity of the patient's gastroenterological disturbance correlates best with the severity of the state of immunological deficiency present. Much more investigation in this field is required to elucidate the relationship.

TODDLER'S DIARRHOEA

In the first edition of this book, this disorder, variously known as toddler's diarrhoea, non-specific diarrhoea, or the irritable colon syndrome (Davidson and Wasserman, 1966), was excluded as there appeared to be no evidence that the condition was associated with any abnormality of the small intestine *per se*. However, Tripp *et al.* (1978) have found evidence that, although the small intestinal mucosa in these children is morphologically normal, there is a significant increase in specific enzyme activity for adenyl cyclase, and also for Na^+-K^+-ATP-ase in small intestinal biopsies taken from children with this syndrome. They suggest that this increase is a response of normal villous cells to crypt cell secretion. This could be mediated via prostaglandins, high plasma Prostaglandin F Levels having been found in children with this syndrome (Hamdi and Dodge, 1978). Whether the colon is also functionally abnormal is not yet clear.

Burke and Anderson (1975) have described this disorder as being the largest group of young children referred for investigation because of persistent or intermittent looseness and frequency of stools in westernised communities.

Toddler's diarrhoea usually has its onset between the age of six and twenty months. Often, the child has previously been constipated, and sometimes has had infantile colic. In most children the diarrhoea ceases spontaneously between the ages of two and four years, sometimes earlier. The stool pattern is, typically, a large stool early in the day, formed or partly formed, followed by the passage of smaller looser stools containing undigested vegetable material and mucus. The passage of undigested food is characteristic; indeed, one popular name for the syndrome stemming from this observation is 'the peas and carrots syndrome'. Despite the diarrhoea the child grows and develops completely normally. Psychosomatic factors may be important as suggested by the higher proportion of children coming from families of the professional classes. Often the mother may become preoccupied with every stool the child passes, the loose stools causing severe anxiety despite the child's evident general well-being.

Detailed investigation such as small intestinal biopsy are indicated only when there is some doubt about the child's nutritional status or the presence of other symptoms. However, giardiasis and sucrase-isomaltase deficiency can be confused with this disorder.

Management is reassurance and explanation. No specific treatment either drug or dietetic is of proven value.

INTRACTABLE DIARRHOEA OF INFANCY

In 1968, Avery and his colleagues described a severe syndrome of infantile intractable diarrhoea with the following features:

1. Diarrhoea of more than two weeks duration.
2. Age less than three months.
3. Three or more stool cultures negative for bacterial pathogens.
4. All were managed with intravenous fluids.
5. Despite hospital management, diarrhoea was persistent and intractable.
6. There was a high mortality.

The author recognises three variants of a chronic infantile diarrhoea syndrome, which he designates 'intractable'. This word is used in accordance with the Oxford dictionary definition of 'intractable', i.e. 'not easily dealt with'. These three variants are: (1) the intractable diarrhoea of Avery, i.e. chronic diarrhoea persisting despite intravenous fluids and nil by mouth; (2) chronic diarrhoea that disappears on intravenous fluids and nil by mouth, only to recur when oral feeding is resumed; (3) chronic diarrhoea that has been managed by a variety of elimination diets but still persists. Thus, the intractable diarrhoea syndrome of infancy embracing these three groups is a heterogeneous syndrome and is also of diverse aetiology.

Aetiology

This syndrome may result from a variety of disorders which are listed in Table 12.3. Often no cause may be established.

In most of these entities the small intestine is significantly involved but the large intestine may be also.

Immunological Abnormalities in Intractable Diarrhoea

Systemic Abnormalities of Immunity

Lymphocytes. Defects of lymphocyte function, of both humoral and cellular immunity have been described in this syndrome, e.g. abnormalities of serum immunoglobulins reflecting B cell function; low IgG and low IgA levels and defects of cellular immunity; T-cell deficiency. Indeed, an important feature of many children with T-cell deficiency is intractable diarrhoea (Katz and Rosen, 1976). It is also a feature of combined immunodeficiency. Chronic diarrhoea and, on occasion, intractable diarrhoea, are in fact common complications of many immunological diseases of childhood. Sometimes a clear-cut and treatable cause for this diarrhoea can be demonstrated, e.g. secondary infestation with *Giardia lamblia* (*see* chapter 8), but often the mechanism for the severe diarrhoea is quite obscure.

Table 12.3
Differential diagnosis of intractable diarrhoea of infancy

Surgical causes—
    Hirschsprung's disease with enterocolitis
    Ruptured viscus with peritonitis or peritoneal abscess
    Incomplete obstruction
    Stagnant loop syndrome
    Post-enteritis syndrome
    Secondary lactose intolerance
    Cow's milk protein intolerance
    Soy protein intolerance
    Coeliac crisis
Immunodeficiency states—
    combined immune deficiency
    T-cell deficiency
    defective opsonisation
Selective inborn errors of absorption—
    congenital chloridorrhoea
    glucose-galactose malabsorption
    congenital lactase deficiency
Tumours—neuroblastoma, ganglioneuroma
Acrodermatitis enteropathica
Lymphangiectasia
Necrotising enterocolitis
Non-specific enterocolitis
Idiopathic

Phagocytes. Recently, defective opsonisation has been recognised as an important and treatable cause of this syndrome. The capacity of phagocytes to ingest foreign material and to kill and to digest it is a basic component of the defence response of man, but before phagocytosis occurs there must be opsonisation, which is the process of making bacteria and other cellular organisms susceptible to phagocytosis.

Opsonisation of bacteria and other particles involves activation of complement, and such activity can proceed either by the classic (antibody dependent) or the alternate (antibody-independent) pathway. Recently, increasing attention has been paid in immunology to phagocyte function, and defective opsonisation (Soothill and Harvey, 1976) has now been demonstrated as a rare but important cause of the syndrome of intractable diarrhoea, which may respond rapidly to plasma infusions.

Distinction Between Primary and Secondary Immunological Abnormalities

One strange feature of some children with intractable diarrhoea is that, despite their severe secondary malnutrition, they may not have the sort of secondary immunological abnormalities that have been described in primary malnutrition, e.g. diminished skin reactivity to common antigens and reduced ability to sensitisation with dinitrochlorobenzene (DNCB). In practice, it may be very important to distinguish primary and secondary immunodeficiency states associated with intractable diarrhoea, since approach to treatment of these two deficiency states is radically different. Blood transfusion may be dangerous in the former (risk of graft versus host reaction), and so reliable identification of primary defects is vital. Prognosis is much poorer in this group. Wood, 1978, personal communication.

The response of lymphocytes to non-specific mitogens, namely phytohaemagglutinin (PHA) and poke weed mitogen may allow a distinction to be made between primary and secondary problems. Transformation with PHA may be depressed in both syndromes but the poke weed mitogen response is absent in primary immunodeficiency states only.

Local Immune Abnormalities

Intractable Diarrhoea with an Enteropathy

An enteropathy is a common, albeit non-universal, finding in these children (Shwachmann et al.). Avery and his colleagues in 1968, described a non-specific entercolitis in 6 out of 20 of his original cases.

In an autopsy study of 13 children with histological 'enteritis', 2 children with intractable diarrhoea syndrome had a severe enteropathy, and when viewed with the dissecting microscope after autolysis, short, thick ridges and ulcers were seen along the gut (Walker-Smith, 1972).

An immune abnormality may play an important part in the pathogenesis of such an enteropathy, which may be the result of a hypersensitivity reaction to a variety of antigens, e.g. food antigens, bacterial antigens or possibly viral antigens. On occasion it seems to be a sequel to acute gastroenteritis, i.e. it may be a variant of the post-enteritis syndrome referred to in chapter 6. The pathogenesis of diarrhoea in those without diarrhoea is unknown but may be related to the factors discussed in pathogenesis of post-enteritis syndrome (*see* chapter 6).

Management of Intractable Diarrhoea

The management of intractable diarrhoea in infancy is one of the most difficult problems in the whole of paediatric gastroenterology. The first step is to exclude a surgically remediable cause such as an appendix abscess, malrotation, Hirschsprung's disease, and a stagnant loop associated with atresia or surgery to the small intestine (*see* Table 12.3). The second step is to investigate for possible medical causes of the syndrome, particularly the disorders that are simply treated with an elimination diet. In particular, the importance of testing stools, properly collected with Clinitest tablets for reducing substances cannot be overstressed (*see* chapter 3). Stool chromatography may be a useful adjunct, particularly if there have been recent changes of feed. If the infant is not too small or too ill, a small intestinal biopsy early on may be a useful investigation to decide whether or not an enteropathy is present, indicating the likelihood of a food sensitive enteropathy; it also allows an assay for enzyme activity. It can be a useful guide to management. Medium chain triglycerides (MCT) may be preferable to long chain triglycerides (LCT) if enteropathy is present. At the same time, duodenal contents may be sampled for bacterial culture, aerobically and anaerobically.

Seriously Ill Infant requiring IV Fluids. Clinically, one is often presented with a very sick marasmic infant who may also be dehydrated, and who may already have been given a wide variety of different therapeutic feeds without success. In these circumstances treatment must be started immediately and the investigation proceeds *pari passu* with therapy. The first step in management is to set up an intravenous infusion to correct dehydration and any electrolyte disturbance that may be present, including acidosis.

It is usually best to have a period of bowel rest overnight or for 24 hours and to observe whether the diarrhoea stops or continues. There are then two options open: (1) dietary manipulation, (2) total intravenous alimentation. Intractable diarrhoea, as described by

Avery *et al.*, i.e. diarrhoea continuing despite nil by mouth and after rehydration and correction of electrolyte disturbances, is a great problem. If it occurs, a period of total intravenous alimentation is then indicated with nil by mouth, and it should be continued at least until, hopefully, the diarrhoea eventually ceases, as in fact it usually does. A decision to continue on intravenous alimentation when once the diarrhoea has ceased will depend upon the previous history and the child's degree of undernutrition. If nutrition is poor, and the likelihood of relapse after return to oral feeding seems at all likely from the preceding history, the regime should continue. Otherwise, a day after cessation of diarrhoea one may elect to introduce a dietary regime. There is experimental evidence in animals that prolonged nil by mouth leads to atrophy of the small intestinal mucosa (Hughes *et al.*, 1977). Whether this occurs in man is still uncertain. Oral feeds should be introduced very carefully, and intravenous fluids continued as augmented alimentation for a time, until it is clear that the infant can tolerate oral feeding.

Less Seriously Ill Infant not requiring IV Fluids. Returning to the infant who does not require intravenous feeding, a feed that is free of cow's milk should be given and, in general, a diet that is also free of gluten is usually prescribed. As a group, these infants can be divided again into the more severe and the less severe. The more severely ill should be given a 5 per cent glucose and electrolyte mixture (GEM)—*see* Table 12.6—for 12 to 24 hours, provided there is no previous history of monosaccharide intolerance. An alternative is to start with a quarter-strength comminuted chicken feed plus 5 per cent gastrocaloreen, a glucose polymer, and minerals (*see* Appendix). If the GEM is tolerated, quarter-strength comminuted chicken may be added, and then, later, supplemented with gastrocaloreen to boost caloric intake.

If there is a history of previous monosaccharide intolerance, feeding with quarter-strength comminuted chicken is recommended, with addition of 1 per cent glucose or caloreen, and 1 per cent fructose, up to 8 to 10 per cent total carbohydrate, with daily graded increments of 1 per cent of each sugar. This diet should be given in small frequent feeds two or three-hourly, sometimes hourly, bearing in mind that the baby must not be overtaxed if the feed is not given via a gastric tube. Unfortunately, feeding based on comminuted chicken meat is difficult to introduce into an intragastric feeding tube because it is a suspension, but with other feeds the continuous intragastric method may be helpful. If the regime is tolerated by the infant, as it usually is, the feed can be increased in strength step-wise, raising the protein content in quarter increments until the comminuted chicken meat is full strength. Table A1 gives one particular recipe of a solution made up to full strength.

Ketovite tablets and liquid must be added to provide vitamins; also a mineral mixture. The feeds are slowly built up over a period of ten days or more. In some children, intravenous fluids may be useful as augmented alimentation during this regrading. Caloric content can be increased by adding Prosparol, an emulsion of long-chain tryglyceride, and further carbohydrate as gastrocaloreen. The aim should be to provide 180–200 Kcal/kg/day. MCT can be used when there is an enteropathy, but MCT is not so good calorifically as LCT. A similar regime may be followed after a period of total intravenous alimentation, as it is phased out.

Turning now to the less severely ill infant, a formula such as Pregestimil, containing glucose, medium chain triglyceride and a casein hydrolysate, may be used. This particular formula has the drawback of having a high osmolality, and so may not be tolerated by some infants (*see* Table A3). A new modified formula of Pregestimil (3240D), with lower osmolality, containing some long chain triglycerides and a glucose polymer, is preferable.

The advantages such formulae have over that based on comminuted chicken meat is that they are complete feeds, and are far simpler to make up, thus leaving less room for error. Education and language are important here. In an immigrant community, such as that found in the East End of London, this may be crucial.

Close monitoring of stools for consistency, volume, reducing substance content, etc., is as vital as is monitoring of daily weight gain. Management of this kind has led to some improvement in mortality rates for intractable diarrhoea, but despite the regimes described they are still unacceptably high. If such dietary regimes fail and on biopsy an enteropathy is found, steroids may have a place in management, and even lymphocyte stimulating drugs such as levamisole may be used. Further research into the management of this syndrome is urgently required. Those who have diarrhoea from birth and also have a history of an affected sibling have a poor prognosis (Larcher *et al.*, 1977).

SMALL INTESTINAL DISEASE IN CHILDREN WITH MALNUTRITION

Terminology

The term protein-calorie malnutrition has been used to describe all forms of inadequate protein and calorie intake in pre-school children, but now the term protein-energy deficiency is the one that is recommended (Wharton, 1977). It embraces kwashiorkor and marasmus as well as the forms of malnutrition in between these two extremes.

Diarrhoea and Malnutrition

Diarrhoea is common in children with protein-energy deficiency. Gastroenteritis is a frequent association of this syndrome in under-privileged communities. Recurrent attacks may play an important part in its genesis and delayed recovery after acute gastroenteritis may pave the way for its development (Williams, 1962) (*see* chapter 6).

The diarrhoea associated with malnutrition may be due to sugar malabsorption, most often to a disaccharide intolerance, but some-times, in severe cases, to monosaccharide malabsorption (e.g. glucose malabsorption) or, on occasion, to a complete monosaccharide malab-sorption of glucose and fructose (Wharton, 1968) (*see* chapter 7). This sugar intolerance is a temporary phenomenon but there is a wide difference in its duration. Clinically, sugar intolerance, i.e. sugar malabsorption requiring specific treatment, usually ceases to be a problem within three weeks of admission to hospital with acute protein-energy deficiency (Wharton, 1975). Follow-up studies of carbohydrate absorption have, however, shown that lactose absorp-tion may take more than a year before it returns to normal after recovery (Bowie *et al.*, 1967). Because of the risk of lactose intolerance in children with protein-energy deficiency there is considerable controversy concerning the role of milk and milk products in prog-rammes intended to eliminate malnutrition. On the one hand, some workers, for example Bowie (1975) in South Africa, recommend milk products, stressing that they are usually the cheapest and often the only widely available source of protein; on the other hand, other workers such as Suharjano *et al.* (1975), in Indonesia, have suggested that giving lactose may be harmful in severely malnourished children. Mitchell *et al.* (1977) have shown that there are advantages in giving an isocaloric lactose hydrolysate of milk to undernourished Australian aboriginal children.

From all this it seems clear that each community in which protein-energy deficiency exists will need to decide on the most appropriate form of nutrition for its own children.

Carbohydrate malabsorption in these children seems to be related to the presence of a small intestinal enteropathy that leads to reduced disaccharidase activity.

The Small Intestinal Enteropathy of Malnutrition

A small intestinal enteropathy has been attributed to protein-energy deficiency *per se*. Indeed, studies of small intestinal biopsies taken from children with protein-energy deficiency have shown significant mucosal abnormalities (Amin, Walia and Ghai, 1969; Barbazet *et al.*, 1967; Brunser *et al.*, 1966; Burman, 1965; Stanfield, Hutt and Tunnicliffe, 1965), but the severity of the enteropathy described has varied in each tropical country from which the reports have emanated, ranging from mild, partial villous atrophy to a completely flat mucosa. In particular, Brunser *et al.* in Chile, and Barbazet *et al.* to a lesser extent in South Africa have each demonstrated more severe abnormalities than did Burman in Kenya, Stanfield *et al.* in Uganda, and Amin *et al.* in India. Indeed, Burman concluded that the small intestinal abnormalities in kwashiorkor were relatively minor. Yet Brunser found a completely flat small intestinal mucosa in 7 out of 10 children with kwashiorkor in Chile, but he found an essentially normal mucosa in children with marasmus, apart from some reduction in mucosal thickness and the mitotic index, whereas Amin *et al.* in India found more severe changes in marasmus than in kwashiorkor. In any event, regardless of severity, these mucosal abnormalities found in protein-energy deficiency appear to improve with treatment when followed by serial biopsies.

The morphological abnormalities of the small intestinal mucosa described above, must be considered in relation to the small intestinal mucosal morphology of children and adults from tropical countries who are not overtly malnourished. At birth, in both tropical and non-tropical countries, finger-like villi are common, but in early infancy changes occur particularly in the proximal small intestine (*see* chapter 3). In non-tropical countries, broad villi described as leaf-like, tongue-like or like thin-ridges become predominant in the proximal small intestine, spreading distally to a variable extent. In tropical countries, ridge-like villi and convolutions predominate (Wharton,

1977). These changes persist and may even tend to become more severe in adult life in tropical countries whereas in temperate countries finger-like villi re-appear and are predominant in the proximal small intestine of normal healthy adults. This difference in morphology of the small intestine between children and adults in tropical and temperate countries has already been remarked upon in chapter 3. It has been remarked that the morphology of normal small intestinal mucosa in childhood from temperate countries bears some resemblance to morphology of symptom-free adults in tropical countries.

All this means that care must be taken in attributing the morphological changes described above to protein-energy deficiency *per se*. The best evidence that the partial villous atrophy most often described in this syndrome is related to the malnutrition process, stems from the observed improvement with treatment by serial biopsy in individual patients and the fact that protein-deficient monkeys develop partial villous atrophy (Deo and Ramalingaswami, 1964).

In view, then, of this finding of a small intestinal enteropathy attributed to protein-energy deficiency in countries where both coeliac disease and protein-energy deficiency co-exist, differentiation between the two disorders may be very difficult. Such countries include Turkey, Pakistan, and the Sudan. Indeed, it seems probable that in such countries the diagnosis of coeliac disease has been made all too infrequently in the past. With the use of small intestinal biopsy and modern criteria for diagnosis, Suliman (1978) in the Sudan, has shown that coeliac disease is a commoner problem than formerly appreciated. Nevertheless, for genetic reasons, related to HLA antigen status, as referred to in chapter 4, in most countries where protein-energy deficiency is common, coeliac disease appears to be rare.

Chile is another country where both protein-energy malnutrition and coeliac disease do occur, owing to the mixed ethnic origins of the population. There, coeliac disease is an important cause of malabsorption (Danus, Chuaqui and Vallejos, 1971; Guiraldes, Gutiérrez and Latorre, 1977). However, in practice, many of these children are often first regarded as suffering from 'primary' malnutrition with 'secondary malabsorption'. As a result, children diagnosed as having coeliac disease have a higher mean age than in Britain (mean of 5·4, in 1977, with a range of 15 months to 14 years, Guiraldes, 1978). This is due to delay in referral to a gastroenterological centre, which means that, from a practical point of view, most children in this older group, (pre-school or school age children) in Chile, who have a flat mucosa prove to have coeliac disease. If children were biopsied at a younger age this might be different, i.e. other causes of a flat mucosa such as cow's milk protein intolerance might then be recognised. Danus and colleagues (1971), in Chile, published a follow-up study of a group of children, followed for some years, who presented with diarrhoea and a kwashiorkor-like type of malnutrition. He biopsied all of them and found that 50 per cent had an abnormal small intestinal mucosa and 50 per cent did not. He then followed them for some further years and found that all those with an abnormal mucosa thrived on a gluten-free diet and relapsed when gluten was reintroduced, i.e. they had coeliac disease, whereas the other 50 per cent improved on a normal diet, and coeliac disease was excluded.

It is clear that small intestinal mucosal damage of a significant degree may be found in protein-energy deficiency, and it may contribute to the severity of the clinical picture, but its importance in an individual patient is at present hard to assess without the ready availability of facilities for gastroenterological investigation and for long-term follow-up. In countries like Chile and the Sudan these facilities have shown that protein-energy deficiency and coeliac disease can be confused with each other. Hopefully, in time, with the help of individual governments and international agencies, the small intestinal enteropathy of protein-energy deficiency, perhaps the most preventable of diseases of the small intestine in childhood, will disappear. Further research may lead to the recognition of other causes for enteropathies in individual patients which are at present attributed to protein-energy deficiency.

SMALL INTESTINAL LYMPHOSARCOMA

This is the commonest primary malignant tumour of the small intestine in childhood, but it is nonetheless an extremely rare condition. The term lymphosarcoma is now often replaced by lymphocytic lymphoma. This, in turn, may be subdivided into well differentiated lymphomas, i.e. the malignant cell is well differentiated (small lymphocyte) or poorly differentiated lymphomas, i.e. the malignant cell is poorly differentiated (lymphoblast). Another classification of these tumours has also been suggested based on the presence of T-cells or B-cells. This may have prognostic significance.

In childhood, this neoplasm usually affects the ileo-caecal region. Boys are affected most often, and between the ages of one and five years. The disorder may present with abdominal pain and vomiting and sometimes with features of partial intestinal obstruction, and even

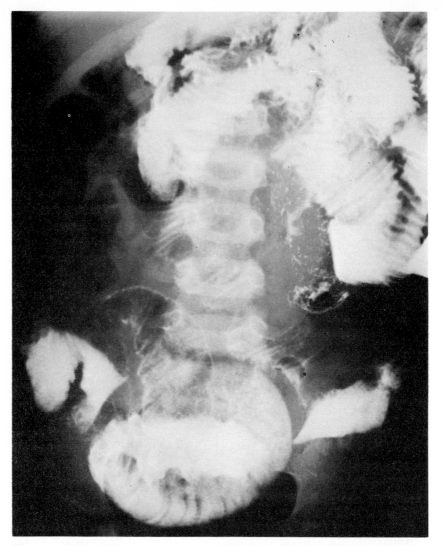

Fig. 12.5. Barium follow-through of a child with small intestinal lymphosarcoma.

with intussusception. It can also present in a manner similar to coeliac disease with steatorrhoea and iron deficiency anaemia (Newman *et al.*, 1975). On examination an abdominal mass may be palpated.

Bate, Walker-Smith and Malpas (1978) have reviewed the gastrointestinal manifestations of 11 children with lymphoma seen over a twelve-month period at St Bartholomew's Hospital, ending in September 1976. Gastrointestinal involvement was found in 9 children.

The small intestine was primarily involved in 2 children, both of whom presented with ascites and intestinal obstruction at age 6 and 9 years respectively. The former also had an intestinal perforation. Another child had secondary involvement of the proximal ileum by lymphoma.

The diagnosis is usually made on barium study, although sometimes a laparotomy may be necessary to clinch the diagnosis. Barium follow-through in these children will usually show disruption of the ileum and the caecum, with coarse irregularity of the barium contour (Bartram and Chrispin, 1973). It is usually possible to differentiate the lesion from Crohn's disease which also affects the ileo-caecal region.

Up till recently the prognosis in this disorder has been very poor, survival for more than one year after diagnosis being very uncommon. Careful staging of the extent of the malignancy, combined with appropriate surgical treatment, radiotherapy and chemotherapy may now offer some hope for these unfortunate children.

DEFECT OF INNERVATION OF THE SMALL INTESTINE

Although small intestinal smooth muscle tissue has intrinsic motility and rhythmicity, organised forward peristalsis is dependent upon an intact myenteric plexus. Tanner, Smith and Lloyd (1976) have described a syndrome of functional obstruction of the small intestine due to peristaltic failure associated with faulty development of the myenteric plexus. The syndrome is also associated with pyloric hypertrophy, short, small intestine and malrotation. In the normal adult myenteric plexus there are two types of neurone, distinguished by their affinity for silver stains. They are termed argyrophil and argyrophobe. Argyophil cells control organised peristalsis and ensure that the bolus moves forward at the correct speed, while argyrophobe cells secrete the transmitter under the control of the argyrophil cells which makes the muscle fibres contract or relax.

In the syndrome described above argyrophil ganglion cells and their processes are absent or much reduced. A similar lack of argyrophil neurones, but specifically in the pylorus, has been described in children with hypertrophic pyloric stenosis (Rintoul and Kirkman, 1961). In the absence of such innervation, smooth muscle of the small intestinal wall contracts spontaneously and rhythmically, but segmentation is not co-ordinated and the food bolus does not move on properly and there is work hypertrophy of the smooth muscle. The diagnosis of this syndrome is likely to be made only at laparotomy, when the markedly thickened bowel wall may suggest the diagnosis. If an ileostomy is performed 2 to 3 cm of ileum should be obtained for histological study with silver staining.

Appendix

SPECIAL MILKS

A number of special or therapeutic milks are mentioned in this book. As these change from time to time, reference is recommended to the manufacturers' product data for the latest information and also to the text of Francis (1975), but for convenience, a brief summary of some special milks used in UK, USA and Australia are listed with the name of the manufacturer in Table A1—

Table A1

Name	Manu-facturer	Properties	Supple-ments
'Milks' for sugar malabsorption			
Nutramigen	Mead Johnson	Casein hydrolysate formula with sucrose and starch as carbohydrate in UK and USA and glucose in Australia	Not necessary
Al 110	Nestlé	Casein, butter fat, corn oil formula with glucose as carbohydrate	Not necessary
Galactomin 17	Cow and Gate	Washed casein with vegetable fats giving full fat content and glucose as carbohydrate (CHO)	Ketovite liquid, Ketovite tablets †Trace elements or 6 to 12 Cow and Gate vitamin mineral tablets* plus vitamins A & D
Galactomin 18	Cow and Gate	As 17 but reduced fat	As 17

Name	Manu-facturer	Properties	Supple-ments
Galactomin 19	Cow and Gate	As 18 but fructose as carbohydrate	As 17
CF₁	Nestlé (Australia)	Milk based formula totally free of carbohydrate	Carbohydrate must be added after brief period of carbohydrate restriction
CHO-free	Syntex (USA)	Milk-protein free, carbohydrate free formula	As above
'Milks' for cow's milk protein intolerance			
Pro-Sobee (liquid)	Mead Johnson	Soy protein isolate formula with sucrose and corn syrup solids as carbohydrate	Not necessary
Sobee (powder)	Mead Johnson	Soya flour formula with sucrose and corn syrup solids as CHO	Not necessary
Velactin	Wander	Soya flour formula with added glucose and starch as carbohydrate, arachis oil and methionine	Vitamin A, D, C
Isomil	Ross	Soya formula with sucrose and corn syrup solids	Not necessary
Medium chain triglyceride 'Milks'			
Pregestimil	Mead Johnson	Hydrolysed casein, glucose, starch, medium chain triglycerides and some corn oil	Not necessary
Portagen	Mead Johnson	Sodium caseinate and corn syrup with sucrose as CHO and medium chain triglycerides and some corn oil	Not necessary

* These contain traces (70 mg/tablet) of sucrose.
† Aminogran mineral mixture new formula (Allen and Hanbury) may be used for trace metals.

OTHER DIETETIC PRODUCTS

A formula made by a combination of chicken meat puree, glucose polymer or glucose and/or fructose, an emulsion of long chain-triglycerides (Prosparol) i.e. 50 per cent Arachis oil emulsion in water, or medium chain triglyceride oil, complete minerals including trace elements and vitamins (as Ketovite liquid and tablets) may sometimes be of value in children with intractable diarrhoea, the post-enteritis syndrome, and massive small intestinal resection. Comminuted chicken (Cow and Gate) provides a suitable basis for this feeding. Table A2 indicates the constituents of full-strength feed, and Table A3 details of full feeding based on this regimen.

Table A2
Constituents of full-strength feed based on comminuted chicken meat—Permission of Francis

Constituents	Amount in 100 ml
Protein (contained in comminuted chicken)	3·75 g
Fat (contained in chicken)	1·65 to 4·15 g
Gastrocaloreen or glucose or fructose	5·0 g
Sodium*	1·85 mmol
Potassium*	2·32 mmol
Calcium*	1·75 mmol
Other minerals	—
Total energy provided:	approx. 211 kilojoules

* values derived from comminuted chicken and mineral mixture.
Conversion SI to traditional Units Energy 4·18 kilojoules ≈ 1 kcal.

Gastrocaloreen (Scientific Hospital Supplies) is a glucose polymer of low osmolality which may be a useful supplement to boost the calorie intake of a child. Osmolality of an infant feed may be of critical importance and Table A4 lists these for some important feeds. Carbohydrates in particular have an important role in the osmolality of a particular feed. The higher their molecular weight, the lower the osmotic pressure of a solution containing a given number of calories, e.g. a 20 per cent solution of dextrose or caloreen (the glucose polymer) provides 800 calories/litre, but their osmotic effect is dramatically different. The osmolarity of dextrose is 1,110 mosmols/litre, and that of caloreen is 240 mosmols/litre. The consequences of giving a hyperosmolar solution are obvious, namely excessive amounts of water being drawn into the lumen of the small intestine, with consequent metabolic disturbances. Such solutions may even damage the small intestinal mucosa. Hence, caloreen has a decided advantage over glucose.

Table A3
Details of full feeding based on chicken meat (permission of Francis)

Constituents	Amounts in feed
Comminuted chicken	To supply 6 g protein/kg/day but no more than 10 g protein/kg/day
Gastrocaloreen	10 g/100 ml of feed
Fat (from Prosparol and comminuted chicken)	4·15 g/100 ml of feed
Aminogran mineral mixture	1·5 g/kg day (provided quantities do not exceed 1 g/100 ml of feed or total of 8 g/day)
Calcium (from comminuted chicken mineral mixture, and added calcium gluconate)	at least 1·25 mmol/100 ml of feed or minimum of 12·5 mmol/day
Feed volume	200 ml/kg/day
Total energy provided	750 or more kiljoules/kg/day (180 or more kcal/kg/day)

Table A4
Osmolalities of feeds (permission of Francis)

Feed		Approx. Feed Osmolality (mmol/kg)
10 g gastrocaloreen	⎫ ⎧ comminuted	285
5 g gastrocaloreen	⎪ ⎪ chicken	204
5 g glucose + 5 g fructose	+ minerals	830
2·5 g glucose + 2·5 g fructose	⎭ ⎩	470
Breast milk		286
Galactomin 18		240
Gold Cap SMA/S26		289
Prosobee		246
Nutramigen		513
Pregestimil		677
3240 D Pregestirnil		360

It is possible to use alternative ingredients to comminuted chicken to produce a similar feed. This is listed in Table A5.

Table A5
Alternative ingredients for the comminuted chicken feed or similar (permission of Francis)

Protein	50 g comminuted chicken ‡ can be replaced * with
	(a) 11·5 g (cooked weight) lean chicken ‡ or rabbit meat
	(b) 14 g (cooked weight) lean lamb or beef†
Protein + Fat	50 g comminuted chicken + 5 ml Prosparol can be replaced with 25 g cooked egg (yolk and white) *
Carbohydrate	5 g gastrocaloreen can be replaced with
	(a) 5 g glucose ⎱ or combination
	(b) 5 g fructose ⎰ of both
	(c) 7 g pure honey

* Bacterial contamination of frozen chicken and other proteins necessitates careful cooking, and aseptic preparation is essential. Home prepared puree meat mixtures are difficult to get through an infant feeding bottle teat due to the fibre size of meat.
† lamb is higher in fat and energy than chicken or rabbit, but a coarser meat fibre.
‡ chicken fat is higher in essential fatty acids than other meats.

Bibliography

CHAPTER 1

Booth, C. C. (1968) The effect of location along the small intestine on absorption of nutrients. In *Handbook of Physiology* (ed. Code, C.F.) Section 6, Ch. 76, p. 1513. Washington: American Physiological Society.

Brown, W. R., Savage, D. C., Dubois, R. S., Alp, M. H., Mallony, A., and Kern, F. (1972) Intestinal microflora of immunoglobulin-deficient and normal human subjects. *Gastroenterology*, **62,**1143.

Bullen, J. J., Rogers, H. J., and Weigh, L. (1972) Iron-binding proteins in milk and resistance to *Escherichia coli* infection in infants. *British Medical Journal*, **1,**69.

Cebra, J. J., Kamat, R. Gearhart, P., Robertson, S. M., and Tseng, J. (1977) The secretory IgA system of the gut. In Immunology of the Gut. *Ciba Foundation Symposium*, **46, 5.**

Cornes, J. S. (1965) Number, size and distribution of Peyer's patches in the human small intestine. *Gut*, **6, 225.**

Counahan, R. and Walker-Smith, J. A. (1976) Stool and Urinary Sugars in Normal Neonate. *Archives of Disease in Childhood*, **51, 517.**

Fairclough, P. D. (1978) Jejunal absorption of water and electrolytes in man: the effects of amino acids, peptides and saccharides. MD Thesis, London University.

Ferguson, A. and Parrott, D. M. V. (1972) Growth and development of 'antigen-free' grafts of fetal mouse intestine. *Journal of Pathology*, **106, 95.**

Ferguson, A. (1974) Lymphocytes in coeliac disease. Coeliac Disease. Second International Symposium, Leyden (Ed. Hekkens, W. Th. J. M. and A. S. Peña). Leyden. Stenfert Kroese, p. 265.

Ferguson, A. (1976) Celiac disease and gastrointestinal food allergy. Immunological aspects of the liver and gastrointestinal tract. MTP Press. p. 153.

Ferguson, A. and MacDonald, T. T. (1977) Effects of delayed hypersensitivity on the small intestine. In Immunology of the Gut. *Ciba Foundation Symposium*, **46, 305.**

Fordtran, J. S., Rector, F. R., and Ewton, M. F. (1965) Permeability characteristics of the human small intestine. *Journal Clinical Investigation*, **44,** 1935.

Fordtran, J. S., Rector, F. C., and Locklear, T. W. (1967). Water and solute movement in the small intestine of patients with sprue. *Journal of Clinical Investigation*, **46**, 287.

Goldblum, R. M. Ahlstedt, S., Carlsson, B., Hanson, L. A., Jodal, V., Lidin-Janson, G., and Sohl-Akerlund, A. (1975) Antibody forming cells in human colostrum after oral immunization. *Nature*, **257**, 797.

Gracey, M. (1977) Aspects of enteric disease in malnourished children. *Newer Horizons in Tropical Pediatrics* (ed. Suraj Gupte) Delhi: Jaypee Brothers, p. 176.

Gracey, M., Burke, V., and Anderson, C. M. (1969) Association of monosaccharide malabsorption with abnormal intestinal flora. *Lancet*, **ii**, 384.

Halpern, M. S. and Koshland, M. E. (1970) Novel subunit in secretory IgA. *Nature*, **228**, 1276.

Harfouche, J. K. (1970) The Importance of Breast Feeding. *Journal of Tropical Paediatrics*, **16**, 133.

Harries, J. T. (1976) The problem of bacterial diarrhoea. Acute diarrhoea in childhood. *Ciba Foundation Symposium* 42, Excerpta Medica: Elsevier. North-Holland.

Heremans, J. F., Heremans, M. T., and Schultze, M. E. (1959) Isolation and description of a few properties of B_2A—globulin of human serum. *Clinica Chemica Acta*, **4**, 96.

Hindocha, P. and Harrison, B. M. (1977) Immunoglobulin levels in gastroenteritis. *British Paediatric Immunology Group*.

Holborow, J. and Lessof, M. (1978) Immunological mechanisms in health and disease. *Medicine*, **1**, 37.

Johnstone, J. M. (1968) Mechanisms of fat absorption. In *Handbook of Physiology* (ed. Code, C. F.) Section, 6, Ch. 70, p. 1353. Washington: American Physiological Society.

Katz, J. (1971) The effect of the diagnosis of coeliac disease on the family. *Medical Journal of Australia*, **1**, 823.

Katz, A. J. and Rosen, F. S. (1977) Gastrointestinal complications of immunodeficiency syndromes. In Immunology of the Gut. *Ciba Foundation Symposium*, **46**, 243.

Matthews, T. H. J., Nair, C. D. G., Lawrence, H. K., and Tyrrell, D. J. A. (1976) Antiviral activity in milk of possible clinical importance. *Lancet*, **ii**, 1387.

Menzies, I. S. (1972) Intestinal permeability in coeliac disease. *Gut*, **13**, 847.

Morin, C. and Davidson, M. (1967) Paediatric gastroenterology. *Gastroenterology*, **52**, 565.

Owen, R. L. and Jones, A. L. (1974) Epithelial cell specialization within human Peyer's patches; an ultrastructural study of intestinal lymphoid follicles. *Gastroenterology*, **66**, 189.

Parrott, D. M. V. (1976) The gut as a lymphoid organ. *Clinics in Gastroenterology*, **5**, 211.

Phillips, A. D., Rice, S. J., France, N. E., and Walker-Smith, J. A. (1978) Bacteria on duodenal lymph follicle from child with diarrhoea. *Lancet*, **i**, 454.

Sakula, J. and Shiner, M. (1957) Coeliac disease with atrophy of the small intestine mucosa. *Lancet*, **ii**, 876.

Schlesinger, J. J. and Covelli, H. D. (1977) Evidence for transmission of lymphocyte responses to tuberculin by breast-feeding. *Lancet*, **ii**, 529.

Silk, D. B. A. (1976) Intestinal absorption 2. Protein, Fluids and Vitamins. *Hospital Update*, **2**, 553.

Silk, D. B. A., Chung, Y. C., Kim, Y. S., Borger, K., Conley, K., and Spiller, G. R. (1976) Comparison of oral feeding of peptide and amino acid meals to normal human subjects. *Gastroenterology*, **70**, 937.

Silk, D. B. A. (1977) Amino acid and peptide absorption in man. In *Ciba Foundation Symposium* 50 (New Series), pp. 15–36. Amsterdam: Elsevier Scientific Publishing Co.

Silverberg, M. and Davidson, M. (1970) Pediatric gastroenterology. *Gastroenterology*, **58**, 229.

Simhon, A. and Mata, L. (1978) Anti-rotavirus antibody in human colostrum. *Lancet*, **i**, 39.

Strauss, E. W. (1966) Electron microscopic study of intestinal fat absorption in vitro from mixed micelles containing linolenic acid, mono-olein and bile salt. *Journal of Lipid Research*, **7**, 307.

Swarbrick, E. T., Stokes, C. K. and Soothill, J. F. (1979) The absorption of antigens after immunisation and the simultaneous induction of specific systemic tolerance. *Gut*, in press.

Taylor, B., Norman, A. P., Orgel, H. A., Stokes, C. R., Turner, M. W., and Soothill, J. F. (1973) Transient IgA deficiency and pathogenesis of infantile atopy. *Lancet*, **ii**, 111.

Tomasi, T. B., Jr., Tan, E. M., and Solomon, A. (1965) Characteristics of immune system common to certain external secretions. *Journal of Experimental Medicine*, **121**, 101.

Walker, W. A. (1976) Antigen absorption from the small intestine and gastrointestinal disease. *Pediatric Clinics of North America*, **22**, 731.

Walker, W. A. and Hong, R. H. (1973). Immunology of the gastrointestinal tract. *Journal of Pediatrics*, **83**, 517.

Williams, C. D. (1962) Malnutrition. *Lancet*, **ii**, 342.

Wood, C. B. S. (1974) Immunology in Childhood. In *Modern Trends in Paediatrics*, p. 255, London: Butterworth.

CHAPTER 3

Alpers, D. H. and Seetharam, B. (1977) Pathophysiology of disease involving intestinal brush-border proteins. *New England Journal of Medicine*, **296**, 1047.

Biempica, L., Toccalino, M., and O'Donnell, J. C. (1968) Cytochemical and ultrastructural studies of the intestinal mucosa of children with coeliac disease. *American Journal of Pathology*, **52**, (795–823).

Bowdler, J. D. and Walker-Smith, J. A. (1969) Le rôle de la radiologie dans le diagnostic de L'intolérance au lactose chez l'enfant. *Annales de Radiologie*, **12**, 467.

Brown, A. L., Jr. (1962) Microvilli of the human jejunal epithelial cell. *Journal of Cell Biology*, **12**, (623–627).

Burgess, E. A. (1974) Personal communication.

Burgess, E. A., Levin, B., Mahalanabis, D., and Tonge, R. E. (1964) Hereditary sucrose intolerance: levels of sucrase activity in jejunal mucosa. *Archives of Disease in Childhood*, **39, 431**.

Burke, V., Kerry K. R., and Anderson, C. M. (1965) The relationship of dietary lactose to refractory diarrhoea in infancy. *Australian Paediatric Journal*, **1**, 147.

Campbell, C., Williams, C., and Walker-Smith, J. A. (1978) Diagnosis of childhood Crohn's disease; value of colonoscopy. *Gut*, **19, 958**.

Chanarin, I. (1975) The folate content of foodstuffs and the availability of different folate analogues for absorption. *Getting most out of food*, No. 10. Van den Berghs and Jurgens Limited.

Chapman, B. L., Henry, K., Paice, F., Stewart, J. S., and Coghill, N. F. (1973) A new technique for examining intestinal biopsies. *Gut*, **11**, 903.

Creamer, B. and Leppard, P. (1965) Post-mortem examination of a small intestine in the coeliac syndrome. *Gut*, **6, 466**.

Crosby, W. H. and Kugler, H. W. (1957) Intraluminal biopsy of the small intestine: the intestinal biopsy capsule. *American Journal of Digestive Diseases*, **2**, 236.

Davidson, G. P. and Townley, R. R. W. (1977) Structural and Functional Abnormalities of the Small Intestine and Nutritional Folic Acid Deficiency in Infancy. *Journal of Pediatrics*, **90.** 590.

de Peyer, E., France, N. E., Phillips, A. D., and Walker-Smith, J. A. (1978) Quantitative Evaluation of Small Intestinal Morphology in Childhood in press.

de Silva, M. (1971) Radiological investigation of small bowel disease in children. *Medical Journal of Australia*, **1**, 819.

Dormondy, K. M., Waters, A. H., and Mollin, D. L. (1963) Folic acid deficiency in coeliac disease. *Lancet*, i, 632.

Dunnill, M. S. and Whitehead, R. (1972) A method for the quantitation of small intestinal biopsy specimens. *Journal of Clinical Pathology*, **25**, 243.

Ferguson, A., Maxwell, J. D., and Carr, K. E. (1969) Progressive changes in the small-intestinal villous pattern with increasing length of gestation. *Journal of Pathology*, **99**, 87.

Ferguson, A. and Murray, D. (1971) Quantitation of intraepithelial lymphocytes in human jejunum. *Gut*, **12**, 988.

Ferguson, A. (1977) Intraepithelial lymphocytes of the small intestine. *Gut*, **18**, 921.

Ford, J. E. and Scott, K. J. (1968) The folic acid activity of some milk foods for babies. *Journal of Dairy Research*, **36**, 447.

Haworth, E. M., Hodson, C. J., Pringle, E. M., and Young, W. F. (1968) The value of radiological investigations of the alimentary tract in children with coeliac syndrome. *Clinical Radiology*, **19**, 65.

Holmes, R., Hourihane, D. O., and Booth, C. C. (1961) Dissecting microscope appearances of jejunal biopsy specimens from patients with idiopathic steatorrhoea. *Lancet*, i, 81.

Holzel, A. (1967). Sugar malabsorption due to deficiencies of disaccharidase activities and of monosaccharide transport. *Archives of Disease in Childhood*, **42**, 341.

Jewett, T. C., Duszynoki, D. O., and Allen, J. E. (1970) The visualization of Meckel's diverticulum with 99 m Tc pertechnetate. *Surgery*, **68**, 567.

Kerry, K. R. and Anderson, C. M. (1964) A ward test for sugar in the faeces. *Lancet*, i, 981.

Kilby, A. (1976) Paediatric small intestinal biopsy capsule with two ports. *Gut*, **17**, 158.

Laws, J. W. and Neale, G. (1966) Radiological diagnosis of disaccharidase deficiency. *Lancet* ii, 139.

LeBlond, C. P. and Walker, B. E. (1956) Absorption. *Physiological Review*, **36**, 255.

Leonidas, J. C. and Germann, D. R. (1974) Technetium—99 m pertechnetate imaging in diagnosis of Meckel's diverticulum. *Archives of Disease in Childhood*, **49**, 21.

Loehyr, C. A. and Creamer, B. (1966) Post-mortem study of small intestinal mucosa. *British Medical Journal*, **1**, 827.

Manuel, P., France, N. E., and Walker-Smith, J. A. (1979) Patchy Enteropathy. *Gut*, in press.

Menzies, I. S. (1973) Quantitative estimation of sugars in blood and urine by paper chromatography using direct densitometry. *Journal of Chromatography*, **81**, 109.

Padykula, Helen A. (1962) Recent Functional Interpretations of Intestinal Morphology. *Federation Proceedings*, **21**, (873–879).

Phillips, A. D., France, N., and Walker-Smith, J. (1977) The structure of the enterocyte in relation to its position on the villus—an electron microscopical study. *Acta Paediatrica Belgica*, **30**, 196.

Read, A. E., Gough, K. R., Bones, J. A., and McCarthy, C. F. (1962) An improvement to Crosby peroral intestinal capsule. *Lancet*, i, 894.

Robbards, M. (1973) Changes in plasma nephelometry after oral fat loading in children with normal and abnormal jejunal morphology. *Archives of Disease in Childhood*, **48**, 656.

Roy-Choudry, D., Cooke, W. T., Tan, D. T., Banwell, J. G., and Smith, B. J. (1966) Jejunal biopsy: criteria and significance. *Scandinavian Journal of Gastroenterology*, **1**, 57.

Rubin, C. E., Brandberg, L. L., Phelps, P. C., and Taylor, H. C. (1960) Studies of coeliac sprue, *Gastroenterology*, **38**, 28.

Rubin, C. E. and Dobbins, W. O. (1965) Peroral biopsy of the small intestine. A review of its diagnostic usefulness. *Gastroenterology*, **49**, 676.

Shmerling, D. H., Forrer, J. C. W., and Prader, A. (1970) Faecal fat and nitrogen in healthy children and in children with malabsorption or maldigestion. *Pediatrics*, **46**, 690.

Shiner, Margot (1974) Electron Microscopy of Jejunal mucosa. In *Clinics in Gastroenterology*, **3**, 33.

Soeparto, P., Stobo, E. A., and Walker-Smith, J. A. (1972) The role of chemical examination of the stool in the diagnosis of sugar malabsorption in children. *Archives of Disease in Childhood*, **47**, 56.

Stone, M. C. and Thorp, J. M. (1966) A new technique for the investigation of the low density lipoproteins in health and disease. *Clinica chimica acta*, **14**, 812.

Tamura, T. and Stokstad, E. L. R. (1973) The Availability of Food Folate in Man. *British Journal of Haematology*, **14**, 13.

Toner, P. G. (1968) Cytology of intestinal Epithelial Cells. *International Reviews in Cytology*, **24**, 233.

Trier, J. S. (1964) Studies on small intestinal crypt epithelium II. Evidence for and mechanisms of secretory activity by undifferentiated crypt cells of the human small intestine. *Gastroenterology*, **47**, 480.

Trier, J. S. (1967) Structure of the mucosa of the small intestine as it relates to intestinal function. *Federation Proceedings*, **26**, 1391.

Van de Kamer, J. H., Ten Bokkel Huinink, H., and Weijers, H. A. (1949) Rapid method for the determination of fat in faeces. *Journal of Biological Chemistry*, **177**, 347.

Vanier, T. M. and Tyas, J. F. (1967) Folic acid status in premature infants. *Archives of Disease in Childhood*, **42**, 57.

Visakorpi, J. K. (1970) An international inquiry concerning the diagnostic criteria of coeliac disease. *Acta Paediatrica Scandinavica*, **59**, 463.

Walker, W. A. (1975) Antigen absorption from the small intestine and gastrointestinal disease. *Paediatric Clinics of North America*, **22**, 731.

Walker-Smith, J. A. (1972) Uniformity of dissecting microscope appearances in proximal small intestine. *Gut*, **13**, 17.

Walker-Smith, J. A. and Reye, R. D. K. (1971) Small intestinal morphology in aboriginal children. *Australian and New Zealand Journal of Medicine*, **4**, 477.

W.H.O. Group of Experts (1972) *Nutritional Anaemias*. Technical Report Series No. 503. Geneva.

CHAPTER 4

Albert, E. D., Harms, K., Wank, R., Steinbauer-Rosenthal, I., and Scholz, S. (1973) HL A8 in coeliac disease. Joint meeting of European Societies for Immunology. *1973 Transplant Proceedings*.

al-Hassany, M. (1975) Coeliac disease in Iraqi children. *Journal of Tropical Paediatrics*, **21**, 178.

Anderson, C. M. (1960) Histological changes in the duodenal mucosa in coeliac disease. *Archives of Disease in Childhood*, **35**, 419.

Anderson, C. M. Gracey, M., and Burke, V. (1972) Coeliac disease. Some still controversial aspects. *Archives of Disease in Childhood*, **47**, 292.

Araya, M. and Walker-Smith, J. A. (1975) Specificity of ultrastructural changes in small intestinal epithelium in early childhood. *Archives of Disease in Childhood*, **50**, 844.

Arneil, G. C., Hutchinson, J. H., and Shanks, R. A. (1973) Cited in *Present-day Practice in Infant Feeding*, London: HMSO.

Asquith, P. (1974) Immunology, *Clinics in Gastroenterology*, **3**, 213.

Bennett, T., Hunter, D., and Vaughan, J. M. (1932) Idiopathic steatorrhoea (Gee's disease): a nutritional disturbance associated with tetany, osteomalacia and anaemia. *Quarterly Journal of Medicine*, **1**, 603.

Bernadin, J. E., Saunders, R. M., and Kasarda, D. D. (1976) Absence of carbohydrate in celiac-toxic A-gliadin. *Cereal chemistry*, **53**, 612.

Bitar, J. G., Salem, A. A., and Nasr. A. T. (1970) Coeliac disease from the middle east. *Lebanese Medical Journal*, **23**, 423.

Bloom, S. R. and Polak, J. M. (1978) Gut Hormone Intolerance. *Lancet*, **1**, 550.

Booth, C. C. (1968) Enteropoiesis: Structural and functional relationships of the enterocyte. *Postgraduate Medical Journal*, **44**, 12.

Booth, C. C. (1970) The enterocyte in coeliac disease. *British Medical Journal*, **4**, 14.

Brow, J. R., Parker, F., Weinstein, W. M., and Rubin, C. E. (1971) The small intestinal mucosa in dermatitis herpetiformis. *Gastroenterology*, **60**, 355.

Browning, T. H. and Trier, J. S. (1969) Organ culture of mucosal biopsies of human small intestine. *Journal of Clinical Investigation*, **48**, 1423.

Burman, J., Saelzer, E., Kilbby, A., Mollin, D., and Walker-Smith (1978) Folate studies in children with coeliac disease and post-enteritis syndrome. In press.

Carter, C., Sheldon, W., and Walker, C. (1959) The inheritance of coeliac disease. *Annals of human Genetics*, **23**, 266.

Cooper, B. T., Holmes, G. K. T., and Cooke, W. T. (1978) Intestinal lymphoma associated with malabsorption. *Lancet*, i, 387.

Cornell, H. J. and Rolles, C. J. (1978) Further evidence of a primary mucosal defect in coeliac disease. *Gut*, **19**, 253.

Cornell, H. J. and Townley, R. R. W. (1973) Investigation of possible peptidase deficiency in coeliac disease. *Clinica chimica acta*, **43**, 113.

Cudworth, A. G. and Woodrow, J. C. (1974) HLA antigens and diabetes mellitus. *Lancet*, ii, 1153.

Day, G., Evans, K., and Wharton, B. (1973) Abnormalities of insulin and growth hormone secretion in children with coeliac disease. *Archives of Disease in Childhood*, **48**, 41.

Dicke, W. K. (1950) Coeliakie: een onderzoek naar de nadelige invloed van sommige graansoorte op de lijder aan coeliakie. M.D. Thesis, Utrecht.

Dicke, W. K., Weijers, H. A., and van de Kamer, J. H. (1953) Coeliac disease II. *Acta paediatrica* (Uppsala), **42**. 34.

Dissanayake, A. S., Truelove, S. C., and Whitehead, R. (1974) Lack of harmful effect of oats on small intestinal mucosa in coeliac disease. *British Medical Journal*, **4**, 189.

Doe, W. F., Henry, K., and Booth, C. C. (1974) Complement in coeliac disease. In *Coeliac Disease*, (ed. Hekkens, W. Th. J. M. and Pena, A. S.) Leiden: Stenfert Kroese, In press.

Dormandy, K. M., Waters, A. H., and Mollin, D. L. (1963). Folic Acid Deficiency in Coeliac Disease. *Lancet*, **i**, 632.

Douglas, A. P. and Booth, C. C. (1970). Digestion in Gliadin Peptides by Normal Human Jejunal Mucosa, and by mucosa from patients with adult coeliac disease. *Clinical Science*, **38**, 11.

Douglas, A. P. and Peters, T. J. (1970) Peptide hydrolase activity of human intestinal mucosa in adult coeliac disease. *Gut.* **11**, 15.

Dowd, B. D. and Walker-Smith, J. A. (1974) Samuel Gee, Aretaeus and the coeliac affection. *British Medical Journal*, **2**, 45.

Egan-Mitchell, B., Fottrell, P. F., and McNicholl, B. (1978) Prolonged gluten tolerance in treated coeliac disease. In *Perspectives in Coeliac Disease.* (ed. McNicholl, B., McCarthy, C. F., and Fottrell, P. F.) Lancaster: MTP Press Limited, p. 25.

Ezoke, W., Hekkens, W. Th. J. M., and Hobbs, J. R. (1974) Antibodies in the sera of coeliac patients which can co-opt K-cells to attack gluten-labelled targets. In *Coeliac Disease* (ed. Hekkens, W. Th. J. M. and Pena, A. S.) Leiden: Stenfert Kroese. p. 176.

Falchuk, Z. M. and Katz, A. J. (1978) Organ culture model of gluten-sensitive enteropathy. In *Perspectives in Coeliac Disease.* Third International Coeliac Symposium (ed. McNicholl, B., McCarthy C. F., and Fottrell, P. F.) Lancaster: MTP Press, p. 65.

Falchuk, Z. M. and Strober, W. (1972) Increased jejunal immunoglobulin synthesis in patients with nontropical sprue as measured by a solid phase immunoabsorption technique. *Journal of Laboratory and Clinical Medicine*, **79**, 1004.

Falchuk, Z. M., Rogentine, G. N., and Strober, W. (1972) Predominance of histocompatibility antigen HL-A8 in patient with gluten-sensitive enteropathy. *Journal of Clinical Investigation*, **51**, 1602.

Ferguson, A. (1976) Coeliac disease and gastrointestinal food allergy. In *Immunological Aspects of the Liver and Gastrointestinal Tract*, Lancaster: MTP Press.

Ferguson, A. (1977) Intraepithelial lymphocytes of the small intestine. *Gut*, **18**, 921.

Fink, S. and Laszlo, D. (1957) A metabolic study following oral calcium, 45 administrations in a patient with nontropical sprue. *Gastroenterology*, **32**, 689.

Frazer, A. C. (1956) Growth defect in coeliac disease. *Proceedings of the Royal Society of Medicine*, **49**. 1009.

Gardiner, A., Porteous, N., and Walker-Smith, J. A. (1972). The effect of coeliac disease on the mother child relationship. *Australian Paediatric Journal*, **8**, 39.

Gardner, A. J., Mutton, K. J., and Walker-Smith, J. A. (1973) A family study of coeliac disease. *Australian Paediatric Journal*, **9**, 18.

Gee, S. J. (1888) On the coeliac affection. *St Bartholomew's Hospital Reports*, **24**, 17.

Gerrard, J. W. and Lubos, M. C. (1967) *Paediatric Clinics of North America*, **14**, 73.

Gibbons, R. A. (1889) The coeliac affection in children. *Edinburgh Medical Journal*, **35**, 321.

Gough, K. R., Read, A. E., and Naish, J. M. (1962) Intestinal reticulosis as a complication of idiopathic steatorrhoea. *Gut*, **3**, 232.

Halsted, C. H., Reisenauer, A. M., Romers, J. J., Contor, D. S., and Ruebner, B. (1977) Jejunal perfusion of simple and conjugated folates in celiac sprue. *Journal of Clinical Investigation*, **59**, 933.

Hamilton, J. R., Lynch, M. J., and Reilly, B. J. (1969) Active coeliac disease in childhood. *Quarterly Journal of Medicine*, **38**, 135.

Harris, O. D., Cooke, W. T., Thomson, H. and Waterhouse, J. A. H. (1967) Malignancy in adult coeliac disease and idiopathic steatorrhoea. *American Journal of Medicine*, **42**, 899.

Hekkens, W. Th., Haex, A. J., Willighagen, R. G. L. (1970) In *Coeliac Disease* (ed. Booth, C. C. and Dowling H.), Edinburgh and London: Churchill Livingstone.

Hekkens, W., Th. J. M. (1978) Protein chemistry and toxicity overview. In *Perspectives in Coeliac Disease*. Third International Coeliac Symposium. (ed. McNicholl, B., McCarthy, C. F. and Fottrell, P. F.) Lancaster: MTP Press, p. 3.

Hoffbrand, A. V., Douglas, A. P., Fry, T., and Stewart, J. S. (1970) Malabsorption of dietary folate (pteroylglutamates) in adult coeliac disease and dermatitis herpetiformus. *British Medical Journal*, **4**, 85.

Hoffman, H. N., Wollaeger, E. E. and Greenberg, E. (1966) Discordance for nontropical sprue in a monozygotic twin pair. *Gastroenterology*, **51**, 36.

Holdsworth, C. D. and Dawson, A. M. (1965) Absorption of fructose in man. *Proceedings of the Society for Experimental Biology and Medicine*, **118**, 142.

Holmes, G. K. T., Stokes, P. L., Sorahan, T. M., Prior, P., Waterhouse, J. A. H. M., and Cooke, W. T. (1976) Coeliac disease Gluten-free diet and malignancy, *Gut*, **17**, 612.

Jos, J. and Charbonnier, L. (1976) *In vitro* toxicity of wheat gluten fractions and subfractions on coeliac intestinal mucosa. *Acta Paediatrica Belgium*, **29**, 261.

Jos, J., Charbonnier, L. Mougenot, J. F., Mossé, J., and Rey, J. (1978) Isolation and characterisation of the toxic fraction of wheat gliadin in coeliac disease. In

Perspectives in Coeliac Disease. Third International Coeliac Symposium. (ed. McNicholl, B., McCarthy, C. F. and Fottrell, P. F.) Lancaster: MTP Press. p. 75.

Kasarda, D. D., Qualset, C. O., Mecham, D. K., Goodenberger, D. M., and Strober, W. (1978) A test of toxicity of bread from wheat lacking alpha gliadins coded by the 6A chromosome. In *Perspectives in Coeliac Disease* (ed. McNicholl, B., McCarthy, C. F., and Fottrell, P. E.) Lancaster: MTP Press, p. 62.

Kendall, M. J., Cox, P. S., Schneider, W., and Hawkins, C. F. (1972) Gluten subfractions in coeliac disease. *Lancet,* ii, 1065.

Kenrick, K. G. and Walker-Smith, J. A. (1970) Immunoglobulins and dietary protein antibodies in childhood coeliac disease. *Gut,* 11, 635.

Keunig, J. J., Peña, A. S. van Leeuwen, A., van Hoof, J. P., and van Rood (1976) HLA–DW3 associated with coeliac disease. *Lancet,* i, 506.

Kilby, A., Walker-Smith, J. A., and Wood, C. B. S. (1975) Small intestinal mucosa in cow's milk allergy. *Lancet,* i, 53.

Killman, S. A. (1964) Effect of deoxyuridine on incorporation of Tritiated Thymidine: Difference between normoblasts and megaloblasts. *Acta Medica Scandinavica,* 175, 483.

Kowlessar, O. D. (1967) Effect of wheat proteins in coeliac disease. *Gastroenterology,* 52, 893.

Kuitunen, P., Pelkonen, P., Perkkio, M., Savilahts, E., and Visakorpi, K. (1977) Transient Gluten Intolerance. *Acta Paediatrica Belgica,* 30, 250.

Kuman, P. J., Silk, B. A., Marks, J. Clark, M. L., and Dawson, A. M. (1973) Treatment of dermatitis herpetiformis with corticoids and a gluten-free diet. A study of jejunal morphology and function. *Gut,* 14, 208.

Lancaster-Smith, M., Kumar, P., and Clark, M. L. (1974) Immunological phenomena following gluten challenge in the jejunum of patients with adult coeliac disease and dermatitis herpetiformis. In *Coeliac Disease,* (ed. Hekkens, W. Th. J. M., and Peña, A. S.) Leiden: Stenfert Kroese. p. 173.

Lindberg, T., Berg, N. D., Bonulf, S., and Jakobsson, I. (1978) Liver damage in coeliac disease or other food intolerance in childhood. *Lancet,* i, 390.

Lloyd-Still, J. D., Grand, R. J., Kon-Taik Khaw, M. D., and Swachmann, H. (1972) The use of corticosteroids in coeliac crisis. *Journal of Pediatrics,* 81, 1074.

Mann, D. L., Katz, S. I., Nelson, D. L., Abelson, L. D., and Strober, W. (1976) Specific B-cell antigens associated with gluten-sensitive enteropathy and dermatitis herpetiformis. *Lancet,* i, 110.

Manuel, P., France, N. E., Walker-Smith, J. A. (1979) Patchy Enteropathy. *Gut,* in press.

McNeish, A. S., Harms, K., Rey, J., Shmerling, D. H., Visakorpi, J., and Walker-Smith, J. A. (1979) Re-evaluation of diagnostic criteria for coeliac disease. Archives of Disease in Childhood. In press.

McNeish, A. S. and Nelson, R. (1974) Coeliac disease in one of monozygotic twins. *Clinics in Gastroenterology,* 3, 143.

McNeish, A. S., Rolles, C. J., Nelson, R., Kyaw-Myint, T. O., Mackintosh, P., Williams, A. F (1974) Factors affecting the differing racial incidence of coeliac disease. In *Coeliac Disease* (ed. Hekkens, W., Th. J. M., and Peña, A. S.) Leiden: Stenfert Kroese. p. 330.

Marks, J., Shuster, S., and Watson, A. J. (1966) Small bowel changes in dermatitis herpetiformis. *Lancet*, ii, 1280.

Meeuwisse, G. W. (1970) Diagnostic creteria in coeliac disease. *Acta paediatrica Scandinavica*, 59, 461.

Mortimer, P. E., Stewart, J. S., Norman, A. P., and Booth, C. C. (1968) Follow-up of coeliac disease, *British Medical Journal*, 2, 7.

Nelson, R., McNeish, A. S., and Anderson, C. M. (1973) Coeliac disease in children of Asian immigrants. *Lancet*, i, 348.

Packer, S. M., Charlton, V., Keeling, J. W., Risdon, A., Ogilivie, D., Rowlatt, R. J., Larcher, V. F., and Harries, J. T. (1978) Gluten challenge in treated coeliac disease. *Archives of Disease in Childhood*.

Paulley, J. W. (1954) Observations on the aetiology of idiopathic steatorrhoea. *British Medical Journal*, ii, 1318.

Phelan, J. J., McCarthy, C. F., Stevens, F. M., McNicholl, B., and Fottrell, P. F. (1974) The nature of gliadin toxicity in coeliac disease: a new concept. Coeliac Disease. *Proceedings of the Second International Coeliac Symposium.* (ed. Hekkens, W. Th. J. M., and Peña, A. S.) Leiden: Stenfert Kroese. p. 60.

Phelan, J. J., Stevens, F. M., McNicholl, B. Comerford, F. R., Fottrell, P. F., and McCarthy, C. F. (1978) The detoxification of gliadin by the enzyme clearage of a side-chain substituent. In *Perspectives in Coeliac Disease*. Third International Coeliac Symposium. (ed. McNicholl, B., McCarthy, C. F., and Fottrell, P. F.) Lancaster: MTP Press, p. 33.

Polak, J. M., Pearse, A. G. E., van Norden, S., Bloom, S. R., and Rossiter, M. A. (1973) Secretin cells in coeliac disease. *Gut*, 14, 870.

Prader, A., Tanner, J. M., and von Harnack, G. A. (1963) Catch-up growth following illness or starvation. *Journal of Pediatrics*, 62, 646.

Prader, A., Shmerling, D. H., Zachmann, M., and Biro, Z. (1969) Catch-up growth in coeliac disease, *Acta paediatrica Scandinavica*, 58, 311.

Rolles, C. J., Kendall, M. J., Nutter, S., and Anderson, C. M. (1973) One hour blood-xylose screening-test for coeliac disease. *Lancet*, ii, 1043.

Rossipal, E. (1978) Investigation of the cellular immunity in infants and children with coeliac disease using the DNCB test. In *Perspectives in Coeliac Disease*. (ed. McNicholl, B., McCarthy, C. F., and Fottrell, P. E.) Lancaster: MTP Press Limited, p. 377.

Rubin, C. E., Brandborg, L. L., Phelps, P. C., and Taylor, H. C. (1960) Studies of coeliac sprue. *Gastroenterology*, 38, 28.

Rubin, W., Fauci, A. S., Sleisenger, M. H., and Jeffries, G. H. (1965) Immunofluorescent studies in adult celiac disease. *Journal of Clinical Investigation*, 44, 475.

Sakula, J. and Shiner, M. (1957) Coeliac disease with atrophy of the small intestine mucosa. *Lancet*, **ii**, 876.

Savilahti, E. (1972) Intestinal immunoglobulins in children with coeliac disease. *Gut*, **13**, 958.

Schmitz, J., Jos, J., and Rey, J. (1978) Transient mucosal atrophy in confirmed coeliac disease. In *Perspectives in Coeliac Disease*. (ed. McNicholl, B., McCarthy, C. F., and Fottrell, P. F.) Lancaster: MTP Press Limited, p. 259.

Seah, P. P., Fry, L., Holborow, E. J., Rossiter, M. A., Doe, W. F., Magalhaes, A. F., and Hoffbrand, A. V. (1973) Antireticulin antibody: incidence and diagnostic significance. *Gut*, **4**, 311.

Segall, E. (1974) Oats and coeliac disease. *British Medical Journal*, **4**, 589.

Shiner, M. and Ballard, J. (1972) Antigen-antibody reactions in the jejunal mucosa in childhood coeliac disease after gluten challenge. *Lancet*, **i**, 1202.

Shmerling, D. H. and Shiner, M. (1970) The response of the intestinal mucosa to the intraduodenal instillation of gluten in patients with coeliac disease. In *Coeliac Disease* (ed. Booth, C. C. and Dowling, R. H.) Edinburgh and London: Churchill Livingstone. p. 64.

Shmerling, D. H. (1969) An analysis of controlled relapses in gluten-induced coeliac disease. *Acta Paediatrica Scandinavica*, **58**, 311.

Shmerling, D. H. (1978) Questionaire of the European Society for Paediatric Gastroenterology and Nutrition on Coeliac Disease. In *Perspectives in Coeliac Disease* (ed. McNicholl, B., McCarthy, C. F., and Fottrell, P. F.) Lancaster: MTP Press Limited. p. 245.

Sinaasappel, M. and Hekkens, W. Th. J. M. (1978) Alterations of the jejunal mucosa after short term instillation of gliadin fractions in children with coeliac disease. In *Perspectives in Coeliac Disease* (ed. McNicholl, B., McCarthy, C. F., and Fottrell, P. F.) Lancaster: MTP Press Limited, p. 257.

Sladen, G. E. and Kumar, P. J. (1973) Is the xylose test still a worthwhile investigation? *British Medical Journal*, **3**, 223.

Stokes, P. L., Asquith, P., Holmes, G. K. T., Mackintosh, P., and Cooke, W. T. (1972) Histocompatibility antigens associated with adult coeliac disease. *Lancet*, **ii**, 162.

Strober, W. (1976) Gluten-sensitive enteropathy. In *Clinics in Gastroenterology*. (ed. Wright, R.) Eastbourne: W. B. Saunders Company Ltd.

Suliman, G. I. (1978) Coeliac disease in Sudanese children, *Gut*, **19**, 121

Townley, R. R. W. and Anderson, C. M. (1967) Coeliac disease: A review. *Ergebnisse der inneren Medizin und Kinderheilkunde*, **26**, 1.

Trier, J. S. (1974) Organ culture of intestinal mucosa. In *Coeliac Disease* (ed. Hekkens, W. Th. J. M. and Peña, A. S.) Leyden: Stenfert Kroese.

Tripp, J. H., Manning, J. A., Muller, D. P. R., Walker-Smith, J. A., O'Donoghue, D. P., Kumar, P. J., and Harries, J. T. (1978) Mucosal adenylate cyclase and sodium-potassium stimulated adenosine triphosphatase in jejunal biopsies of adults and children with coeliac disease. Gastroenterology and Nutrition on Coeliac Disease. *Perspectives in Coeliac Disease* (ed. McNicholl, B., McCarthy, C. F., and Fottrell, P. F.) Lancaster: MTP Press Limited, p. 245.

Vanderschueren-Lodeweyckx, M., Wolter, R., Molla, A., Eggermont, E., and Eeckels, R. (1973) Plasma growth hormone in coeliac disease. *Helvetica paediatrica acta,* **28,** 349.

Walker-Smith, J. A. (1972) Transient gluten intolerance. *Archives of Disease in Childhood,* **47,** 155.

Walker-Smith, J. A. (1973) Discordance for childhood coeliac disease in monozygotic twins. *Gut,* **14,** 374.

Walker-Smith, J. A. and Grigor, W. A. (1969) Coeliac disease in a diabetic child. *Lancet,* **i,** 1021.

Walker-Smith, J. A. (1977) A fresh look at coeliac disease. *Newer Horizons in Tropical Pediatrics* (ed. S. Gunte) Delhi: Jaypee Brothers.

Walker-Smith, J. A. and Kilby, A. (1977) Small intestinal enteropathies. In *Essentials of Paeditric Gastroenterology.* Edinburgh and London: Churchill Livingstone.

Walker-Smith, J. A., Kilby, A., and France, N. E. (1978) Reinvestigation of children previously diagnosed as coeliac disease. In *Perspectives in Coeliac disease.* (ed. McNicholl, B., McCarthy, C. F., and Fottrell, P. F.) Lancaster: MTP Press Limited, p. 267.

Wall, A. J., Douglas, A. P., Booth, C. C., and Pearse, A. G. E. (1970) Response of the jejunal mucosa in adult coeliac disease to oral prednisolone, *Gut,* **11,** 7.

Weiser, M. M. and Douglas, A. P. (1976) An alternative mechanism for gluten toxicity in coeliac disease. *Lancet,* **i,** 567.

Weiser, M. M. and Douglas, A. P. (1978) Cell surface glycosyl-transferases of the enterocyte in coeliac disease. In *Perspectives in Coeliac Disease.* Third International Coeliac Symposium. (ed. McCarthy and McNicholl) Lancaster: MTP Press Limited. p. 451

Wright, N. A. and Watson, A. J. (1974) The morphogenesis of the flalavillous mucosa of coeliac disease. In *Coeliac Disease.* (ed. Hekkens, W. Th. J. M. and Peña, A. S.) Leiden: Stenfert Kroese. p. 151.

Young, W. and Pringle, E. M. (1971) 110 children with coeliac disease. *Archives of Disease in Childhood,* **46,** 421.

CHAPTER 5

Ament, M. E. and Rubin, C. E. (1972) Soy protein—another cause of the flat intestinal lesion. *Gastroenterology,* **62,** 227.

Anderson, A. F. and Schloss, O. M. (1923) Allergy to cow's milk in infants with nutritional disorders. *American Journal of Diseases of Children,* **26,** 451.

Anderson, K. J., McLaughlan, P., Devey, M. E., and R. R. A. Coombs (1979) Anaphylactic sensitivity of guinea-pigs drinking different preparations of cow's milk and infant formulae. Clinical experimental immunology. In press.

Barnes, G. L. and Townley, R. R. W. (1973) Duodenal mucosal damage in 31 infants with gastroenteritis. *Archives of Disease in Childhood*, **48**, 343.

Bleumink, E. (1974) Allergies and toxic protein in food. In *Coeliac Disease* (ed. Hekkens, W. Th. J. M. and Peña, A. S.). Leyden: Stenfert Kroese. p. 46.

Buisseret. (1978) Common manifestations of cow's milk allergy in children. *Lancet*, **i**, 301.

Chandra, R. K. (1976) Immunological consequences of malnutrition including fetal growth retardation, in Food and Immunology. *Swedish Nutrition Foundation Symposium XIII*. Stockholm: Almqvist and Eiksell International.

Coombs, R. R. A., Devey, Madeleine E., and Anderson, Karen J. (1979) 'Refractoriness to anaphylactic shock after continuous feeding of cows' milk to guinea-pigs'. *Clinical Experimental Immunology*. In press.

Delire, M., Cambiaso, C. L., and Masson, P. L. (1978) Circulatory immune complexes in infants fed on cow's milk. *Nature*, **272**, 632.

de Peyer, E. and Walker-Smith, J. A. (1977) Cow's milk intolerance presenting as necrotizing enterocolitis. *Helvetica Paediatrica Acta*, **32**, 509.

Devey, Madeleine E., Anderson, Karen J., Coombs, R. R. A., Henschel, M. J., and Coates, Marie E. (1976) 'The modified anaphylaxis hypothesis for cot death: Anaphylactic sensitization in guinea-pigs fed cow's milk'. *Clinical Experimental Immunology*, **26**, 542.

Dicke, W. K. (1952) De subacute, chronische en recidiverende darmstoornis van de kleuter. *Nederlandsch tijdschrift voor geneeskunde*, **96**, 860.

Egan-Mitchell, B., Fottrell, P. F., and McNicholl, B. (1978) Prolonged gluten tolerance in treated coeliac disease. Perspectives in Coeliac Disease. (ed. McNicholl, B., McCarthy, C. F., and Fottrell, P. F.) Lancaster: MTP Press Limited, p. 25.

Ferguson, A. (1976) Coeliac disease and gastrointestinal food allergy. In *Immunological Aspects of the Liver and Gastrointestinal Tract*. Lancaster: MTP Press.

Finkelstein, H. (1905) Kuhmilch als Ursach Akuter Ernahrungstoerungen bei Saeuglingen. *Montasschrift für Kinderheilkunde*, **4**, 65.

Fontaine, J. L., and Navarro, J. (1975) Small intestinal biopsy in cow's milk protein allergy in infancy, *Archives of Disease in Childhood*, **50**, 357.

Frier, S., Kletter, B., Gery, I., Lebenthal, E., and Geifman, M. (1969) Intolerance of milk protein, *Journal of Pediatrics*, **75**, 623.

Gell, P. G. H. and Coombs, R. R. A. (1968) Classification of allergic reactions responsible for hypersensitivity and disease. In *Clinical Aspects of Immunology*. (ed. Gell, P. G. H. and Coombs, R. R. A.) Blackwell: Oxford and Edinburgh, p. 575.

Gerrard, J. W., Lubos, M. C., Hardy, L. W., Holmind, B. A. and Webster, D. (1967) Milk allergy: clinical picture and familial incidence. *Canadian Medical Associations Journal*, **97**, 780.

Glaser, J. and Johnstone, D. C. (1953) Prophylaxis of allergy in the newborn. *Journal of the American Medical Association*, **153**, 620.

Goldman, A. S., Anderson, D. W., Sellers, W., Saperstein, S., Kniker, W. T., and Halpern, S. R. (1963) Milk allergy. *Pediatrics*, **32**, 425.

Gruskay, F. L. and Cook, R. E. (1955) The gastrointestinal absorption of unaltered protein in normal infants and in infants recovering from diarrhoea. *Pediatrics*, **16**, 763.

Gryboski, J. D. (1967) Gastrointestinal milk allergy in infants. *Pediatrics*, **40**, 354.

Halpern, S. R. (1963) Milk allergy. *Pediatrics*, **32**, 425.

Harrison, B. M., Kilby, A., Walker-Smith, J. A., France, N. E., and Wood, C. B. S. (1976) Cow's milk protein intolerance: a possible association with gastroenteritis. lactose intolerance and IgA deficiency. *British Medical Journal*, **1**, 1501.

Harrison, M. (1974) Sugar malabsorption in cow's milk protein intolerance. *Lancet*, **i**, 360.

Hill, L. W. and Stuart, H. C. (1929) A soy-bean food preparation for feeding infants with milk allergy. *Journal of the American Medical Association*, **93**, 986.

Iyngkaran, N., Robinson, N. J., Sumithran, E., Lam, S. K., Putchucheary, S. D. and Yadav, M. (1978) Cow's milk protein-sensitive enteropathy. An important factor in prolonging diarrhoea in acute infective enteritis in early infancy. *Archives of Disease in Childhood*, **53**, 150.

Katz, A. J., Goldman, H. and Grand, R. J. (1977) Gastric mucosal biopsy in eosinophilic (allergic) gastroenteritis. *Gastroenterology*, **73**, 705.

Kilby, A., Walker-Smith, J. A. and Wood, C. B. S. (1976) Small intestinal mucosa in cow's milk allergy. *Lancet*, **i**, 53.

Koivikko, A. (1973) IgA deficiency and infantile atopy. *Lancet*, **ii**, 668.

Kuitunen, P., Rapola, J., Savilahti, E. and Visakorpi, J. K. V. (1973) Response of the jejunal mucosa to cow's milk in the malabsorption syndrome with cow's milk intolerance. *Acta paediatrica Scandinavica*, **62**, 585.

Kuitunen, P., Visakorpi, J. K., Savilahti, E., and Pelkonen, P. (1975) Malabsorption syndrome with cow's milk intolerance clinical findings and course in 54 cases. *Archives of Disease in Childhood*, **50**, 351.

Kuitunen, P., Pelkonnen, P., Perkkio, M., Savilahtie, E. and Visakorpi, J. K. (1977) Transient Gluten Intolerance. *Acta Paediatrica Belgica*, **30**, 250.

Lippard, V. W., Schloss, O. M. and Johnson, P. A. (1936) Immune reactions induced in infants by intestinal absorption of incompletely digested cow's milk proteins. *American Journal of Disease in Childhood*, **51**, 562.

Liu, Hsi-Yen, Taso, M. U. and Moore, B. (1967) Bovine milk protein induced malabsorption of lactose and fat in infants. *Gastroenterology*, **62**, 227.

Matthews, T. S. and Soothill, J. F. (1970) Complement activation after milk feeding in children with cow's milk allergy. *Lancet*, **ii**, 893.

McNeish A. S. (1974) The role of lactose in cow's milk intolerance. *Acta paediatrica Scandinavica*. **63**, 652.

McNeish, A. S., Rolles, C. J., and Arthur, L. J. H. (1976) Criteria for Diagnosis of

Temporary Gluten Intolerance. Archives of Disease in Childhood. **51**, 275.

McNicholl, B., Egan-Mitchell, B., and Fottrell, P. F. (1974) Varying Gluten Susceptibility in Coeliac Disease. Coeliac Disease—Proceedings of the Second International Coeliac Symposium, (ed. Hekkens, W. Th. J. M. and Peña, A. S.) Leiden: Stenfert Kroese, p. 413.

Meeuwisse, G. (1970) Diagnostic criteria in coeliac disease. *Acta paediatrica Scandinavica*, **59**, 461.

Mendoza, J., Meyers, J., Snyder, R. (1970) Soy-bean sensitivity: Case report. *Pediatrics*, **46**, 774.

Montreuil, J. (1971) *Annales de la nutrition et de l'alimentation*, **25**, A1–37.

Nusslé, D., Bozic, C., Cox, J., Deleze, G., Roulet, M., Fete, R., and Megevana, A. (1978). Non-Coeliac Gluten Intolerance in Infancy. Perspectives in Coeliac Disease, (ed. McNicholl, B., McCarthy, C. F. and Fottrell, P. F.) Lancaster: MTP Press, Limited, p. 277.

Parish, W. E., Barrett, A. M., Coombs, R. R. A., Gunther, Mavis and Camps, F. E. (1960) 'Hypersensitivity to milk and sudden death in infancy', *Lancet*, **ii**, 1106.

Peltonen, M. E., Kassanen, A. and Peltonen, T. E. (1955) *Annales paediatriae Fenniae*, **1**, 119.

Schloss. O. M. A. (1911) A case of allergy to common foods. *American Journal of Diseases of Children*, **3**, 341.

Schmitz, J., Jos, J., and Rey, J. (1978) Transient mucosal atrophy in confirmed coeliac disease. *Perspectives in Coeliac Disease*. (ed. McCarthy and McNicholl) Proceedings of Third International Coeliac Symposium. Galway. Lancaster: MTP Press. p. 259.

Shiner, M., Ballard, J., and Smith, M. E. (1975). The small intestinal mucosa in cow's milk allergy. *Lancet*, **i**, 136.

Shmerling, D. H. (1978), Questionnaire of the European Society for Paediatric Gastroenterology and Nutrition on Coeliac Disease. Perspectives in Coeliac Disease. (ed. McNicholl, B., McCarthy, C. F., and Fottrell, P. F.) Lancaster: MTP Press Limited, p. 245.

Silverberg, M. and Davidson, M. (1974) Milk (Bovine) protein gastrointestinal hypersensitivity associated with cosinophilic gastroenteropathy in children. *Acta paediatrica Scandinavica*. **63**, 654.

Silverman, A., Roy, C. C., and Cozzeto, F. J. (1971) In *Paediatric Clinical Gastroenterology*, p. 552, St. Louis: The C. V. Mosby Company.

Swarbrick, E. T., Stokes, L. K. and Soothill, J. (1979) The absorption of antigens after immunisation and the simultaneous induction of specific tolerance. *Gut*, in press.

Taylor, B., Norman, A. P., Orgel, H. A., Stokes, C. R., Turner, M. W. and Soothill, J. (1973) Transient IgA deficiency and pathogenesis of infantile atopy. *Lancet*, **ii**, 111.

Visakorpi, J. K. (1970) An international enquiry concerning the diagnostic criteria of coeliac disease. *Acta paediatrica Scandinavica*, **59**, 463.

Visakorpi, J. K. and Immonen, P. (1967) Intolerance to cow's milk and wheat gluten in the primary malabsorption syndrome in infancy. *Acta paediatrica Scandinavica*, **56,** 49.

Waldmann, T. A., Wochner, R. D., and Lasterl (1967) Allergic gastroenteropathy. A cause of excessive gastrointestinal protein loss. *New England Journal of Medicine*, **276,** 761.

Walker-Smith, J. A. (1970) Transient gluten intolerance. *Archives of Disease in Childhood*, **45,** 523.

Walker-Smith, J. A., Kilby, A., and France, N. E. (1978) Reinvestigation of Children Previously Diagnosed as Coeliac Disease. Perspectives in Coeliac Disease. (ed. McNicholl, B., McCarthy, C. F., and Fottrell, P. F.) Lancaster: MTP Press Limited, p. 267.

Walker-Smith, J. A. and Reye, R. D. K. (1971) Small intestinal morphology in aboriginal children. *Australia and New Zealand Journal of Medicine*, **4,** 477.

CHAPTER 6

Araya, M., Silink, S. J., Nobile, S. and Walker-Smith, J. A. (1975). Blood vitamin levels in children with gastroenteritis. Australian and New Zealand Journal of Medicine, **5,** 239.

Avigad, S., Manuel, P., Bampoe, V., Walker-Smith, J. A. and Shiner M. (1978). Small intestinal mucosal antibodies against antigens of non-pathogenic luminal or mucosal bacteria in young children with and without diarrhoea. *Lancet*, **i,** 1130.

Banatvala, J. E. (1975) Acute diarrhoea in childhood. *Ciba Foundation Symposium*, **42,** 232.

Barnes, G. L. and Townley, R. R. W. (1973) Duodenal mucosal damage in 31 infants with gastroenteritis. *Archives of Disease in Childhood*, **48,** 343.

Barnes, G. L. (1973) Studies in infantile gastroenteritis, M.D. thesis Department of Paediatrics, University of Otago, Dunedin, New Zealand.

Biddulph, J. and Pangkatana, P. (1971) Weanling diarrhoea. Papua and New Guinea *Medical Journal*, **14,** 7.

Bishop, R. F., Davidson, G. P., Holmes, I. H., and Ruck, B. J. (1973) Virus particles in epithelial cells of duodenal mucosa from children with acute non-bacterial gastroenteritis. *Lancet*, **ii,** 1281.

Bishop, R. F., Davidson, G. P., Nolmes, I. H., and Ruck, B. J. (1974) Detection of a new virus by electron microscopy of faecal extracts from children with acute gastroenteritis. *Lancet*, **i,** 149.

Bishop, R. F., Cameron, D. J. S., Barnes, G. P., Holmes, I. H., and Ruck, B. J. (1976) The aetiology of diarrhoea in newborn infants. *Ciba Foundation Symposium* 42 (new series) Acute diarrhoea in childhood. Elsevier Excerpta Medica North-Holland.

Blacklow, N. R., Dolin, R., Fedson, D. S., Dupont, H., Northrup, R. S., Hornick, R. B. and Chanock, R. M. (1972) Acute infectious non-bacterial gastroenteritis:

aetiology and pathogenesis. *Annals of Internal Medicine*, **76**, 993.

Bortulussi, R., Szymanski, M., Hamilton, R. (1974) Studies on the etiology of acute infantile diarrhoea. *Pediatric Research*, **8**, 379.

Bray, J. (1945) Isolation of antigenically homogenous strains of Bacterium coli neapolitum from summer diarrhoea of infants. *Journal of Pathology and Bacteriology*, **57**, 239.

Braun, O. H. (1974) Bray's discovery of pathogenic *E. coli* as a cause of infantile gastroenteritis. *Archives of Disease in Childhood*, **49**, 668.

Bullen, C. L. and Willis, A. T. (1971) Resistance of the breast fed infant to gastroenteritis. *British Medical Journal*, **3**, 338.

Burke, V., Kerry, K. R. and Anderson, C. M. (1965) The relationship of dietary lactose to refractory diarrhoea in infancy. *Australian Paediatric Journal*, **1**, 147.

Carr, M. E., Donald, G., McKendrick, W., and Spyridakis, T. (1976) The clinical features of infantile gastroenteritis due to rotavirus. *Scandinavica Journal of Infectious Disease*, 8, 241.

Caul, E. O., Paver, W. K., and Clarke, S. K. R. (1975) Coronavirus particles in faeces from patients with gastroenteritis. *Lancet*, **i**, 1192.

Chantemesse, A. and Widal, F. (1888) Sur les microbes de la dysenteric epidemique. *Bulletin de l'Academic de médicine* (Paris), **19**, 522.

Chatterjee, A., Mahalanabis, D., Jalan, K. N., Maitra, T. K., Agarwal, S. K. Bagchi, D. K., and Indra, S. (1977) Evaluation of a sucrose/electrolyte solution for oral rehydration in acute infantile diarrhoea. *Lancet*, **i**, 1333.

Chrystie, I. L., Totterdell, B., Baker, M. J., Scopes, J. W., and Banatvala, J. E. (1975) Rotavirus infections in a maternity unit. *Lancet*, **ii**, 79.

Colle, E., Aroub, E., and Raile, R., (1958) Hypertonic dehydration (hypernatraemia): the role of feedings high in solute *Pediatrics*, **2**, 5.

Creamer, B. and Leppard, P. (1965) Post-mortem examination of a small intestine in the coeliac syndrome. *Gut*. **6**, 466.

Curry, J. (1976) Infecting dose of salmonella. *Lancet* i, 1296.

Darrow, D. C., Pratt, E. L., Flett, J., Gawble, A. H. and Wiese, H. F. (1949) Disturbances of water and electrolytes in infantile diarrhoea. *Pediatrics*, **5**, 129.

Davidson, G. P., Bishop, R. F., Townley, R. R. W., Holmes, I. H., and Ruck, B. J. (1975a) Importance of a new virus in acute sporadic enteritis in children. *Lancet*, **i**, 242.

Davidson, G. P., Goller, I., Bishop, R. F., Townley, R. R. W., Holmes, I. H., and Ruck, B. J. (1975a) Immunofluorescence in duodenal mucosa of children with acute enteritis due to a new virus. Journal of Clinical Pathology, 28, 263.

Davies, D. P., Ansari, B. M., Mandal, B. K. (1977) Hypernatraemia and gastroenteritis, *Lancet*, **i**, 252.

Dixon, J. (1965) Effect of antibiotic treatment on the duration of excretion of *Salmonella typhimurium* by children. *British Medical Journal*, **2**, 1343.

Dorman, D. (1968) Personal communication.

Dorman, D. (1972) Personal communication.

Dupont, H. L., Formal, S. B., Hornick, R. B., Snyder, M. J., Libonati, J. P., Sheahan, D. P., Labrec, E. H., and Kalpas, J. P. (1971) Pathogenesis of *Escherichia coli* diarrhoea. *New England Journal of Medicine,* **285,** 1.

Feldman, R. A., Kamath, K. R., Sundar Rao, P. S. S., and Webb, J. K. G. (1969) Infection and disease in a group of south Indian families. *American Journal of Epidemiology,* **289,** 364.

Feldman, R. A., Bhat, P., and Kamath, K. R. (1970) Infection and disease in a group of south Indian families. IV. Bacteriologic methods and a report of the frequency of enteric bacterial infections in pre-school children. *American Journal of Epidemiology,* **92,** 367.

Fenner, F. (1971) Infectious disease and social change. *Medical Journal of Australia,* **1,** 1043.

Ferguson, A., McClure, J. P., and Townley, R. R. W. (1976) Intraepithelial lymphocyte counts in small intestinal biopsies from children with diarrhoea. *Acta Paediatrica Scandinavica,* **65,** 541.

Ferguson, A. and Snodgrass, D. P. (1978) Intestinal Architecture and epithelial cell kinetics during and after experimental rotavirus infection in lambs. *Acta Paediatrica Belgica.* **31,** 109.

Field, M. (1971) Intestinal secretion: effect of cyclic AMP and its role in cholera. *New England Journal of Medicine,* **2854,** 1137.

Field, M. (1978) Effect of enterotoxins. Joint meeting of North American Society for Pediatric Gastroenterology and European Society for Paediatric Gastroenterology and Nutrition.

Finberg, L. F. (1970) The management of the critically ill child with dehydration secondary to diarrhoea. *Pediatrics,* **45,** 1029.

Finberg, L. F. (1973) Hypernatraemic (hypertonic) dehydration in infants. *New England Journal of Medicine,* **289,** 196.

Flewett, T. H., Bryden, A. S., and Davies, H. (1973) Virus particles in gastroenteritis, *Lancet,* **ii,** 1497.

Flewett, T. H. (1976a) Diagnosis of enteritis virus. *Proceedings of the Royal Society of Medicine,* **69,** 693.

Flewett, T. H. (1976b) Implications of recent virological researches. *Ciba Foundation Symposium* 42 (new series) Acute diarrhoea in childhood. Elsevier Excerpta Medica North-Holland.

Fonteyne, J., Zusis, G., Lambert, J. P. (1978) Recurrent rotavirus gastroenteritis, *Lancet,* **i,** 983.

Formal, S. B., Gemski, P., Gianella, R. A., and Takeuchi, A. (1976) Studies on the pathogenesis of enteric infections caused by invasive bacteria. Acute diarrhoea in childhood. *Ciba Foundation Symposium* 42, new series. Elsevier, Excerpta Medica. North Holland P 27.

French, T., Falhalla, L., Bird, R., Manuel, P. D., Cutting, W. A. M., and Walker-Smith, J. A. (1969) Rota virus in Childhood: Further clinical observations. In press.

Gamble, J. L. (1953) Early history of fluid replacement therapy. *Pediatrics*, **11**, 554.

Garrow, J. S., Smith, R., and Ward, E. E. (1968) In *Electrolyte metabolism in severe infantile malnutrition*. London: Pergamon Press.

Gianella, R. A., Gots, R. E., Charnex, A. N., Greenough, B., and Formal, S. B. (1975) Pathogenesis of salmonella-mediated fluid secretion. Alteration of adenylate cyclase and inhibition by indomethacin. *Gastroenterology*, **69**, 1238.

Giles, C., Sangster, G., and Smith, J. (1949) Epidemic gastroenteritis in infants in Aberdeen during 1947. *Archives of Disease in Childhood*, **24**, 45.

Gilles, R. G., Monif, M. D., and Hood, C. I. (1970) Ileocolitis associated with measles (Rubella). *American Journal of Diseases of Children*, **120**, 245.

Gould, S. (1977) MD Thesis.

Gracey, M. (1973) Enteric Disease in Young Australian Aborigines. *Australian and New Zealand Journal of Medicine*, **3**, 576.

Gribbin, M., Walker-Smith, J. A., and Wood, C. B. S. (1976) A twelve month prospective survey of admissions to the gastroenteritis unit of a children's hospital. *Acta Paediatrica Belgica*, **29**, 69.

Gribbin, M., Walker-Smith, J. A., and Wood. C. R. S. (1973) Delayed recovery following acute gastroenteritis, *Acta Paediatrica Belgica*, **29**, 167.

Gribbin, M., Walker-Smith, J. A., and Wood, C. B. S. (1976) Gastroenteritis and its sequelae: A prospective review of experience in a children's hospital. *Acta Paediatrica Scandinavica*, **64**, 145.

Hamilton, J. R., Gall, D. G., Butler, D. G., and Middleton, P. J. (1976) Viral gastroenteritis: recent progress, remaining problems. Ciba Foundation Symposium 42, (new series). Acute diarrhoea in childhood. Elsevier Excerpta Medica North-Holland.

Hansen, J. D. L. (1968) Features and treatment of kwashiorkor at the Cape. *Calorie deficiencies and protein deficiencies. Proceedings of a colloquim*, p. 33. London: Churchill.

Harrison, B. M., Kilby, A., Walker-Smith, J. A., France, N. E., and Wood, C. B. S. (1976) Cow's milk protein intolerance: A possible association with gastroenteritis, lactose intolerance and IgA deficiency. *British Medical Journal*, **1**, 1501.

Hirschorn, N., McCarthy, B. J., Ranney, B., Hirschorn, M. A., Woodward, S. T., Lacapa, A., Cash, R. A., and Woodward, W. E. (1973) *Ad libitum* oral glucose-electrolyte therapy for acute diarrhoea in Apache children. *Journal of Pediatrics*, **83**, 562.

Holmes, I. H., Ruck, B. J., and Bishop, R. F. (1975) Infantile enteritis viruses: morphogenesis and morphology. *Journal of Virology* **16**, 937.

Holmes, I. H., Rodger, S. M., Schnagl, R. P., Ruck, B. J., Gust, I. D., Bishop, R. F., and Barnes, G. L. (1976) Is lactase the receptor and uncoating enzyme for infantile enteritis (rota) viruses? *Lancet*, i, 1387.

Hutchins, P., Matthews, T. H. J., Manly, J. A. E. Lawrie, B., and Walker-Smith, J. A. (1978) Comparison of oral sucrose and glucose electrolyte solutions in the out-patient management of acute gastroenteritis in infancy. *Lancet*, i, 1211.

Ironside, A. G. (1973) Gastroenteritis in infancy. *British Medical Journal*, 1, 284.

Ironside, A. G., Tuxford, A. F. and Heyworth, B. (1970) A survey of infantile gastroenteritis. *Biritsh Medical Journal*, 3, 20.

Jelliffe, D. B. and Jelliffe, E. F. (1978) The weanling's dilemma, *Lancet* 1, 611.

Kapikian, A. Z., Cline, W. L., and Mebus, C. A. (1975) New complement-fixation test for the human reovirus-like agent of infantile gastroenteritis. *Lancet*, i, 1956.

Kilby, A., Walker-Smith, J. A., and Wood, C. B. S. (1976) Studies on the Immunoglobulin containing Cells and Intraepithelial Lymphocytes in the Small Intestinal Mucosa of Infants with the Post-gastroenteritis Syndrome. *Australian Paediatric Journal*, 12, 241.

Kingston, M. E. (1973) Biochemical disturbances in breast fed infants with gastroenteritis and dehydration. *Journal of Pediatrics*, 82, 1073.

Kretchmer, N. (1969) Child health in the developing world. *Paediatrics*, 43, 4.

Kunin, A. S., Surawicz, B., and Sims, E. A. H. (1962) Decrease in serum potassium concentration and the appearance of arrhythmias during infusion of potassium with glucose in potassium depleted patients. *New England Journal of Medicine*, 266, 288.

Kurtz, J. B., Lee, T. W., and Pickering, D. (1977) Astrovirus associated gastroenteritis in a children's ward. *Journal of clinical Pathology*, 30, 948.

Levine, M. M., Bergquist, E. G., Nalin, D. R., Waterman, D. H., Horwick, R. B., Young, C. R., and Sotman, S. (1978) Escherichia coli strains that cause diarrhoea but do not produce heat-labile or heat-stabile enterotoxins and are non-invasive. *Lancet*, i, 1119.

Madeley, C. R. and Cosgrove, B. P. (1975) 28 nm particles in faeces in infantile gastroenteritis. *Lancet*, ii, 451.

Mayrhofer, G. (1977) Sites of synthesis and localization of IgE in rats infested with Nippostrongylus brasiliensis. *Immunology of the Gut. Ciba Foundation Symposium* 46. Elsevier. Excerpta Medica North Holland, p. 155.

Lambeth, L. and Mitchell, J. H. (1975) Transmission of human rotavirus gastroenteritis to a monkey. *Australian paediatric journal* 11, 127.

Latta, T. (1831–32) View of rationale and results of treatment of cholera by aqueous and saline injections, *Lancet*, 2, 274.

Lucas, D. R., Bird, R., Cutting, W. and Walker-Smith, J. A. (1979) Temporary monosaccharide intolerance complicating winter gastroenteritis in infancy. In preparation.

Madeley, C. R., Cosgrove, B. P., Bell, E. J., and Fallow, R. J. (1975) Stool viruses in babies in Glasgow. *Journal of Hygiene* 78, 261.

Maiya, P. P., Pereira, S. M., Mathan, M., Bhat, P., Albert, M. J., and Baker, S. J. (1976) Acute gastroenteritis in infancy and early childhood in Southern India. *Archives of Disease in Childhood*, **52**, 482.

Maki, M., Gronroos, P., Wesikari, T., and Visakorpi, J. K. (1978) The Invasiveness of Yersinia enterocolitica in acute diarrhoea. *Acta Paediatrica Belgica*, **31**, 108.

Manuel, P. (1978) Unpublished data.

Marshall, W. and Walker-Smith, J. A. (1977). Unpublished observations.

Matthews, T. H. J., Nair, C. D. G., Lawrence, M. K., Tyrrell, D. J. A. (1976) Antiviral activity in milk of possible clinical importance. *Lancet*, **ii**, 1387.

Mavromichalis, J., Evans, N., McNeish, A. S., Bryden, A. S., Davies, H. A., and Flewett, T. H., (1977) Intestinal damage in rotavirus and adenovirus gastroenteritis assessed of D-xylose malabsorption. *Archives of Disease in Childhood*, **52**, 549.

McClelland, D. B. L. and Gilmour, H. (1976) In *Immunology of the Gut. Ciba Foundation Symposium* 46 (new series). Elsevier Excerpta Medica North-Holland Amsterdam, p. 362.

McNeish, A. S., Fleming, J., Turner, P., and Evans, N. (1975) Mucosal adherence of human enteropathogenic Escherichia coli. *Lancet*, **ii**, 946.

Middleton, P. J., Szymanski, M. T. and Abbott, G. D., (1974) Orbivirus acute gastroenteritis in infancy. *Lancet*, **i**, 1241.

Middleton, P. J., Petric, M., and Hewitt, C. M. (1976) Counterimmunoelectroosmophoresis for the detection of infantile gastroenteritis virus (orbi-group) antigen and antibody. *Journal of Clinical Pathology*, **29**, 191.

Moenginah, P. A. Suprapto, Soenarto, J., Bachtin, M., Sutrisno, D. Sutaryo, and Rohde, J. E. (1975) *Lancet*, **ii**, 323.

Moffett, H. L., Shulenberger, H. K. and Burkholder, E. R. (1968) Epidemiology and aetiology of severe infantile diarrhoea. *Journal of Pediatrics*, **72**, 1.

Moore, E. E. M. (1974) *Shigella sonnei* septicaemia in a neonate. *British Medical Journal*, **1**, 22.

Murphy, A. M., Albery, M. and Crewe, E. (1977) Rotavirus infections of neonates. *Lancet*, **ii**, 1149.

Nelson, J. D. and Haltalin, R. C. (1971) Accuracy of diagnosis of bacterial diarrhoeal disease by clinical features. *Journal of Pediatrics*, **78**, 519.

Oates, R. K. (1973) Infant feeding practices. *British Medical Journal*, **2**, 762.

Paver, W. K., Caul, E. O., Ashley, C. R. and Clarke, S. K. R. (1973) A small virus in human faeces. *Lancet*, **i**, 237.

Portnoy, B. L., Dupont, H. L., Pruitt, D., Abdo, J. A. and Rodriguez, J. T. (1976) Drugs and diarrhoea. *JAMA* **16**, 844.

Rahilly, P. M., Shepherd, R., Challis, D., Walker-Smith, J. A. and Manly, J. (1976) Clinical comparison between glucose and sucrose additions to a basic electrolyte mixture in the outpatient management of acute gastroenteritis in children. *Archives of Disease in Childhood*, **51**, 152.

Reiman, H. A., Hodges, J. H. and Price, A. H. (1945) Epidemic diarrhoea, nausea and vomiting of unknown cause. *Journal of American Medical Association*, **127**, 1.

Robinson, J. E., Harvey, B. A. and Soothill, J. F. (1978) Phagocytosis and killing of bacteria and yeast by human milk cells after opsonization in aqueous phase of milk. *British Medical Journal*, **1**, 1443.

Rodriguez, W. J., Kim, H. W., Arrobio, J. O., Brandt, C. D., Chanock, R. M., Kapikian, A. Z., Wyatt, R. G. and Parrott, R. H. (1977) Clinical features of acute gastroenteritis associated with human reovirus-like agent in infants and young children. *Journal of Pediatrics*, **91**, 188.

Rohde, J. E. and Northrup, R. S. (1976) Taking science where the diarrhoea is, *Ciba Foundation Symposium* 42 (new series). *Acute Diarrhoea in Childhood*. Elsevier Excerpta Medica North-West Holland 358.

Ryder, R. W., Sack, D. A., Kapikian, A. Z., McLaughlin, J. C., Chakraborty, J. and Rahman, A. S. (1976) Enterotoxigenic escherichia coli and reovirus-like agent in rural Bangladesh. *Lancet*, **i**, 659.

Schreiber, D. S., Blacklow, N. R. and Trier, J. S. (1975) Lesion of the Proximal Small Intestine in Acute Infectious Nonbacterial Gastroenteritis. *New England Journal of Medicine*, **288**, 1318.

Schreiber, D. S., Trier, J. S., and Blacklow, N. R. (1977) Recent advances in viral gastroenteritis. *Gastroenterology*, **73**, 174.

Sheehy, T. W., Artenstein, M. S. and Green, R. W. (1964) Small intestinal mucosa in certain viral diseases. *Journal of the American Medical Association*, **190**, 1023.

Shepherd, R. W., Truslow, S., Walker-Smith, J. A., Bird, R., Cutting, W., Darnell, R. and Barker, C. M. (1975) Infantile gastroenteritis: a clinical study of reovirus-like agent infection. *Lancet*, **ii**, 1082.

Shiga, K. (1898) Ueber den Dysenteriebacillus (bacillus dysenteriae). *Zentralblatt für Bacteriologie*, **24**, 913.

Sinha, A. K., and Tyrell, D. A. (1973) Changes in the clinical pattern of gastrointestinal infection in North West London. *British Journal Clinical Practice*, **27**, 45.

Sivakumar, B. and Reddy, V. (1972) Absorption of labelled Vitamin A in children during infection. *British Journal of Nutrition*, **27**, 299.

Skirrow, M. B. (1977) Campylobacter enteritis: a "new" disease. *British Medical Journal*, **2**, 9.

Soothill, J. F. (1976) Breast-feeding: the immunological argument. *British Medical Journal*, **1**, 1466.

Spence, L., Fanvel, M., and Bouchard, S. (1975) Test for reovirus-like agent. *Lancet*, **ii**, 322.

Spencer, I. W. F. and Coster, M. E. E. (1969) The epidemiology of gastroenteritis in infancy. *South African Medical Journal*, **2**, 1391.

Stoliar, O. A., Pelley, R. P., Kaniecki-Green, E., Klaus, M. H. and Carpenter, C. C. J. (1976) Secretory IgA against enterotoxins in breast-milk. *Lancet*, **i**, 1258.

Sunshine, P. and Kretchmer, N. (1964) Studies of small intestine during development. *Pediatrics,* **34,** 38.

Suprapti, R., Nafsiah, T. and Rumini, M. (1968) Microbiological parasitic and epidemiological considerations on infantile diarrhoeal disease. *Paediatrica Indonesiana,* **8,** 133.

Suzuki, H. and Konno, T. (1975) Reovirus-like particles in jejunal mucosa of a Japanese infant with acute infectious nonbacterial gastroenteritis. *Tohoku journal of experimental medicine,* **115,** 199.

Tallett, S. MacKenzie, C., Middleton, P., Kerzner, B. and Hamilton, R. (1977) Clinical, laboratory and epidemiologic features of a viral gastroenteritis in infants and children. *Paediatrics,* **60,** 217.

Tan, G. S., Townley, R. R. W., Davidson, G. P., Bishop, F. R., Holmes, I. H., and Ruck, B. J. (1974) Virus in faecal extracts from children with gastroenteritis. *Lancet,* **i,** 110.

Tauwers. S., De. Boeck, M. and Butzler (1978) Compylobater enteritis in Brussells. *Lancet,* **i,** 604.

Torres-Pinedo, R. L., Lavastida, M., and Rivera, C. L. (1966) Studies on infant diarrhoea. A comparison of the effects of milk feeding and intravenous therapy upon the composition and values of the stool and urine. *Journal of Clinical Investigation* **45,** 469.

Tripp, J. H., Wilmers, M. J. and Wharton, B. A., (1977) Gastroenteritis: a continuing problem of child health in Britain. *Lancet,* **ii,** 233.

Vantrappen, G., Agg, H. O., Ponette, E., Geboes, K., and Bertrand, P. H. (1977) Yersinia enteritis and enterocolitis: gastroenterological aspect. *Gastroenterology,* **72,** 220.

Von Bonsdorff, C. H., Hovi, T., Makela, P., Hovi, L., Tevalvoto-Aarnio, M. (1976) Rotavirus associated with acute gastroenteritis in adults. *Lancet,* **ii,** 432.

Walker, A. C. and Marshall, W. (1977) Unpublished data.

Walker, A. C. (1971) The aboriginal child: gastroenteritis. *Ross Conference of Aboriginal Child,* Sydney.

Walker-Smith, J. A. (1972) Gastroenteritis. *Medical Journal of Australia,* **1,** 329.

Walker-Smith, J. A., Kamath, K. R. and Stobo, E. A. (1972) Some observations on monosaccharide malabsorption. *Australian Paediatric Journal,* **8,** 157.

Walker-Smith, J. A. (1975) Diseases of the small intestine in childhood. 1st Ed. Pitman Medical, Tunbridge Wells, p. 139.

Walker-Smith, J. A. (1978) Rotavirus Gastroenteritis. *Archives of Disease in Childhood,* **53,** 355.

Weil, M. H. (1969) A unified guide to parenteral fluid therapy. *Journal of Pediatrics,* **75,** 1.

Weil, M. H. (1973) Editorial Comment. *Journal of Pediatrics,* **82,** 1079.

Whaley, P. and Walker-Smith, J. A. (1977) Hypernatraemia and gastroenteritis.

Lancet, **i**, 51.

Wharton, B. A. (1968) Difficulties in the initial treatment of kwashiorkor. *Calorie deficiencies and protein deficiencies. Proceedings of a colloquium,* p. 147. London: Churchill.

Wheatley, D. (1968) Incidence and treatment of infantile gastroenteritis in general practice. *Archives of Disease in Childhood,* **43**, 53.

W.H.O. World Health Statistics Report 1974, **27**, 563.

Willians Smith, H. (1976) Neonatal Escherichia Coli Infections in Domestic Mammals: Transmissibility of Pathogenic Characteristics Acute Diarrhoea in Childhood. *Ciba Foundation Symposium* **42**, page 45.

Yolken, R. H., Kim, H. W., Clen, T., Wyatt, R. G., Kalica, A. R., Chanock, R. M. and Kapikian, A. Z. (1977) Enzyme-linked immunosorbent assay (ELISA) for detection of human reovirus-like agent of infantile gastroenteritis *Lancet,* **ii**, 263.

Zahorsky, J., Hyperemesis Hiemis, or the Winter Vomiting Disease. *Archives of Paediatrics (1929)* **64**, 391.

Zoppi, G., De Ganello, A., and Gaburro, D. (1977) Persistent Post-enteritis Diarrhoea. *European Journal of Paediatrics,* **126**, 225.

CHAPTER 7

Ament, M. E. and Perera, D. R. (1973) Sucrase-isomaltase deficiency—a frequently misdiagnosed disease. *Journal of Pediatrics,* **83**, 721.

Antonowicz, I., Lebenthal, E., and Shwachmann, H. (1978) Disaccharidase activities in small intestinal mucosa in patients with cystic fibrosis, *Journal of Pediatrics,* **92**, 214.

Arthur, A. B., Clayton, B., Cottom, D. G., Seakins, J. W. T., and Platt, J. W. (1966) Importance of disaccharide intolerance in the treatment of coeliac disease. *Lancet,* **i**, 172.

Auricchio, S., Rubino, A., and Murset, G. (1965) Intestinal glycosidase activities in the human embryo, foetus and newborn. *Pediatrics,* **35**, 944.

Auricchio, S., Dahlquist, A., Murset, G., and Parker, A. (1963) Isomaltose intolerance causing decreased ability to utilize dietary starch. *Journal of Pediatrics,* **62**, 165.

Bates, R., Walker-Smith, J. A., and Stobo, E. A. (1972) *Australian Paediatric Journal,* **8**, 217.

Boellner, S. W., Beard, A. G., and Panos, T. C. (1965) Impairment of intestinal hydrolysis of lactose in newborn infants. *Pediatrics,* **36**, 542.

Bolin, T. D., Crane, G. G., and Davis, A. E. (1968) Lactose intolerance in various ethnic groups in South-east Asia. *Australasian Annals of Medicine,* **17**, 300.

Borgstrom, B., Dahlqvist, A., Lundh, G., and Sjovall, J. (1957) Studies of intestinal digestion and absorption in the human. *Journal of Clinical Investigation,* **36**, 1521.

Burgess, E. A., Levin, B., Mahalanabis, D., and Tonge, R. E. (1964) Hereditary sucrose intolerance: levels of sucrase activity in jejunal mucosa. *Archives of Disease in Childhood*, **39**, 431.

Burke, V., Kerry, K. R., and Anderson, C. M. (1965) The relationships of dietary lactose to refractory diarrhoea in infancy. *Australian Paediatric Journal*, **1**, 147.

Burke, V. and Anderson, C. M. (1966) Sugar intolerance as a cause of protracted diarrhoea following surgery of the gastrointestinal tract in neonates. *Australian Paediatric Journal*, **2**, 114.

Burke, V. and Danks, D. M. (1966) Monosaccharide malabsorption in young infants. *Lancet*, **i**, 1177.

Cook, G. C. (1967) The practical significance of lactase deficiency in childhood. *Journal of Tropical Paediatrics*, **13**, 85.

Crane, R. K. (1962) Hypothesis for mechanism of intestinal active transport of sugars. *Federation Proceedings*, **21**, 891.

Dahlqvist, A., Auricchio, S., Semenza, G. and Prader, A. (1963) Human intestinal disaccharidases and hereditary disaccharide intolerance. *Journal of Clinical Investigation*, **42**, 556.

Davidson, A. G. F. and Mullinger, M. (1970) Reducing substances in neonatal stools detected by Clinitest. *Pediatrics*, **46**, 632.

Dawson, A. M. (1970) The absorption of disaccharides. In *Modern Trends in Gastroenterology*, (ed. Card, W. I. and Creamer, B.) Ch. 6, p. 105. London: Butterworth.

Douwes, A. C., Fernander, J. and Degenhart, H. J. (1978) Lactose tolerant test in children: diagnostic value of blood glucose determination challenged by expiratory hydrogen measurement. *Archives of Disease in Childhood*, **53**, 939.

Dubois, R. S., Roy, C. C., Fulginiti, V. A., Merrill, D. A. and Murray, R. L. (1970) Disaccharidase deficiency in children with immunological defects. *Journal of Pediatrics*, **76**, 377.

Durand, P. (1958) Lattosuria idiopatica in una paziente con diarrea cronica ed acidosi. *Minerva pediatrica*, **10**, 706.

Fordtran, J. S. and Ingelfinger, F. J. (1968) Absorption of water, electrolytes and sugars from the human gut. In *Handbook of Physiology*, (ed. Code, C. F.) Section 6, Ch. 74, p. 1457. Washington: American Physiological Society.

Gracey, M., Burke, V., and Anderson, C. M. (1969) Association of monosaccharide malabsorption with abnormal intestinal flora. *Lancet*, **ii**, 384.

Gracey, M., Burke, V., and Oshin, A. (1972) Active intestinal transport of D-fructose. *Biochimica et biophysica acta*, **266**, 397.

Gracey, M. and Burke, V. (1973) Sugar-induced diarrhoea in children. *Archives of Disease in Childhood*, **48**, 331.

Gray, G. M. (1970) Carbohydrate digestion and absorption. *Gastroenterology*, **58**, 96.

Gray, G. M. (1975) Carbohydrate digestion and absorption. *New England Journal of Medicine*, **292**, 1225.

Habte, D., Sterk, G. G., and Hjalmarsson, B. (1973) Lactose malabsorption in Ethiopian children. *Acta paediatrica Scandinavica*, **62**, 649.

Harrison, M. (1974) Sugar malabsorption in cow's milk protein intolerance. *Lancet*, **i**, 360.

Harrison, M. and Walker-Smith, J. A. (1977) Reinvestigation of lactose intolerant children: lack of correlation between continuing lactose intolerance and small intestinal morphology, disaccharidase activity, and lactose tolerance test. *Gut*, **18**, 48.

Holzel, A., Schwarz, V., and Sutcliffe, K. W. (1959) Defective lactose absorption causing malnutrition in infancy. *Lancet*, **i**, 1126.

Holzel, A. (1967) Sugar malabsorption due to deficiency of disaccharidase activities and monosaccharide transport. *Archives of Disease in Childhood*, **42**, 341.

Kerry, K. R. and Anderson, C. M. (1964) A ward test for sugar in faeces. *Lancet*, **i**, 981.

Kerry, K. R. and Townley, R. R. W. (1965) Genetic aspects of sucrase-isomaltase deficiency. *Australian Paediatric Journal*, **1**, 223.

Kilby, A., Burgess, E. A., Wigglesworth, S. and Walker-Smith, J. A., (1978) Sucrase-isomaltase deficiency: a follow-up report. *Archives of Disease in Childhood*, **53**, 677.

Launiala, K. (1968) The mechanism of diarrhoea in congenital disaccharide malabsorption. *Acta paediatrica Scandinavica*, **57**, 420.

Launiala, K., Kuitunen, P., and Visakorpi, J. K. (1966) Disaccharidases and histology of duodenal mucosa in congenital lactose malabsorption. *Acta paediatrica* (Uppsala), **55**, 257.

Laws, J. W. and Neale, G. (1966) Radiological diagnosis of disaccharidase deficiency. *Lancet*, **ii**, 139.

Levin, B., Abraham, J. M., Burgess, E. A., and Wallis, P. G. (1970) Congenital lactose malabsorption. *Archives of Disease in Childhood*, **45**, 173.

Lifshitz, F. (1977) Carbohydrate problems in paediatric gastroenterology. *Clinics in Gastroenterology*, **6**, 415.

Lindquist, B., Meeuwisse, G. W. and Melin, K. (1962) Glucose-galactose malabsorption. *Lancet*, **ii**, 666.

Lindquist, B. L. and Wranne, L. (1976) Problems in analysis of faecal sugar. *Archives of Disease in Childhood*, **31**, 189.

Lucas, D., Manuel, P., and Walker-Smith, J. A. (1978) In preparation.

Maffei, H. V. L., Metz, G., Bampoe, V., Shiner, M., Herman, S., and Brook, C. G. D. (1977) Lactose intolerance, detected by the hydrogen breath test, in infants and children with chronic diarrhoea. *Archives of Disease in Childhood*, **52**, 766.

McMichael, H. B., Webb, J., and Dawson, A. M. (1965) Lactose deficiency in adults: a cause of 'funtional' diarrhoea. *Lancet*, **i**, 717.

Meeuwisse, G. W. (1970) Glucose-galactose malabsorption. Studies on renal glucosuria. *Helvetica Paediatrica Acta*, **25**, 13.

Metz, G., Gassull, M. A., Seeds, A. R., Blendis, L. M., and Jenkins, D. J. (1976) A simple method of measuring breath hydrogen in carbohydrate malabsorption by end expiratory sampling. *Clinical Science and Molecular Medicine*, **50**, 237.

Miller, D. and Crane, R. K. (1961) The digestive function of the epithelium of the small intestine. 1. An intracellular locus of disaccharide and sugar phosphate ester hydrolysis. *Biochimica et biophysica acta* (Amst.), **52**, 281.

Mitchell, J. D., Brand, J., and Halbisch, J. (1977) Weight-gain inhibition of lactose in Australian aboriginal children. *Lancet*, **i**, 500.

Muller, M., Walker-Smith, J. A., Shmerling, D. H., Curtius, H., and Prader, A. (1969) Lactulose: a gas-liquid chromatography method of determination and evaluation of its use to assess intestinal mucosal damage. *Clinica chimica acta*, **24**, 45.

Newcomer, A. D. and McGill, D. B. (1966) Lactose tolerance tests in adults with normal lactase activity. *Gastroenterology*, **50**, 340.

Phillips, A. D., Avigad, S., Sacks, J., Rice, S., and Walker-Smith, J. A. (1978) Disaccharidases and microvillous surface area. *Acta Paediatrica Belgica*.

Prader, A., Shmerling, D. H., and Hadorn, B. (1966) Disaccharides and coeliac disease. *Lancet*, **i**, 435.

Schaub, J. and Lentze, M. (1973) Sugars, lactic acid and pH in faeces of children. A useful diagnostical approach for gastrointestinal disorders. *Zeitblatt für kinderheilkunde*, **115**, 141.

Semenza, G., Auricchio, S., and Rubino, A. (1965) Multiplicity of human intestinal disaccharidases. 1. Chromatography separation of maltases and of two lactases. *Biochimica et biophysica acta* (Amst.), **96**, 487.

Soeparto, P., Stobo, E. A., and Walker-Smith, J. A. (1972) Role of chemical examination of the stool in diagnosis of sugar malabsorption in children. *Archives of Disease in Childhood*, **47**, 56.

Todd, R. M. (1974) Sugars in breast milk and artificial formulae. *BPA Council/ MEIU Joint-meeting*.

Walker-Smith, J. A. (1973) Screening tests for sugar malabsorption. *Journal of Pediatrics*, **82**, 893.

Weijers, H. A., van de Kamer, J. H., Dicke, W. K., and Ijsseling, J. (1961) Diarrhoea caused by deficiency of sugar splitting enzymes. 1. *Acta paediatrica* (Uppsala), **50**, 55.

Wharton, B. A. (1968) Difficulties in the initial treatment of kwashiorkor. *Calorie Deficiencies and Protein Deficiencies. Proceedings of a Colloquium*, p. 147. London: Churchill.

CHAPTER 8

Giardiasis

Ament, M. E. and Rubin, C. E. (1972) Relation of giardiasis to abnormal intestinal structure and function in gastrointestinal immunodeficiency syndrome. *Gastroenterology*, **62**, 216.

Ament, M. E. (1972) Diagnosis and treatment of giardiasis. *Journal of Pediatrics*, **80**, 633.

Barbezat, G. O., Bowie, M. D., Kaschula, R. O. C. and Hansen, J. D. L. (1967) Studied on the small intestinal mucosa of children with protein-calorie malnutrition. *South African Medical Journal*, **41**, 1031.

Barbieri, D., de Brito, T., Hoshino, S., Nascimento, O. B., Martins Campos, J. V., Guarentei, G., and Marcondes, E. (1970) Giardiasis in childhood. *Archives of Disease in Childhood*, **45**, 466.

Carswell, F., Gibson, A. A. M. and McAllister, T. A. (1973) Giardiasis and coeliac disease. *Archives of Disease in Childhood*, **48**, 414.

Court, J. N. and Stanton, C. (1959) The incidence of *Giardia lamblia* infestation of children in Victoria. *Medical Journal of Australia*, **2**, 438.

Leon-Barua, R. and Lumbreras-Cruz, H. (1968). The possible role of intestinal bacterial flora in the genesis of diarrhoea and malabsorption associated with parasitosis. *Gastroenterology*, **55**, 559.

Ochs, H. D., Ament, M. E. and Davis, S. D. (1972) Giardiasis with malabsorption in X-linked agammaglobulinaemia. *New England Journal of Medicine*, **7**, 341.

Powell, S. L. (1968) Metronidazole: An anti-infective agent of growing importance. *Medicine Today*, **2**, 44.

Strongyloidiasis

Booth, C. C. (1965) Physiopathology of intestinal malabsorption. In *Recent Advances in Gastroenterology* (ed. Badenoch, J. and Brooke, B. N.) p. 162. London: Churchill.

De Paola, D., Dias, L. B. and da Silva, J. R. (1962) Enteritis due to *Strongyloides stercoralis*. *American Journal of Digestive Diseases*, **7**, 1086.

Walker-Smith, J. A., McMillan, B., Middleton, A. W., Robertson, S. and Hopcroft, A. (1969) Strongyloidiasis causing small bowel obstruction in an aboriginal infant. *Medical Journal of Australia*, **2**, 1263.

APPENDICES

Francis, D. E. M. (1975) In Diets for Sick Children, 3rd edn. Oxford and Edinburgh: Blackwell Scientific Publications.

Francis, D. E. M. (1978) *Journal of Human Nutrition*. Treatment of Multiple Malabsorption Syndrome of Infancy, **32**, 270.

Larcher, V. F., Shepherd, R., Francis, D. E. M. and Harris, J. T. (1977) Protracted Diarrhoea in Infancy. *Archives of Disease in Childhood*, **52**, 597.

CHAPTER 9

Apley, J. (1975) The Child with Abdominal Pains. 2nd. Edition. Blackwell, Oxford.

Bender, S. W. (1977) Crohn's disease in children: initial symptomatology. *Acta Paediatrica Belgica*, **30**, 193.

Brooke, B. N., Hoffman, D. C., and Swarbrick, E. T. (1969) Azathioprine for Crohn's disease. *Lancet*, **ii,** 612.

Campbell, C., (1978) Personal communication.

Chrispin, A. R. and Tempany, E. (1967) Crohn's disease of the jejunum in children. *Archives of Disease in Childhood*, **42,** 631.

Crohn, B. B., Ginzburg, L., and Oppenheimer, G. D. (1932) Regional ileitis: a pathologic and clinical entity. *Journal of the American Medical Association*, **99,** 1323.

Crohn, B. B. and Yarnis, H. (1958) *Regional ileitis.* Second edition, New York.

Dunne, W. T., Cook, W. J., and Allan, R. N. (1977) Enzymatic and Morphometric evidence for Crohn's disease as a diffuse lesion of the gastrointestinal tract. *Gut*, **18,** 290.

Dvorak, A. M., Monahan, R. A., Osage, J. E., and Dickersin, G. R. (1978) Mast-cell degranulation in Crohn's Disease. *Lancet*, **i,** 498.

Dyer, N. and Dawson, A. D. M. (1973) Malnutrition and malabsorption in Crohn's disease with reference to the effect of surgery. *British Journal of Surgery*, **60,** 136.

Green, F. H. and Fox, H. (1973) A study by immunofluorescence of the intestinal mucosa in ulcerative colitis and Crohn's disease. *Journal of Medical Microbiology*, **6,** 18.

Green, J. R. B., O'Donoghue, D. P., Edwards, C. R. W., and Dawson, A. M. (1977) A case of apparent hypopituitarism complicating chronic inflammatory bowel disease in childhood and adolescence. *Acta Paediatrica Scandinavica*, **66,** 643.

Gryboski, J. D., Katz, J., Sangree, M. H., and Herskovic, T. (1968) Eleven adolescent girls with severe anorexia. *Clinical Pediatrics*, **7,** 684.

Hadfield, G. (1939) The primary histological lesion of regional ileitis. *Lancet*, **ii,** 773.

Henderson, A. and Hishon, S. (1978) Crohn's disease responding to oral disodium cromoglycate. *Lancet*, **i,** 109.

Hildebrand, H. and Ursing, B. (1977) Treatment of Crohn's disease in adolescence with metronidazole. A pilot study. *Acta Paediatrica Belgica*, **30,** 195.

James, A. H. (1977) Breakfast and Crohn's disease. *British Medical Journal*, **1,** 943.

Lennard-Jones, J. E. (1970) Crohn's disease. In *Modern Trends in Gastroenterology*, ed. Card, W. L. and Creamer, B. London: Butterworth.

Marshall, W. and Walker-Smith, J. A. (1978) Personal communications.

McCaffery, T. D., Nast, R., Lawrence, A. M., and Kirsner, J. B. (1974) Severe growth retardation in children with inflammatory bowel disease. *Pediatrics*, **45,** 386.

Miller, D. S., Keighley, A. C., and Langman, M. J. S. (1974) Changing patterns in epidemiology of Crohn's disease. *Lancet*, **ii,** 691.

Mitchell, D. N. and Rees, R. J. W. (1970) A transmissible agent from sarcoid tissue. *Lancet*, **ii,** 81.

Morson, B. C. (1968) Histopathology of Crohn's disease. *Proceedings of the Royal Society of Medicine,* **61,** 79.

Navarro, J., Ricour, C., Mougenot and Duhamel, J. F. (1977) Constant rate enteral alimentation in Crohn's Disease (at hospital and at home). *Acta Paediatrica Belgica,* **30,** 195.

O'Donoghue, D. P. and Dawson, A. M. (1977) Crohn's disease in childhood. *Archives of Disease in Childhood,* **52,** 627.

Ricour, C., Navarro, J., Duhamel, J. F., and Mougenot, J. F. (1977) Total parenteral nutrition in Crohn's Disease. *Acta Paediatrica Belgica,* **30,** 195.

Scadding, J. G. (1967) *Sarcoidosis.* London: Eyre and Spottiswoode.

Silverman, F. N. (1966) Regional enteritis in children. *Australian Paediatric Journal,* **2,** 207.

Vantrappen, G., Ghoos, Y. Rutgeerts, P., and J. Janssens (1977) Bile acid studies in uncomplicated Crohn's disease. *Gut,* **18,** 730.

Wallis, S. M. and Walker-Smith, J. A. (1976) An unusual case of Crohn's disease in a West Indian Child. *Acta Paediatrica Scandinavica,* **65,** 749.

Whorwell, P. J., Phillips, C. A., Beeken, W. L., Little P. K., and Roessner, K. D. (1977) Isolation of reovirus-like agents from patients with Crohn's disease. *Lancet,* **i,** 1169.

Williams, C., Campbell, C. and Walker-Smith, J. A. (1978) Diagnosis of Crohn's disease in childhood. In preparation.

Willoughby, J. M. T., Kumar, P., Beckett, J., and Dawson, A. M. (1971) Controlled trial of azathioprine in Crohn's disease. *Lancet,* **ii,** 944.

CHAPTER 10

Barnard, C. N. (1956) The genesis of intestinal atresia. *Surgical Forum,* **7,** 393.

Bayes, B. J. and Hamilton, J. R. (1969) Blind loop syndrome in children. Malabsorption secondary to intestinal stasis. *Archives of Disease in Childhood,* **44,** 76.

Burke, V. and Anderson, C. M. (1966) Sugar intolerance as a cause of protracted diarrhoea following surgery of the gastrointestinal tract in neonates. *Australian Paediatric Journal,* **2,** 219.

Challacombe, D. N., Richardson, J. M., and Anderson, C. M. (1974) Bacterial microflora of the upper gastrointestinal tract in infants without diarrhoea. *Archives of Disease in Childhood,* **49,** 264.

Challacombe, D. N., Richardson, J. M., Rowe, B., and Anderson, C. M. (1974) Bacterial microflora of the upper gastrointestinal tract in infants with protracted diarrhoea. *Archives of Disease in Childhood,* **49,** 270.

Cook, R. C. M. and Rickham, P. P. (1969) Neonatal intestinal obstruction due to milk curds. *Journal of Pediatric Surgery,* **4,** 599.

de Peyer, E. and Walker-Smith, J. A. (1977) Cow's milk intolerance presenting as necrotizing enterocolitis. *Helvetica Paediatrica Acta*, **32,** 509.

Dickson, J. A. A. (1970) Apple peel small bowel: an uncommon variant of duodenal and jejunal atresia. *Journal of Pediatric Surgery*, **5,** 595.

Dickson, J. A. S. (1972) The acute abdomen in infancy. *Practitioner*, **209,** 170.

Dickson, J. A. S., Lewis, C. T., and Swain, V. A. J. (1974) Milk bolus obstruction in the neonate. *British Pediatric Association Annual Meeting, 1974*.

Dickson, J. S. (1975) Necrotizing enterocolitis in the newborn infant. Report of the sixty-eighth Ross Conference on Pediatric Research.

Engel, R. R., Virning, N. L., Hunt, C. E., and Levitt, M. D. (1973) Origin of mural gas in necrotixing enterocolitis. *Pediatric Research*, **7,** 292.

Frantz, I. D., L'Heureux, P., Engel, R. R., and Hunt, C. E. (1975) Necrotizing enterocolitis. *Journal of Pediatrics*, **86,** 259.

Fromm, H. and Hoffman, A. F. (1971) Breath test for altered bile-acid metabolism. *Lancet*, **ii,** 621.

Gorbach, S. L., Plaut, A. G., Nahas, L., Weinstein, L., Spanknebel, G., and Levitan, R. (1967) Studies of intestinal microflora. *Gastroenterology*, **53,** 856.

Gracey, M., Burke, V., and Anderson, C. M. (1969) Association of monosaccharide malabsorption with abnormal small intestinal flora. *Lancet*, **ii,** 384.

Gracey, M. and Burke, V. (1973) Sugar-induced diarrhoea in children. *Archives of Disease in Childhood*, **48,** 331.

Grob-Vontobel, V. (1969) Uber einen erfolgreich behandelten Fall mit multiplen Dunndarmatresien. *Helvetica Paediatrica Acta*, **2,** 136.

Gross, R. E. (1953) *The surgery of Infancy and Childhood* First edition. Philadelphia and London: Saunders.

Hamilton, J. D., Dyer, N. H., Dawson, A. M., O'Grady, F. W., Vince, A., Fenton, J. C. B., and Mollin, D. L. (1970) Assessment of significant bacterial overgrowth in the small bowel. *Quarterly Journal of Medicine*, **39,** 265.

Herbst, J. J. (1975) Report of the sixty-eighth Ross conference on Paediatric Research, Ross Laboratories, Columbus, Ohio.

Holder, T. M. and Leape, L. I. (1968) The acute surgical abdomen in the neonate. *New England Journal of Medicine*, **278,** 605.

Howard, F., Flynn, D. M., Bradley, J., Noone, P., Szawathowski, M. (1977) Necrotizing enterocolitis. *Lancet*, **ii,** 1099.

Kilby, A., Walker-Smith, J. A., and Dickson, J. S. (1975) Stagnant loop syndrome with evidence of bile salt deconjugation. *Proceedings of the Royal Society of Medicine*, **68,** 417.

Lloyd, J. R. (1969) The aetiology of gastrointestinal perforations in the newborn. *Journal of Pediatric Surgery*, **4,** 77.

Louw, J. H. (1959) Congenital intestinal atresia and stenosis in the newborn. Observation on its pathogenesis and treatment. *Annals of the Royal College of Surgeons of England*, **25,** 209.

Middleton, A. W. (1969) Vomiting in the first month of life. *Bulletin of the Post-Graduate Committee in Medicine University of Sydney*, **25**, 56.

Mishalany, H. G. and Najjar, M. D. (1968) Familial jejunal atresia: three cases in one family. *Journal of Pediatrics*, **73**, 753.

Nixon, H. H. (1955) Intestinal obstruction in the newborn. *Archives of Disease in Childhood*, **30**, 13.

Noblett, H. R. (1969) Treatment of uncomplicated meconium ileus by Gastrografin enema. A preliminary report. *Journal of Pediatric Surgery*, **4**, 190.

Rowe, M. I. (1975) Necrotizing enterocolitis in the newborn infant. Microcirculation reactions to asphyxia. Report of the sixty-eight Ross Conference on Paediatric Research, Ross Laboratories, Columbus, Ohio.

Santulli, T. V. and Blanc, W. A. (1961) Congenital atresia of the intestine—pathogenesis and treatment. *Annals of Surgery*, **154**, 939.

Silverman, A., Roy, C. C. and Cozzetto, J. (1971) *Paediatric clinical gastroenterology*. St. Louis: The C. V. Mosby Company.

Tandler, J. (1902) as cited by Louw (1959) *Morphologisches Jahrbuch*, **29**, 187.

Young, D. G. and Wilkinson, A. W. (1968) Abnormalities associated with neonatal duodenal obstruction. *Surgery*, **63**, 832.

CHAPTER 11

Asatoor, A. M., Cheng, B., Edwards, K. D. G., Lant, A. F., Matthews, D. M., Milne, M. D., Navab, F., and Richards, A. J. (1970) Intestinal absorption of two dipeptides in Hartnup disease. *Gut*, **11**, 380.

Dowling, R. H. and Booth, C. C. (1966) Functional compensation after small bowel resection in man. Demonstration by direct measurement. *Lancet*, ii, 146.

Dudrick, S. J. (Cited by Parkinson and Walker-Smith) 1972.

Goldenberg, J. and Cummins, A. J. (1963) The effect of pH on the absorption rate of glucose in the small intestine of humans. *Gastroenterology*, **45**, 189.

Greenberger, N. J. and Skillman, T. G. (1969) Medium chain triglycerides. *Journal of the American Medical Association*, **280**, 1045.

Hamilton, R., Reilly, B. J. and Morecki, R. (1969) Short small intestine associated with malrotation: a newly described congenital cause of intestinal malabsorption. *Gastroenterology*, **56**, 124.

Harries, J. T. (1971) Intravenous feeding in infants. *Archives of Disease in Childhood*, **46**, 855.

Kern, F., Struthers, J. E. and Attwood, W. L. (1963) Lactose intolerance as a cause of steatorrhoea in an adult. *Gastroenterology*, **45**, 477.

Klein, R. E., Habicht, J. P. and Yarborough, C. (1971) Effects of protein-calorie malnutrition on mental development. *Advances in Pediatrics*, **18**, 75.

Lawler, W. H. and Bernard, H. R. (1962) Survival of an infant following massive resection of the small intestine. *Annals of Surgery*, **153**, 204.

Linder, A. M., Jackson, W. P. U. and Linder, G. C. (1953) Small gut insufficiency following intestinal surgery. Further clinical and autopsy studies of man surviving three and half years with seven inches of small intestine. *South African Journal of Clinical Science*, **4**, 1.

McCollum, J. P. K., Ogilvie, D., Muller, D. P. R., Manning, J., Packer, S. and Harries, J. T. (1975) Hyperoxaluria in children with hepatic, pancreatic and intestinal dysfunction. *Archives of Disease in Childhood*, **50**, 824.

McMahon, R. A. (1966) Massive resection of intestine in *Australian and New Zealand Journal of Surgery*, **35**, 202.

Moe, P. J. (1964) Intestinal function after massive resection of the small intestine in the newborn. *Acta paediatrica* (Uppsala), **53**, 578.

Parkinson, R. S., Kern, I. B., and Bowring, A. C. (1972) Intravenous alimentation in the neonate and infant. *Medical Journal of Australia*, **1**, 1182.

Parkinson, R. S. and Walker-Smith, J. A. (1973) Short small-bowel syndrome. *Medical Journal of Australia*, **2**, 205.

Porus, R. L. (1965) Epithelial hyperplasia following massive small bowel resection in man. *Gastroenterology*, **48**, 753.

Potts, W. J. (1955) Pediatric surgery. *Journal of the American Medical Association*, **157**, 627.

Sedgewick, C. E. and Goodman, A. A. (1971) Short bowel syndrome. *Surgical Clinics of North America*, **51**, 675.

Silk, D. B. A., Marrs, T. C., Addison, J. M., Burston, M. D., Clark, M. L. and Matthews, D. M. (1973) Absorption of amino acids from an animo acid mixture stimulating casein and atryptic hydrolysate of casein in man. *Clinical Science and Molecular Medicine*, **45**, 715.

Strauss, E., Gerson, C. D. and Yalow, R. S. (1974) Hypersecretion of gastrin associated with short bowel syndrome. *Gastroenterology*, **66**, 175.

Valman, B. (1974) Long term prognosis after resection of the ileum in childhood. *Archives of Disease in Childhood*, **48**, 79.

Valman, H. B., Oberholzer, V. G. and Palmer, T. (1976) Hyperoxaluria after resection of ileum in childhood. *Archives of Disease in Childhood*, **48**, 121.

Valman, H. B. (1976) Diet and growth after resection of ileum in childhood. *Journal of Pediatrics*, **88**, 41.

Walker-Smith, J. A. and Wyndham, N. (1967) Total loss of mid-gut. *Medical Journal of Australia*, **1**, 857.

Wilmore, D. W. (1969) Short bowel syndrome. A comprehensive approach to patient management. *Journal of the Kansas City Medical Society*, **70**, 233, 280.

Wilmore, D. W. and Dudrick, S. J. (1968) Growth and development of an infant receiving all nutrients exclusively by vein. *Journal of the American Medical Association*, **20**, 860.

Wilmore, D. W., Dudrick, S. J., Daly, J. M. and Vars, H. M. (1971) The role of nutrition in the adaption of the small intestine after massive resection. *Surgery Gynecology and Obstetrics*, **132**, 673.

Wilmore, D. W. (1972) Factors correlating with a successful outcome following extensive intestinal resection in newborn infants. *Journal of Pediatrics*, **80**, 88.

Wilmore, D. W. (1972) Factors correlating with a successful outcome following extensive intestinal resection in newborn infants. *Journal of Pediatrics*, **80**, 88.

Winawer, S. J., Broitman, S. A. and Wolochow, D. A. (1966) Successful management of massive small-bowel resection based on assessment of absorption defects and nutritional needs. *New England Journal of Medicine*, **274**, 72.

Young, W. F., Swain, V. A. J. and Pringle, E. M. (1969) Long-term prognosis after major resection of small bowel in infancy. *Archives of Disease in Childhood*, **44**, 465.

CHAPTER 12

Acrodermaritis enteropathica

Aggett, P. J., Atherton, D. J., Delves, H. T., Thorn, J. M., Bangham, A., Clayton, B. E., and Harries, J. T. (1978) Studies in Acrodermatitis enteropathica. *Proceedings of the IIIrd International Symposium on Trace Element Metabolism in Man and Animals* (ed. M. Kirchgeisner) Technical University of Munich: Fieising.

Barnes, P. M. and E. J. Moynahan (1973) Zinc deficiency in acrodermatitis enteropathica: multiple dietary intolerance treated with synthetic diet. *Proceedings of Royal Society of Medicine*, **66**, 327.

Evans, G. W. and Johnson, P. E. (1976) Zinc-binding factor in acrodermatitis enteropathica. *Lancet*, **ii**, 1310.

Evans, G. W. and Johnson, P. E. (1977) Zinc Binding Factor in Acrodermatitis Enteropathica. *Lancet*, **i**, 52.

Kelly, P., Davidson, G. P., Townley, R. R. W., and Campbell, P. E. (1976) Reversible intestinal mucosal abnormality in acrodermatitis enteropathica. *Archives of Disease in Childhood*, **51**, 219.

Lombeck, I., von Bassewitz, D. B., Becker, K., Tinschmann, P., and Kastner, H. (1974) Ultrastructural findings in acrodermatitis enteropathica. *Pediatric Research*, **8**, 82.

Moynahan, E. J. (1974) Acrodermatitis enteropathica: a lethal inherited human zinc deficiency disorder. *Lancet*, **ii**, 399.

Protein-losing enteropathies

Tift, W. L. (1977) Protein-losing enteropathies. Essentials of Paediatric Gastroenterology (ed. J. T. Harries), London: Churchill Livingstone.

Waldman, T. A., Wochner, R. D., Laster, L., and Gordon, R. S. (1967) Allergic gastroenteropathy. A cause of excessive gastrointestinal protein loss. *New England*

Journal of Medicine, **276,** 761.

Walker-Smith, J. A., Mistilis, S. M., and Skyring, A. P. (1967) The use of Cr^{51}Cl$_3$ in the diagnosis of protein-losing enteropathy. *Gut,* **8,** 116.

Small intestinal lymphangiectasia

Jarnum, S. (1963) *Protein-losing gastroenteropathy.* Oxford: Blackwell.

Jarnum, S. and Petersen, V. P. (1961) Protein-losing enteropathy. *Lancet,* i, 417.

McKendry, J. B. J., Lindsay, W. K., and Gerstein, M. C. (1957) Congenital defects of the lymphatics in infancy. *Pediatrics,* **19,** 21.

Mistilis, L. P., Skyring, A. P., and Stephen, D. C. (1965) Intestinal lymphangiectasia—a mechanism of enteric loss of protein and fat. *Lancet,* i, 77.

Mistilis, L. P. and Skyring, A. P. (1966) Intestinal lymphangiectasia: therapeutic effect of lymph venous anastomosis. *American Journal of Medicine,* **40,** 634.

Petersen, V. P. and Hastrup, J. (1963) Protein-losing enteropathy in constrictive pericarditis. *Acta medica Scandinavica,* **173,** 401.

Schwartz, M. and Jarnum, S. (1959) Gastrointestinal protein loss in idiopathic (hypercatabolic) hypoproteinaemia. *Lancet,* i, 327.

Tift, W. L and Lloyd, J. K. (1975) Intestinal lymphangiectasia. Long-term results with an MCT diet. *Archives of Disease in Childhood,* **50,** 269.

Waldmann, T. A. (1966) Protein-losing enteropathy. *Gastroenterology,* **50,** 422.

Waldmann, T. A., Steinfeld, J. L., Dutcher, T. F., Davidson, J. D., and Gordon, R. S. (1961) The role of the gastrointestinal system in idiopathic hypoproteinaemia. *Gastroenterology,* **41,** 197.

Walker-Smith, J. A., Reye, R. D. K., Soutter, G. B. S., and Kenrick, K. G. (1969) Small intestinal lymphangioma. *Archives of Disease in Childhood,* **44,** 527.

Abetalipoproteinaemia

Fosbrooke, A., Choksey, S., and Wharton, B. (1973) Familial hypobetalipoproteinaemia. *Archives of Disease in Childhood,* **48,** 729.

Lloyd, J. K. (1968) Disorders of the serum lipoproteins. I lipoprotein deficiency states. *Archives of Disease in Childhood,* **43,** 393.

Salt, H. B., Wolff, O. H., Lloyd, J. K., Fosbrooke, A. S., Cameron, A. H., and Hubble, D. V. (1960) On having no beta-lipoprotein. *Lancet,* ii, 325.

Selective defects of small intestinal absorption

Baron, D. N., Dent, C. E., Harris, H., Hart, E. W., and Jepson, J. B. (1956) Hereditary pellagra-like skin rash with temporary cerebellar ataxia, constant renal amino-aciduria, and other bizzarre biochemical features. *Lancet,* ii, 421.

Bell, M., Harries, J. T., Wolff, O., Dawson, A. M., and Waters, A. H. (1973) Familial selective malabsorption of vitamin B_{12}. *Archives of Disease in Childhood*, **48**, 896.

Danks, D. M., Stevens, B. J., Campbell, P. E., Gillespie, J. M., Walker-Smith, J. A., Blomfield, J., and Turner, B. (1972) Menkes' kinky-hair syndrome. *Lancet*, **i**, 1100.

Danks, D. M., Cartwright, E., Stevens, B. J., and Townley, R. R. W. (1973) *Science*, **179**, 1140.

Danks, D. M., Camakaris, J., and Stevens, B. J. (1977) The cellular defect in Menkes' syndrome and in mottled mice. *Third International Symposium on Trace Element Metabolism in Man and Animals*. Freising-Weihenstefhan.

Friedman, M., Hatcher, G., and Watson, L. (1967) Primary hypomagnesaemia with secondary hypocalcaemia in an infant. *Lancet*, **i**, 703.

Grasbeck, R., Gordin, R., Kantero, I., and Kuhlback, B. (1960) Selective vitamin B_{12} malabsorption and proteinuria in young people. A syndrome. *Acta Medica Scandinavica*, **167**, 289.

Grover, W. D. and Scrutton, M. C. (1975) Copper infusion therapy in trichopoliodystrophy. *Journal of Pediatrics*, **86**, 216.

Hunt, D. M. (1974) Primary defect in copper transport underlies mottled mutant in the mouse, *Nature*, **249**, 852.

Imerslund, O. (1960) Idiopathic chronic megaloblastic anaemia in children. *Acta paediatrica*, **49**, Suppl., 119.

MacKenzie, I. L., Donaldson, R. M., Trier, J. S. and Mathan, U. L. (1972) Ileal mucosa in familial selective vitamin B_{12} malabsorption. *New England Journal of Medicine*, **286**, 1021.

Menkes, J. H., Alter, M., Steigleder, G. K., Weakley, D. R., and Sung, J. H. (1962) A sex-linked recessive disorder with retardation of growth peculiar hair and focal cerebral and cerebellar degeneration. *Pediatrics*, **29**, 766.

Milne, M. D., Crawford, M. A., Girao, C. B., and Loughridge, L. W. (1960) The metabolic disorder in Hartnup disease. *Quarterly Journal of Medicine*, **29**, 407.

Navab, F. and Asatoor, A. M. (1970) Studies on intestinal absorption of amino acids and a dipeptide in a case of Hartnup disease. *Gut*, **11**, 373.

Rosenberg, L. E., Downing, S., Durant, J. L., and Segal, S. (1966) Cystinuria. *Journal of Clinical Investigation*, **45**, 365.

Stromme, J. H., Nesbakken, R., Normann, T., Skjorten, F., Skyberg, D., and Johannessen, B. (1969) Familial hypomagnesaemia. *Acta Paediatrica Scandinavica*. **58**, 433.

Walker-Smith, J. A., Turner, B., Blomfield, J., and Wise, G. (1973) Therapeutic implications of copper deficiency in Menkes' steely-hair syndrome. *Archives of Disease in Childhood*, **48**, 953.

Immune deficiency syndromes

Brown, W. R., Butterfield, D., Savage, D., and Tada, T. (1972) Clinical microbiological and immunological studies in patients with immunoglobulin deficiencies and gastrointestinal disorders. *Gut*, **13**, 441.

Dubois, R. S., Roy, C. C., Fulginiti, V. A., Merrill, D. A., and Murray, R. L. (1970) Disaccharidase deficiency in children with immunologic defects. *Journal of Pediatrics*, **3**, 377.

Heremans, P. E., Huizenga, K. A., and Hoffman, H. N. (1966) Dysgammaglobulinaemia associated with nodular hyperplasia of the small intestine. *American Journal of Medicine*, **40**, 78.

Katz, A. J. and Rosen, F. (1977) Gastrointestinal complications of immunodeficiency syndromes. Immunology of the Gut. *Ciba Foundation Symposium* **46**, p. 243.

Ochs, H. D. and Ament, M. E. (1976) Gastrointestinal tract and immunodeficiency. Immunological aspects of the liver and gastrointestinal tract. (ed. A. Ferguson and R. N. M. MacSween MTP), p. 83.

Roy, C. C. and Dubois, R. S. (1971) The human gut and immune homeostasis. *Clinical Pediatrics*, **10**, 275.

Savilahti, E., Pelkonen, P., and Visakorpi, J. K. (1971) IgA deficiency in children: a clinical study with special reference to intestinal findings. *Archives of Disease in Childhood*, **46**, 665.

Soothill, J. F. (1977) Genetic and nutritional variations in antigen handling and disease. Immunology of the Gut. *Ciba Foundation Symposium* **46**, p. 225.

Toddler's diarrhoea

Burke, V. and Anderson, C. M. (1975) The Irritable colon syndrome. Paediatric Gastroenterology (ed. Anderson, C. M. and Burke, V.) Oxford: Blackwell.

Davidson, M. and Wasserman, R. (1966) The irritable colon of childhood (chronic non-specific diarrhoea syndrome). *Journal of Pediatrics*, **69**, 1027.

Hamdi, I. and Dodge, J. A. (1978) Prostaglandins in non-specific diarrhoea. *Acta Paediatrica Belgica*, **31**, 106.

Tripp, J. H., Manning, J. A., Muller, D. P. R., Walker-Smith, J. A., O'Donoghue, D. P., Kumar, P. J., and Harries, J. T. (1978) Mucosal adenylate cyclase and sodium-potassium stimulated adenosine triphosphatase in jejunal biopsies of adults and children with coeliac disease. Perspectives in coeliac disease. *3rd International Coeliac Symposium* (Ed. McNicholl, B., McCarthy, C. F., and Fottrell, P. F.) Lancaster. MTP Press, p. 461.

Intractable diarrhoea

Avery, G. B., Villavicencio, O., and Lilly, J. R. (1968) Intractable diarrhoea in early infancy. *Pediatrics*, **41**, 712.

Hughes, C. A., Sabin, E., and Dowling, R. H. (1978) Changes in intestinal structure and function and pancreatic mass during intravenous feeding. *Acta Paediatrica Belgica*, **30**, 197.

Katz, A. J. and Rosen, F. (1977) Gastrointestinal complications of immunodeficiency syndromes. Immunology of the Gut. *Ciba Foundation Symposium* **46**, p. 243.

Shwachmann, H., Lloyd-Still, J. D., Khaw, K-T., and Antonowicz, I. (1973) Protracted diarrhoea of infancy treated by intravenous alimentation. II Studies of small intestinal biopsy results. *American Journal of Diseases of Children*, **125**, 360.

Soothill, J. F. and Harvey, B. A. M. (1976) Defective opsonization. A common immunity deficiency. *Archives of Disease in Childhood*, **51**, 91.

Walker-Smith, J. A. (1972) Small intestinal morphology in childhood. *Arquivos de Gastroenterologia*, **9**, 119.

Small intestinal disease in children with malnutrition.

Amin, K., Walia, B. N. S., and Ghai, O. P. (1969) Small bowel functions and structure in malnourished children. *Indian Journal of Pediatrics*, **6**, 67.

Barbazet, G. O., Bowie, M. D., Kaschula, R. O. C., and Hansen, J. D. L. (1967) Studies on small intestinal mucosa of children with protein-calorie malnutrition. *South Afircan Medical Journal*, **41**, 1031.

Bowie, M. D., Barbezat, G. O., and Hansen, J. D. L. (1967) Carbohydrate absorption in malnourished children. *The American Journal of Clinical Nutrition*, **20**, 89.

Bowie, M. D. (1975) Effect of lactose-induced diarrhoea on absorption of nitrogen and fat. *Archives of Disease in Childhood*, **5**, 363.

Brunser, O., Reid, A., Monckeberg, F., Maccioni, A., and Contreras, I., (1966) Jejunal biopsies in infant malnutrition with special reference to mitotic index. *Pediatrics*, **38**, 605.

Burman, D. (1965) The jejunal morphology in kwashiorkor. *Archives of Disease in Childhood*, **40**, 526.

Chandra, R. K. (1976) Immunological consequences of malnutrition including fetal growth retardation. In Food and Immunology (Swedish Nutrition Foundation Symposium XIII). Stockholm: Almquist and Eiksell International.

Danús, O., Chuaqui, B. and Vallejos, E. (1971) Desnutrición pluricarencial (Kwashiorkor). Estudio histológico de mucosa intestinal y evolucion clínica en 20 niños. *Pediatría (Santiago)* **14**, 141.

Deo, M. G. and Ramalingaswami, V. (1964) Absorption of CO^{58} labelled cyancobalamin in protein deficiency: An experimental study in the rhesus monkey. *Gastroenterology*, **46**, 167.

Guiraldes, E., Gutiérrez, C., and Latorre, J. J. (1977) Biopsia intestinal en enfermedad celíaca. *Revista Médica de Chile*, **105**, 553.

Guiraldes, E. (1978) Personal communication.

Mitchell, J. D., Brand, J., and Halbisch, J. (1977) Weight Gain Inhibition of Lactose in Australian Aboriginal Children. *Lancet*, **i**, 500.

Soothill, J. F. (1977) Genetic and nutritional variations in antigen handling and disease. Immunology of the gut. *Ciba Foundation Symposium* 46, (new series) Amsterdam: Elsevier Excerpta Medica North-Holland, p. 225.

Stanfield, J. P., Hutt, M. S. R., and Tunnicliffe, R. (1965) Intestinal biopsy in kwashiorkor. *Lancet*, **ii,** 519.

Suliman, G. (1978) Coeliac disease in the Sudan. *Gut.* **19,** 121.

Suharjono, Sutejo, and Sunoto (1975) Refeeding with Lactose Free Milk (AI 110 Nestlé) in Children Suffering from Gastroenteritis and Dehydration. Proceedings of First Asian Paediatric Congress, Manila.

Wharton, B. A. (1968) Difficulties in the initial treatment of kwashiorkor. *Calorie Deficiencies and Protein Deficiencies—Proceedings of a colloquium*, p. 147. London: Churchill.

Wharton, B. A. (1975) Gastroenterological problems in children of developing countries. Paediatric Gastroenterology (ed. Anderson, C. M. and Burke, V.) Oxford: Blackwell.

Wharton, B. A. (1977) The effects of malnutrition on structure and function. Essentials of Paediatric Gastroenterology (ed. Harries, J.) London: Churchill Livingstone, 130.

Williams, C. D. (1962) Malnutrition *Lancet*, **ii,** 342.

Small intestinal lymphosarcoma

Bate, C., Walker-Smith, J. A., and Malpas, J. S. (1978) Gastrointestinal Manifestations of Childhood Malignant Disease. In preparation.

Bartram, C. and Chrispin, A. R. (1973) Primary lymphosarcoma of the ileum and caecum. *Pediatric Radiology*, **1,** 28.

Newman, C., Malpas, J., Dickson, J. S., Stansfeld, A., and Walker-Smith, J. A. (1975) Small intestinal lymphosarcoma in a child, a problem in diagnosis and management. In press.

Defect of innervation of the small intestine

Rintoul, J. R. and Kirkman, N. F. (1961) The myenteric plexus in infantile hypertrophic pyloric stenosis. *Archives of Disease in Childhood*, **36,** 474.

Tanner, M. S., Smith, B., and Lloyd, J. K. (1976) Functional intestinal obstruction due to deficiency of argyrophil neurones in the myenteric plexus. *Archives of Disease in Childhood*, **51,** 837.

Index